AF133795

Matrix Metalloproteinases in Health and Disease

Matrix Metalloproteinases in Health and Disease

Editor

Raffaele Serra

MDPI • Basel • Beijing • Wuhan • Barcelona • Belgrade • Manchester • Tokyo • Cluj • Tianjin

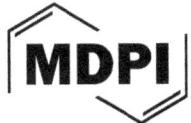

Editor
Raffaele Serra
University Magna Graecia of
Catanzaro
Italy

Editorial Office
MDPI
St. Alban-Anlage 66
4052 Basel, Switzerland

This is a reprint of articles from the Special Issue published online in the open access journal *Biomolecules* (ISSN 2218-273X) (available at: https://www.mdpi.com/journal/biomolecules/special_issues/Matrix_Metalloproteinases_Health_Disease).

For citation purposes, cite each article independently as indicated on the article page online and as indicated below:

LastName, A.A.; LastName, B.B.; LastName, C.C. Article Title. *Journal Name* **Year**, *Article Number*, Page Range.

ISBN 978-3-03943-052-9 (Hbk)
ISBN 978-3-03943-053-6 (PDF)

© 2020 by the authors. Articles in this book are Open Access and distributed under the Creative Commons Attribution (CC BY) license, which allows users to download, copy and build upon published articles, as long as the author and publisher are properly credited, which ensures maximum dissemination and a wider impact of our publications.

The book as a whole is distributed by MDPI under the terms and conditions of the Creative Commons license CC BY-NC-ND.

Contents

About the Editor vii

Raffaele Serra
Matrix Metalloproteinases in Health and Disease
Reprinted from: *Biomolecules* **2020**, *10*, 1138, doi:10.3390/biom10081138 1

Luis Santiago-Ruiz, Ivette Buendía-Roldán, Gloria Pérez-Rubio, Enrique Ambrocio-Ortiz, Mayra Mejía, Martha Montaño and Ramcés Falfán-Valencia
MMP2 Polymorphism Affects Plasma Matrix Metalloproteinase (MMP)-2 Levels, and Correlates with the Decline in Lung Function in Hypersensitivity Pneumonitis Positive to Autoantibodies Patients
Reprinted from: *Biomolecules* **2019**, *9*, 574, doi:10.3390/biom9100574 5

Erika Cione, Elena Piegari, Giuseppe Gallelli, Maria Cristina Caroleo, Elena Lamirata, Francesca Curcio, Federica Colosimo, Roberto Cannataro, Nicola Ielapi, Manuela Colosimo, Stefano de Franciscis and Luca Gallelli
Expression of MMP-2, MMP-9, and NGAL in Tissue and Serum of Patients with Vascular Aneurysms and Their Modulation by Statin Treatment: A Pilot Study
Reprinted from: *Biomolecules* **2020**, *10*, 359, doi:10.3390/biom10030359 17

Jaana Rautava, Ulvi K. Gürsoy, Adrian Kullström, Eija Könönen, Timo Sorsa, Taina Tervahartiala and Mervi Gürsoy
An Oral Rinse Active Matrix Metalloproteinase-8 Point-of-Care Immunotest May Be Less Accurate in Patients with Crohn's Disease
Reprinted from: *Biomolecules* **2020**, *10*, 395, doi:10.3390/biom10030395 29

Elena Rodríguez-Sánchez, José Alberto Navarro-García, Jennifer Aceves-Ripoll, Judith Abarca-Zabalía, Andrea Susmozas-Sánchez, Teresa Bada-Bosch, Eduardo Hernández, Evangelina Mérida-Herrero, Amado Andrés, Manuel Praga, Mario Fernández-Ruiz, José María Aguado, Julián Segura, Luis Miguel Ruilope and Gema Ruiz-Hurtado
Variations in Circulating Active MMP-9 Levels during Renal Replacement Therapy
Reprinted from: *Biomolecules* **2020**, *10*, 505, doi:10.3390/biom10040505 41

David Heinzmann, Moritz Noethel, Saskia von Ungern-Sternberg, Ioannis Mitroulis, Meinrad Gawaz, Triantafyllos Chavakis, Andreas E. May and Peter Seizer
CD147 is a Novel Interaction Partner of Integrin $\alpha M\beta 2$ Mediating Leukocyte and Platelet Adhesion
Reprinted from: *Biomolecules* **2020**, *10*, 541, doi:10.3390/biom10040541 55

Andrea Ferrigno, Laura G. Di Pasqua, Giuseppina Palladini, Clarissa Berardo, Roberta Verta, Plinio Richelmi, Stefano Perlini, Debora Collotta, Massimo Collino and Mariapia Vairetti
Transient Expression of Reck Under Hepatic Ischemia/Reperfusion Conditions Is Associated with Mapk Signaling Pathways
Reprinted from: *Biomolecules* **2020**, *10*, 747, doi:10.3390/biom10050747 65

Shane O'Sullivan, Jun Wang, Marek W. Radomski, John F. Gilmer and Carlos Medina
Novel Barbiturate-Nitrate Compounds Inhibit the Upregulation of Matrix Metalloproteinase-9 Gene Expression in Intestinal Inflammation through a cGMP-Mediated Pathway
Reprinted from: *Biomolecules* **2020**, *10*, 808, doi:10.3390/biom10050808 77

Michele Provenzano, Michele Andreucci, Carlo Garofalo, Teresa Faga, Ashour Michael, Nicola Ielapi, Raffaele Grande, Paolo Sapienza, Stefano de Franciscis, Pasquale Mastroroberto and Raffaele Serra
The Association of Matrix Metalloproteinases with Chronic Kidney Disease and Peripheral Vascular Disease: A Light at the End of the Tunnel?
Reprinted from: *Biomolecules* **2020**, *10*, 154, doi:10.3390/biom10010154 . . . . **91**

Helena Laronha, Inês Carpinteiro, Jaime Portugal, Ana Azul, Mário Polido, Krasimira T. Petrova, Madalena Salema-Oom and Jorge Caldeira
Challenges in Matrix Metalloproteinases Inhibition
Reprinted from: *Biomolecules* **2020**, *10*, 717, doi:10.3390/biom10050717 . . . . **107**

Zhao Liu, Roderick J. Tan and Youhua Liu
The Many Faces of Matrix Metalloproteinase-7 in Kidney Diseases
Reprinted from: *Biomolecules* **2020**, *10*, 960, doi:10.3390/biom10060960 . . . . **169**

About the Editor

Raffaele Serra is an Associate Professor of Vascular Surgery at the Department of Medical and Surgical Sciences, University Magna Graecia of Catanzaro, Italy. In 1999, he graduated in Medicine and Surgery; in 2004, he became Specialist in "Vascular Surgery"; and in 2009, he completed his PhD fellowship in "Clinical and Experimental Biotechnology in Veins and Lymphatics Disease". Since 2017, he has been the Director of Interuniversity Center of Phlebolymphology (CIFL) International Research and Educational Program in Clinical and Experimental Biotechnology at University Magna Graecia of Catanzaro. His clinical and research interests include vascular surgery, general surgery, cardiovascular disease, wound healing and wound care, chronic venous disease, peripheral artery disease, aortic disease, vasculitis, and biotechnology. Prof. Serra has published more than 180 articles in peer-reviewed journals in the field of Vascular Surgery and General Surgery. Moreover, he is also an Editor of several international high-impact factor journals.

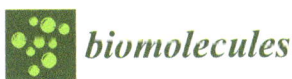

Editorial

Matrix Metalloproteinases in Health and Disease

Raffaele Serra

Department of Medical and Surgical Sciences, University Magna Graecia of Catanzaro, Viale Europa, Catanzaro, 88100 Germaneto, Italy; rserra@unicz.it; Tel.: +393-387-078-043

Received: 28 July 2020; Accepted: 31 July 2020; Published: 1 August 2020

Keywords: matrix metalloproteinases; health; disease

Matrix metalloproteinases (MMPs) are members of an enzyme family and, under normal physiological conditions, are critical for maintaining tissue allostasis. MMPs can catalyze the normal turnover of the extracellular matrix (ECM) and its activity is also regulated by a group of endogenous proteins called tissue inhibitors of metalloproteinases (TIMPs) or other proteins, such as Neutrophil Gelatinase-Associated Lipocalin (NGAL). An imbalance in the expression or activity of the aforementioned proteins can also have important consequences in several diseases, such as cancer, cardiovascular disease, peripheral vascular disease, inflammatory disease, and others. In recent years, MMPs have been found to have an important role in the field of precision medicine as they may serve as biomarkers that may predict an individual's disease predisposition, state, or progression. MMPs are also thought to be a sensible target for molecular therapy [1–4].

This Special Issue includes ten papers: seven original articles and three review articles dealing with a broad range of diseases related to MMPs.

The article by Santiago Ruiz et al [5] showed that several polymorphisms and genes associated with metalloproteinases influence the development of Hypersensitivity Pneumonitis (HP), an inflammatory disease caused by an exaggerated immune response to the inhalation of certain organic particles. Remodeling of the ECM in the airways and pulmonary interstice seem to relate to the worsening of lung function. This study documented that some polymorphisms in the MMP-1 and MMP-2 genes are associated with the risk of hypersensitivity pneumonitis, and, in particular, the MMP-2 polimorphism also correlates with lung function.

The study by Cione E et al. [6] evaluated the expression of MMP-2, MMP-9, and NGAL in the plasma and tissue of patients with aneurysmal disease. In particular, the modulation of these three biochemical indicators, related to vascular remodeling, was also studied in patients under statin treatment. The study deepens the pathophysiology of arterial aneurysms in light of ECM alterations, and suggests that statin treatment may have a role in the prevention of aneurysm growth and subsequent rupture by modulating the effects of MMP-2, MMP-9, and NGAL on ECM alterations, endothelial function, and also reducing inflammation and oxidative stress.

The paper by Rautava J et al. [7] deals with Crohn's disease (CD) a complex inflammatory disease of the gastrointestinal tract, and the tendency of such patients to develop periodontitis, caries, and oral mucosal lesions. The study speculates that the dysregulation of the immune system in CD may have an effect on MMP-8 levels in the oral cavity. In this context, MMP-8 seems to be the key inflammatory mediator in these conditions; In fact, elevated MMP-8 levels have been detected in CD patients both in the intestine and in the oral cavity.

The article by Rodríguez-Sánchez E. et al. [8] explores the variations in circulating active MMP-9 levels during Renal Replacement Therapy (RRT), which is a condition that may be complicated by a chronic state of inflammation and a high mortality risk. The study documented that MMP-9 is an effective marker of vascular dysfunction in patients undergoing RRT.

The study by Heinzmann D et al. [9] explored the recruitment of leukocytes and platelets to activated endothelia as well as platelet–leukocyte interactions in the context of thromboinflammatory mechanisms. In particular, this study highlights that the surface receptor CD147 (basigin, extracellular matrix–metalloproteinase inducer; EMMPRIN) has a role in the host defense from self-derived, as well as invading targets, and it is also a major factor modulating the expression of MMPs. In this context, CD147 seems to have pathophysiological relevance in platelet–leukocyte interactions in thrombosis related mechanisms.

The paper by Ferrigno A et al. [10] studied the involvement of MMPs in hepatic ischemia/reperfusion (I/R) injury. This study showed the precise role of MMPs, in particular MMP-2 and MMP-9, that may contribute to the development of organ dysfunction and injury, especially in the early phase of this condition.

The article by O'Sullivan S. et al. [11] studied the role of MMP-9 in inflammatory bowel disease (IBD) and investigated the mechanism of action of barbiturate-nitrate hybrid compounds and their component parts using models of intestinal inflammation in vitro in order to inhibit the upregulation of MMP-9 gene expression. This study highlights the potential of treating colonic inflammation by means of downregulating MMP-9 activity, and subsequent inflammatory sprout in IBD.

The study by Provenzano M. et al. [12] aimed to examine the role of MMPs in increasing the risk of peripheral vascular disease (PVD) by the specific factors related to Chronic Kidney Disease (CKD). This paper speculates on the possibility of a strict link between PAD and PVD, mediated by MMPs, in particular MMP-2 and MMP-9, and the latter also sustained by an increase in NGAL circulating levels that are also known to be directly related to diabetic status and inversely to estimated glomerular filtration rate (eGFR) levels.

The paper by Laronha H. [13] extensively reviewed the currently reported synthetic inhibitors of MMPs and also provided an accurate description of their properties. In particular, Hydroxamate-Based Inhibitors, Non-Hydroxamate-Based Inhibitors, Catalytic Domain (Non-Zinc Binding) Inhibitors, Allosteric and Exosite Inhibitors, and Antibody-Based Inhibitors are presented and discussed.

The article by Liu Z. et al. [14] reviewed the expression, regulation, novel substrates, and mechanisms of MMP-7 in several kidney diseases. In particular, MMP-7 was found upregulated in acute kidney injury (AKI), CKD, and glomerular diseases and was also predominantly localized in renal tubular epithelia. Furthermore, MMP-7 levels may serve as a noninvasive biomarker for predicting AKI prognosis and monitoring CKD progression.

This Special Issue describes important findings related to MMPs function, and dysregulation in several areas, such as vascular, kidney, and respiratory systems and also highlights the most recent progress on the knowledge and the clinical and pharmacological applications related to the most relevant areas of healthcare.

Conflicts of Interest: The authors declare no conflict of interest.

References

1. Serra, R.; Gallelli, L.; Butrico, L.; Buffone, G.; Caliò, F.G.; De Caridi, G.; Massara, M.; Barbetta, A.; Amato, B.; Labonia, M.; et al. From varices to venous ulceration: The story of chronic venous disease described by metalloproteinases. *Int. Wound J.* **2017**, *14*, 233–240. [CrossRef] [PubMed]
2. Serra, R.; Ielapi, N.; Barbetta, A.; Buffone, G.; Bevacqua, E.; Andreucci, M.; de Franciscis, S.; Gasbarro, V. Biomarkers for precision medicine in phlebology and wound care: A systematic review. *Acta Phlebol.* **2017**, *18*, 52–56.
3. Serra, R.; Ielapi, N.; Barbetta, A.; Andreucci, M.; de Franciscis, S. Novel biomarkers for cardiovascular risk. *Biomark Med.* **2018**, *12*, 1015–1024. [CrossRef] [PubMed]
4. Busceti, M.T.; Grande, R.; Amato, B.; Gasbarro, V.; Buffone, G.; Amato, M.; Gallelli, L.; Serra, R.; de Franciscis, S. Pulmonary embolism, metalloproteinases and neutrophil gelatinase associated lipocalin. *Acta Phlebol.* **2013**, *14*, 115–121.
5. Santiago-Ruiz, L.; Buendía-Roldán, I.; Pérez-Rubio, G.; Ambrocio-Ortiz, E.; Mejía, M.; Montaño, M.; Falfán-Valencia, R. MMP2 Polymorphism Affects Plasma Matrix Metalloproteinase (MMP)-2 Levels,

and Correlates with the Decline in Lung Function in Hypersensitivity Pneumonitis Positive to Autoantibodies Patients. *Biomolecules* **2019**, *9*, 574. [CrossRef] [PubMed]

6. Cione, E.; Piegari, E.; Gallelli, G.; Caroleo, M.C.; Lamirata, E.; Curcio, F.; Colosimo, F.; Cannataro, R.; Ielapi, N.; Colosimo, M.; et al. Expression of MMP-2, MMP-9, and NGAL in Tissue and Serum of Patients with Vascular Aneurysms and Their Modulation by Statin Treatment: A Pilot Study. *Biomolecules* **2020**, *10*, 359. [CrossRef] [PubMed]

7. Rautava, J.; Gürsoy, U.K.; Kullström, A.; Könönen, E.; Sorsa, T.; Tervahartiala, T.; Gürsoy, M. An Oral Rinse Active Matrix Metalloproteinase-8 Point-of-Care Immunotest May Be Less Accurate in Patients with Crohn's Disease. *Biomolecules* **2020**, *10*, 395. [CrossRef] [PubMed]

8. Rodríguez-Sánchez, E.; Navarro-García, J.A.; Aceves-Ripoll, J.; Abarca-Zabalía, J.; Susmozas-Sánchez, A.; Bada-Bosch, T.; Hernández, E.; Mérida-Herrero, E.; Andrés, A.; Praga, M.; et al. Variations in Circulating Active MMP-9 Levels During Renal Replacement Therapy. *Biomolecules* **2020**, *10*, 505. [CrossRef] [PubMed]

9. Heinzmann, D.; Noethel, M.; Ungern-Sternberg, S.V.; Mitroulis, I.; Gawaz, M.; Chavakis, T.; May, A.E.; Seizer, P. CD147 is a Novel Interaction Partner of Integrin αMβ2 Mediating Leukocyte and Platelet Adhesion. *Biomolecules* **2020**, *10*, 541. [CrossRef] [PubMed]

10. Ferrigno, A.; Di Pasqua, L.G.; Palladini, G.; Berardo, C.; Verta, R.; Richelmi, P.; Perlini, S.; Collotta, D.; Collino, M.; Vairetti, M. Transient Expression of Reck Under Hepatic Ischemia/Reperfusion Conditions Is Associated with Mapk Signaling Pathways. *Biomolecules* **2020**, *10*, 747. [CrossRef] [PubMed]

11. O'Sullivan, S.; Wang, J.; Radomski, M.W.; Gilmer, J.F.; Medina, C. Novel Barbiturate-Nitrate Compounds Inhibit the Upregulation of Matrix Metalloproteinase-9 Gene Expression in Intestinal Inflammation through a cGMP-Mediated Pathway. *Biomolecules* **2020**, *10*, 808. [CrossRef] [PubMed]

12. Provenzano, M.; Andreucci, M.; Garofalo, C.; Faga, T.; Michael, A.; Ielapi, N.; Grande, R.; Sapienza, P.; Franciscis, S.; Mastroroberto, P.; et al. The Association of Matrix Metalloproteinases with Chronic Kidney Disease and Peripheral Vascular Disease: A Light at the End of the Tunnel? *Biomolecules* **2020**, *10*, 154. [CrossRef] [PubMed]

13. Laronha, H.; Carpinteiro, I.; Portugal, J.; Azul, A.; Polido, M.; Petrova, K.T.; Salema-Oom, M.; Caldeira, J. Challenges in Matrix Metalloproteinases Inhibition. *Biomolecules* **2020**, *10*, 717. [CrossRef] [PubMed]

14. Liu, Z.; Tan, R.J.; Liu, Y. The Many Faces of Matrix Metalloproteinase-7 in Kidney Diseases. *Biomolecules* **2020**, *10*, 960. [CrossRef] [PubMed]

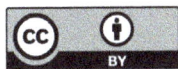

© 2020 by the author. Licensee MDPI, Basel, Switzerland. This article is an open access article distributed under the terms and conditions of the Creative Commons Attribution (CC BY) license (http://creativecommons.org/licenses/by/4.0/).

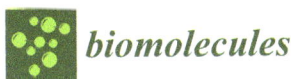

Article

MMP2 Polymorphism Affects Plasma Matrix Metalloproteinase (MMP)-2 Levels, and Correlates with the Decline in Lung Function in Hypersensitivity Pneumonitis Positive to Autoantibodies Patients

Luis Santiago-Ruiz [1,†], Ivette Buendía-Roldán [2,†], Gloria Pérez-Rubio [3], Enrique Ambrocio-Ortiz [3], Mayra Mejía [1], Martha Montaño [4] and Ramcés Falfán-Valencia [3,*]

1. Interstitial Lung Disease and Rheumatology Unit, Instituto Nacional de Enfermedades Respiratorias Ismael Cosío Villegas, Mexico City 14080, Mexico; luissantiago091@gmail.com (L.S.-R.); medithmejia1965@gmail.com (M.M.)
2. Translational Research Laboratory on Aging and Pulmonary Fibrosis, Instituto Nacional de Enfermedades Respiratorias Ismael Cosío Villegas, Mexico City 14080, Mexico; ivettebu@yahoo.com.mx
3. HLA Laboratory, Instituto Nacional de Enfermedades Respiratorias Ismael Cosío Villegas, Mexico City 14080, Mexico; glofos@yahoo.com.mx (G.P.-R.); e_ambrocio@iner.gob.mx (E.A.-O.)
4. Department of Research in Pulmonary Fibrosis, Instituto Nacional de Enfermedades Respiratorias Ismael Cosío Villegas, Mexico City 14080, Mexico; mamora572002@yahoo.com.mx
* Correspondence: rfalfanv@iner.gob.mx; Tel.: +52-55-5487-1700 (ext. 5152)
† These authors contributed equally to this work.

Received: 3 September 2019; Accepted: 26 September 2019; Published: 5 October 2019

Abstract: Among hypersensitivity pneumonitis (HP) patients have been identified who develop autoantibodies with and without clinical manifestations of autoimmune disease. Genetic factors involved in this process and the effect of these autoantibodies on the clinical phenotype are unknown. Matrix metalloproteinases (MMPs) have an important role in architecture and pulmonary remodeling. The aim of our study was to identify polymorphisms in the *MMP1*, *MMP2*, *MMP9* and *MMP12* genes associated with susceptibility to HP with the presence of autoantibodies (HPAbs+). Using the dominant model of genetic association, comparisons were made between three groups. For rs7125062 in *MMP1* (CC vs. CT+TT), we found an association when comparing groups of patients with healthy controls: HPAbs+ vs. HC ($p < 0.001$, OR = 10.62, CI 95% = 4.34–25.96); HP vs. HC ($p < 0.001$, OR = 7.85, 95% CI 95% = 4.54–13.57). This rs11646643 in *MMP2* shows a difference in the HPAbs+ group by the dominant genetic model GG vs. GA+AA, ($p = 0.001$, OR = 8.11, CI 95% = 1.83–35.84). In the linear regression analysis, rs11646643 was associated with a difference in basal forced vital capacity (FVC)/12 months ($p = 0.013$, β = 0.228, 95% CI95% = 1.97–16.72). We identified single-nucleotide polymorphisms (SNPs) associated with the risk of developing HP, and with the evolution towards the phenotype with the presence of autoantibodies. Also, to the decrease in plasma MMP-2 levels.

Keywords: hypersensitivity pneumonitis; metalloproteinases; genetic association; autoantibodies; MMP1; MMP2; SNPs

1. Introduction

Hypersensitivity pneumonitis (HP) is a complex disease caused by an exaggerated immune response to the inhalation of a wide variety of organic particles [1]. Although it has been established that the development of the disease depends on the time of exposure and the antigenic load, only a small proportion of individuals exposed to antigens associated with HP develop the disease, suggesting additional host and environmental factors may play a role in the pathogenesis [2].

In chronic stages, HP is characterized by progressive lung remodeling, which is associated with the loss of functional architecture and an excessive extracellular matrix (ECM) deposition [3]. Therefore, ECM proteins have been previously explored as indicators of disease activity, and as potential biomarkers of diagnosis and prognosis in patients with chronic obstructive pulmonary disease (COPD) and idiopathic pulmonary fibrosis (IPF) [4].

Recently, the existence of hypersensitivity pneumonitis with autoimmune characteristics (HPAF) in a US cohort has been described, determining the prevalence of 15% in the HP patients; in addition, the autoimmunity profile was recognized as an independent predictor of mortality [5]. It is not clear if HPAF patients have different genetic susceptibility characteristics to the non-autoimmunity HP patients. So far there are no genetic studies on the transforming phenotype of HP patients positive to autoantibodies.

Our aim was to identify single nucleotide polymorphisms (SNPs) associated with genetic susceptibility in metalloproteinases genes (*MMP1*, *MMP2*, *MMP9*, and *MMP12*) in HP patients with and without serum autoantibodies, as well as to the progression or development of the disease.

2. Materials and Methods

2.1. Study Population

An analytical, cross-sectional study was conducted. One hundred and thirty-eight patients with Hypersensitivity Pneumonitis (HP) from the Instituto Nacional de Enfermedades Respiratorias Ismael Cosío Villegas (INER), at Mexico City, Mexico were included.

The diagnosis was established according to criteria based upon the presence of HP, either by high-resolution chest tomography, bronchioloalveolar lavage (BAL) with lymphocytosis $\geq$ 40% and/or positive avian antigen. Additionally, in cases without a definitive clinical diagnosis, a lung biopsy was performed to confirm the diagnosis. Subjects with positive serology were included for at least one of the following antibodies: Antinuclear antibodies (ANAs) with a specific pattern of connective tissue disease of any kind (cytoplasmic, nucleolar, centromeric); ANA with pattern homogeneous, fine or coarse mottle, with titles $\geq$ 1:320; at least one antibody in the autoimmunity profiles for myositis or systemic sclerosis; rheumatoid factor $\geq$ 3 times the lower normal limit; Anti-cyclic citrullinated peptide (anti-CCP) $\geq$ 20. Salivary gland biopsy (grade 3–4). All of them without classification criteria according to the American Society of Rheumatology (ACR/EULAR) for connective tissue disease (CTD). A healthy subjects reference group with one hundred and eighty-four controls (HC) were included.

This study was approved by the Institutional Committee for Science and Ethics of the Instituto Nacional de Enfermedades Respiratorias Ismael Cosío Villegas (INER) (approbation codes: B20-15 and C60-17).

2.2. DNA Extraction

We obtained an 8-mL peripheral blood sample from each participant through venipuncture. Blood was collected in tubes with EDTA as an anticoagulant. The DNA extraction was performed using a BDtract DNA isolation kit (Maxim Biotech, Inc. San Francisco, California, USA) and later was quantified with a NanoDrop 2000 (Thermo Scientific, DE, USA). The contamination with organic compounds and proteins was determined by establishing the ratio of 260/240 and 260/280 readings, respectively. The samples were considered free of contaminants in both cases when the ratio was between 1.7 and 2.0.

2.3. Selection of Single Nucleotide Variation

The selection process of the evaluated single-nucleotide polymorphisms (SNPs) included a literature review of previous reports of the genetic association of SNPs in matrix metalloproteinase (MMP) genes associated to respiratory diseases in Caucasian and Asian populations, using the NCBI

(National Center for Biotechnology Information) database, and including scientific articles published between 2007 and 2016.

For the four included genes, tag SNP selection was performed with HaploView version 4.2, using the minor allele frequency (MAF) > 10% and $r^2 \geq 0.80$ in the Caucasian population as a reference. A total of 12 SNPs were selected, and data including chromosome location and polymorphism base change are shown in Table 1.

Table 1. Characteristics of single-nucleotide polymorphisms (SNPs) included.

Gene	SNP	Chr Position	Allele Change	MAF *	Consequence/Gene Location
MMP1	rs470215	chr11:102790368	A>G	G = 0.31373	3' UTR variant
	rs7125062	chr11: 102792772	T>C	C = 0.33799	Intron variant
	rs2071232	chr11:102794938	T>C	C = 0.1993	Intron variant
MMP2	rs243839	chr16:55495499	A>G	G = 0.2914	Intron variant
	rs243835	chr16:55502710	C>T	T = 0.4565	Intron variant
	rs243864	chr16:55478410	T>G	G = 0.1919	2 Kb Upstream variant
	rs11646643	chr16:55484965	A>G	G = 0.3101	Intron variant
MMP9	rs3918253	chr20:46010872	C>T	T = 0.42674	Intron variant
	rs3918278	chr20:46007015	G>A	A = 0.0218	2 Kb Upstream variant
MMP12	rs12808148	chr11:102862432	T>C	C = 0.1190	500 bp Downstream variant
	rs17368659	chr11:102872031	G>T	T = 0.1014	Intron variant
	rs2276109	chr11:102875061	T>C	C = 0.0988	2 Kb Upstream variant

* gnomAD: Allele frequencies are from The Genome Aggregation Database. Cite http://gnomad.broadinstitute.org/ Chr: Chromosome. MAF: Minor allele frequency. UTR: Untranslated region.

2.4. Genotyping

Alleles and genotypes were determined by real-time PCR, 3 µL of DNA were obtained at a concentration of 15 ng/µL. Under the following conditions: 50 °C for 2 min, 95 °C for 10 min, followed by 40 cycles of 95 °C for 15 seconds, and a final cycle of 60 °C for 1 min. The alleles and genotypes of the SNPs were determined by real-time PCR (Real-time PCR System 7300, Applied Biosystems, CA, USA) by allelic discrimination using TaqMan Probes at a concentration of 20× (Applied Biosystems. Foster City CA. USA). In addition, three controls without template (contamination controls) were included for each plate.

2.5. Obtaining Plasma Levels of MMP-2 with ELISA

Based upon the results of the genetic association analysis, plasma MMP-2 protein levels were measured using commercial kits (Elabscience Biotechnology Inc. Houston, TX. USA). Readings were obtained using the iMark™ Microplate Absorbance Reader (Bio-Rad, CA, USA).

2.6. Statistical Analysis

The statistics program SPSS v.21 (SPSS Inc., Chicago, IL, USA) was used to describe the study population and determine the median, minimum and maximum values for each variable, and compared using U de Mann-Whitney. Continuous variables were reported as means with standard deviation (SD) and compared using a Student's *t*-test. Categorical variables were reported as counts and percentages, and compared using Fisher's exact test.

To determine the SNPs associated with the disease's risk, the frequencies of the alleles and genotypes of the study groups were compared, and the odds ratio (OR) was calculated with a 95% confidence interval (CI), using Epi Info version 7.1.5.2 (CDC, GA, USA).

Statistical significance was considered if the *p*-value < 0.05. The ancestral allele was used as the reference for each of the polymorphisms, and was included population data for the frequencies of the

SNPs studied in the HapMap-MEX (Mexican population residing in Los Angeles, California, USA), from the HapMap project (International HapMap Project).

In addition, a linear regression analysis was conducted to investigate the independent effect of the associated genotypes on lung function: Diffusing lung capacity factor for carbon monoxide (DLCO), basal forced vital capacity (FVC) and a difference in basal FVC/12 months.

MMP-2 levels were compared by median values and interquartile ranges for three comparisons: (1) Genotype, (2) the phenotype with positive and (3) negative to autoantibodies phenotype.

3. Results

We included 138 patients with HP for the present study. Thirty-four of these patients had autoantibodies present in serum without classification criteria for CTD. Additionally, a reference group with 184 healthy controls was included. They were paired in gender and age with our corresponding study group. (157 women and 27 men, 54.4 ± 12.78 years of age).

The baseline demographic data and the clinical characteristics of the entire cohort showed that the mean age at the time of HP diagnosis was 51 years (± 11 years); with a BMI of 27 (± 5). Comorbidities included diabetes mellitus (12%) and systemic arterial hypertension (22%). 25% of the patients are former smokers. In the physical examination, the most frequent clinical signs were fever (39%) and digital clubbing (31%). Exposure to the avian antigen (88%) was the most common environmental agent identified.

Comparing the demographic characteristics between HPAbs+ and HP without the presence of autoantibodies (Table 2) both groups were found paired in age and gender. In the HP group, a higher proportion of former smokers was observed (29% vs. 14%, $p = 0.01$), also demonstrating more subjects with systemic hypertension (25.9% vs. 8.8%, $p = 0.002$). There were no differences between the groups with respect to other demographic characteristics and antigen exposure. During the study period, 19% of the entire cohort died. There were no statistically significant differences between the groups with respect to the number of deaths (20% vs. 18%, $p = 0.9$). The number of patients with a decrease of ≥ 10% in the predicted FVC differed between the groups (26.4% in HPAbs+ vs. 5.7% in HP, $p = 0.0001$).

When comparing the respiratory function tests and the clinical laboratory characteristics between both groups (Table 3), those patients with the presence of antibodies (HPAbs+) showed a better FVC predicted and DLCO without being statistically significant.

Table 2. Clinical and demographic characteristics.

Characteristics	HPAbs+ (n = 34)	HP (n = 104)	p-Value
Age, years	52.9 ± 9.3	50.9 ± 11.7	0.3
Sex, female. n (%)	29 (85.2)	89 (85.5)	1.0
BMI, kg/m^2	27.3 ± 5.6	27.9 ± 5.2	0.5
Former smokers. n, (%)	5 (14.7)	30 (29.1)	0.01
Symptoms before diagnosis, months.	24 (1–120)	24 (6–192)	0.1
Antigen exposure			
Avian, n (%)	30 (88.2)	92 (88.4)	1.0
Unknown, n (%)	4 (11.7)	12 (11.5)	1.0
Diabetes mellitus, n (%)	6 (5.7)	10 (9.6)	0.2
Systemic hypertension, n (%)	3 (8.8)	27 (25.9)	0.002
Fever, n (%)	5 (14.7)	10 (9.6)	0.5
Digital clubbing, n (%)	7 (20.5)	26 (25)	0.4
Deceased, n (%)	6 (20)	17 (18)	0.9
≥10% FVC decline, n (%)	9 (26.4)	6 (5.7)	0.0001

HP: Hypersensitivity pneumonitis; Abs: Autoantibodies; mean ± SD; median (minimum and maximum values).

Table 3. Assessment of lung function and main laboratory findings in HP patients.

Characteristics	HPAbs+ (n = 34)	HP (n = 104)	p-Value
FVC % predicted	60 (29–97)	51 (20–98)	0.1
DLCO % predicted	60 (20–125)	41 (16–102)	0.06
pO2, mm Hg	50 (34.7–77.7)	47 (22–71.1)	0.1
Oxygen therapy, n (%)	9 (26)	37 (35)	0.09
PSAP, mm Hg	32 (20–77)	40 (20–90)	0.02
Laboratory blood test			
Optical density for avian antigen	1.45 (0.22–4.40)	0.89 (0.15–3.37)	0.03
White blood cell count, n x 10^3 /mm^3	8.1 (4.7–13.3)	8.1 (2.8–17.8)	0.6
Lymphocytes %	22.6 (12.5–36.5)	20.2 (3.8–77.9)	0.09
Eosinophils %	3.6 (1–12.3)	2.6 (1–18.8)	0.1
Hemoglobin g/dl	15.8 (13.2–20.9)	16 (11.7–21.2)	0.5
Hematocrit %	48.3 (39.4–63.3)	48.8 (35.8-68.7)	0.9
C-reactive protein mg/dl	1.023 (0.121–7.160)	0.541 (0.013–8.920)	0.006
BAL Lymphocytes %	54.5 ± 14.2	46.2 ± 21.2	0.03

HP: Hypersensitivity pneumonitis; Abs: autoantibodies; BAL: Bronchoalveolar Lavage. Mean ± SD; median (minimum and maximum values).

However, those patients with HP showed differences in relation to PSAP, with a higher median compared to the HPAbs+ group (32 mm Hg vs. 40 mmHg $p = 0.002$) required a greater number of patients with supplemental oxygen (26% vs. 35%; $p = 0.09$).

In the laboratory studies, the greater optical density of avian antigen was identified in the HPAbs+ group (1.45 DO vs. 0.89 DO, $p = 0.03$). C reactive protein was also compared as an acute phase reactant in both groups, showing higher levels in patients with HPAbs+ (1.023 mg/dl vs. 0.541 mg/dl, $p = 0.006$). Regarding bronchoalveolar lavage (BAL), the percentage of lymphocytosis was higher in the HPAbs+ group (54.5% vs. 46.2%, $p = 0.03$).

The most expressed antibodies in our study group (Table 4) were the ANA type (50%) showing a higher frequency in their expression with a homogeneous pattern (20%) ≥ 1:320. Followed by others, such as the rheumatoid factor (14.9%) among the most frequently observed.

Table 4. Autoimmune serologic tests.

Characteristics	n (%)
ANA ≥ 1:320	17 (50.0)
Nuclear fine speckled	2 (5.8)
Nuclear coarse speckled	1 (2.9)
Homogeneous nuclear	7 (20.7)
Nucleolar	4 (11.7)
Fibrillar Cytoplasmatic	3 (8.9)
Others	17 (50.0)
RF ≥ 3x upper limit normal	5 (14.9)
Anti-topoisomerase (Scl-70)	2 (5.8)
Anti-Ro (SS-A)	1 (2.9)
Anti-La (SS-B)	2 (5.8)
Anti-dsDNA	4 (11.7)
Anti-CCP ≥ 3x upper limit normal	3 (8.9)

ANA: Anti-nuclear antibody; anti-CCP: Anti-Citrullinated Peptide Antibodies.

3.1. Analysis of Association by Alleles and Genotypes

Alleles associated with risk were identified in the *MMP1* and *MMP2* genes. The T allele for rs7125062 was found associated when comparing groups of patients with healthy subjects: HPAbs+ vs. HC ($p < 0.001$, OR = 3.69, CI 95% = 2.16–6.29); HP vs. HC ($p < 0.001$, OR = 2.97, CI 95% = 1.99–4.09). (Supplementary Table S1). Regarding rs11646643 in *MMP2*, the allele A in frequency was statistically significant when comparing both groups of patients: HPAbs+ vs. HP (p = 0.03, OR = 1.88, CI 95% 1.06–3.33). When compared with healthy subjects, only the HPAbs+ group obtained a statistically significant difference (p = 0.01, OR = 2.35, CI = 95% 1.36–4.05). The group of HP patients showed no difference with the reference group of healthy subjects. (Supplementary Table S1) Allele and genotype frequencies for the three study groups and HapMap-MEX population are included in the Supplementary Tables S2–S4.

Using the dominant model of genetic association, comparisons were made between the three groups. For rs7125062 (CC vs. CT + TT) in the *MMP1* gene, an association was found when comparing both groups of patients with healthy subjects, respectively: HPAbs+ vs. HC (p < 0.001, OR = 10.62, CI 95% = 4.34–25.96) and HP vs. HC (p < 0.001, OR = 7.85, CI 95% = 4.54–13.57). (Table 5).

In addition, grouping all HP patients (HPAbs+ and HP) were compared against HC group, observing an association, (p < 0.001, OR = 8.42, CI 95% = 5.07–13.98). (Supplementary Table S6).

On the other hand, for rs11646643 in *MMP2*, HPAbs+ patients presented a lower frequency in the homozygous GG genotype compared to the HP group (GF = 5.88% vs. 33.65%). The difference was statistically significant when comparing them based on the dominant genetic model GG vs. GA + AA, (p = 0.001, OR = 8.11, CI 95% = 1.83–35.84). A similar effect occurs when comparing the group HPAbs+ vs. HC (p < 0.001, OR = 11.51 CI 95% = 2.67–49.49). (Table 5) Interestingly, the association was significative comparing all HP patients (independently of the serological phenotype) against healthy subjects, respectively: HP (all) vs. HC (p = 0.006, OR = 1.96, CI 95% = 1.21–3.16). (Supplementary Table S6).

For the rest of the SNPs of *MMP1* and *MMP2*, no significant associations were found. There was no association for the *MMP9* and *MMP12* genes. Data for genetic association models for SNPs and genotypes in *MMP9* and *MMP12* genes are shown in Supplementary Tables S7 and S8.

In the linear regression analysis, only rs11646643 (GA+AA) was associated to a difference in basal FVC/12months (p = 0.013, β = 0.228, 95% CI, 95% = 1.97–16.72). No other SNPs or variables were associated.

The genotype and allele frequencies of the 12 evaluated SNPs in Mexicans residing in Los Angeles (HapMap-Mex) are shown in the Supplementary Tables S2–S4.

Genotype frequencies of the two associated SNPs in the HC group were compared to those in the HapMap-Mex. The frequency of the rs7125062 CT genotype in the *MMP1* gene in the HC group was reduced when compared with the population data from the HapMap-Mex (2.17% vs. 58.0%), contrary to observed with the frequency of the CC genotype, which was elevated in the HC group. (Supplementary Table S2).

For the associated SNP in the *MMP2* gene, (rs11646643) the AA genotype frequency in the HC group was similar from the reported in the HapMap-Mex (32.61% vs. 30.0%). Interestingly, the GG and GA genotype frequencies have important differences in their distribution. (Supplementary Table S3).

Table 5. SNPs and associated genotypes in the genes *MMP1* and *MMP2* in patients with hypersensitivity pneumonitis *versus* hypersensitivity pneumonitis with positive autoantibodies.

Gene/Model	SNP/Genotype	Genotype Frequency (%)			HPAbs+ vs. HP			HPAbs+ vs. HC			HP vs. HC		
		HPAbs+ (n = 34)	HP (n = 104)	HC (n = 184)		p	OR (CI 95%)		p	OR (CI 95%)		p	OR (CI 95%)
MMP1	rs7125062												
Codominant	CC	20.59	25.96	73.37			1			1			1
	CT	47.06	49.04	2.17		0.3	1.21 (0.44–3.30)		0.0002	77.1 (20.3–292.6)		<0.001	63.75 (21.25–191.20)
	TT	32.35	25.00	24.46			1.63 (0.54–4.85)			4.7 (1.7–12.8)			2.8 (1.53–5.45)
Dominant	CC	20.59	25.96	73.37			1			1			1
	CT+TT	79.41	74.04	26.63		0.64	1.35 (0.52–3.46)		<0.001	10.62 (4.34–25.96)		<0.001	7.85 (4.54–13.57)
MMP2	rs11646643												
Codominant	GG	5.88	33.65	41.85			1			1			1
	GA	55.88	30.77	25.54		0.04	10.39 (2.2–48.1)		0.007	15.56 (3.46–69.85)		0.2	1.49 (0.82–2.73)
	AA	38.24	35.58	32.61			6.14 (1.2–29.2)			8.34 (1.81–38.38)			1.35 (0.76–2.40)
Dominant	GG	5.88	33.65	41.85			1			1			1
	GA+AA	94.12	66.35	58.15		0.001	8.11 (1.83–35.84)		<0.001	11.51 (2.67–49.49)		0.2	1.41 (0.85–2.34)

HPAbs+: HP patients with autoantibodies positive; HP: hypersensitivity pneumonitis patients without autoantibodies; HC: healthy controls.

3.2. MMP-2 Plasma Levels

Plasma levels of the MMP-2 protein of the HPAbs+ and HP groups were measured by ELISA using commercial kits. There were no significant differences when comparing the levels between patients' groups (132.98 vs. 130.06 ng/ml, $p = 0.8$). However, when these groups were merged and grouped by the rs11646643 genotype (GG vs. GA+AA), there was a statistically significant difference (188.84 vs. 123.39 ng/ml, $p = 0.009$), maintaining this tendency in the same comparisons, but this time intragroup. (Figure 1)

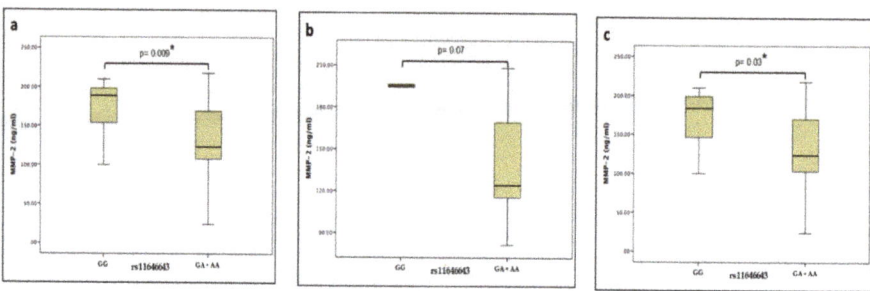

Figure 1. Median values and interquartile ranges of MMP-2 plasma levels in (**a**) genotypes of hypersensitivity pneumonitis (**b**) phenotype with positive autoantibodies (**c**) phenotype negative to autoantibodies.

4. Discussion

In this study we demonstrated that some patients with HP express autoantibodies during clinic evolution without classification criteria for connective tissue disease.

We observed that the presence of autoantibodies establishes an inflammatory phenotype with an elevation of acute phase reactants compared to seronegative HP. However, no differences were observed in respiratory function tests.

There is little knowledge regarding this transforming phenotype with the presence of antibodies present in the serum, as well as the identification of clinical factors associated with poorer results.

In the cohort of patients with HP, most of the subjects were in a chronic phase. The group of subjects with HP (without the presence of antibodies) showed a higher degree of pulmonary hypertension with a decrease in DLCO compared to the seropositive subjects, while in the group with HPAbs+, the levels of avian antigen and C-reactive protein were higher, remarking inflammation and lymphocytosis in the BAL.

We can propose from these differences that the HPAbs+ group develops an inflammatory phenotype, and the presence of autoantibodies could have a detonating role. As in IPF, acute exacerbations can occur in chronic HP conditions, and exposures to inhaled antigens can trigger these exacerbations.

However, despite the avoidance of antigens, progressive pulmonary fibrosis and death may occur, suggesting that additional factors may contribute to the activity of the disease.

In the chronic stages, HP is characterized by a progressive pulmonary remodeling, which is associated with the loss of functional architecture and the excessive deposition of ECM.

Among the metalloproteinases, it has been shown that MMP-1 and MMP-2 play an important role in the remodeling of the respiratory tract, and also are implicated in the degradation of fibrillar collagen, gelatin and collagen type IV, that are the most abundant compounds of the extracellular matrix and the basal membranes [6,7]. Besides, it is known that MMP-1 increases the proliferative and migratory capacities of the epithelial alveolar cells and protects the cells of death [8].

Recently some studies prove that MMP-1 and MMP-2 mediate the suppression induced by interleukin-13 of the expression of the mRNA of elastin in the fibroblasts of the respiratory tract.

MMP-2 also induces the production of collagen, activating the latent transforming growth factor beta-1, an important factor that helps fibrogenesis [9].

In this study of genetic association, we show that two SNPs (of the twelve evaluated in the *MMP1*, *MMP2*, *MMP9* and *MMP12* genes) are associated with genetic susceptibility for HP in Mexican Mestizo population. In the *MMP1* gene, the rs7125062 was associated in the comparations HPAbs+ and HP vs. HC group; while rs11646643 in the *MMP2* gene is associated with the risk of disease and the decline of the lung function in HP; i.e., we can able to identify genetic differences among HPAbs+ and HP patients without autoantibodies.

The rs7125062 was associated in comparisons between groups by serological phenotypes against healthy subjects (HC); In addition, this association was maintained comparing all patients regardless of the phenotype (positive or negative to autoantibodies) against healthy subjects. Observing a tendency of association in relation to the respiratory disease, and not necessarily to the serological phenotype. Regarding rs11646643 of the *MMP2* gene, it is possibly associated with the serological phenotype of the disease. It is possible to perceive due to the increased risk in the respective comparisons: HPAbs+ vs. HP; HPAbs+ vs. HC, (OR = 8.11, OR = 11.51). However, this does not happen to compare the HP vs. HC group.

The modification of the effect on the risk is observed when comparing all patients with HP (regardless of the serological phenotype) against healthy subjects ($p = 0.006$, OR = 1.96), observing the influence of the seropositive phenotype on this association and therefore the role of this SNP.

Just a little proportion of the exposed individuals to an antigen associated with HP will develop the disease, suggesting the existence of another genetic factor associated with the risk. Nowadays there are no studies of the genetic association of rs7125062 and rs11646643 with HP. Therefore, this is the first report of genetic association that involves polymorphism of a single nucleotide with the risk of developing and decline of lung function in the Mexican mestizo population.

In the last SNP, it is located at the GATA-1 (CTATCT) site of the promoter region of the *MMP2* gene [10], that has two sites of the union for the transcription factors AP-2, p53, Sp1 y Sp3 [11]. These transcription factors regulate the transcription rate of the gene and therefore the expression of the protease. Also, there is a tag SNP of the polymorphism rs243865 (-1306 C/T) and rs243866 (-1575G/A) [12], that are found in the gene promoter.

On the other hand, the genetic factor could interact with immunological and environmental factors to influence the individual susceptibility. A similar phenomenon could have been happening with the genotypical frequencies of the group of subjects with autoantibodies in comparison with HP seronegative subjects. The genotype GA+AA of rs11646643 in the *MMP2* gene shows a difference of 27.77% between these two populations, respectively. Curiously this genotype has been correlated to a difference between basal FVC/12 months through of linear regression.

This finding supports the participation of the rs11646643 genotype (GA+AA) in *MMP2* and its association in the lung function decline, independently of the development, or not autoantibodies.

Regarding MMP-2, this is involved in the remodeling of the extracellular matrix in the airways and pulmonary interstice, degrading molecules like collagen type I, III, IV, V, VII y X, gelatin, fibronectin, laminin and aggrecan [13].

In the comparison between the patient groups (HPAbs+ vs. HP), a higher plasmatic level of MMP-2 was identified in those with the GG genotype, suggesting that plasmatic levels were modified in a genotype-dependent mode. In our study, we found that the plasmatic levels of MMP-2 decrease in the subjects with genotype (GA+AA) of rs11646643 in comparison with the subjects genotype (GG). MMP-2 has the capacity of cleaving the chemotactic protein of the monocytes 3 (MCP-3) that allows getting to join to the chemotactic receptors 1, 2 and 3 without activating them. This characteristic suggests that the MMP2 decrease contributes to the persistent inflammatory response, not allowing the modification MCP-3 [14].

The variation in the levels of MMPs is affected by the course and progression of the disease; interestingly, the association seems to be in function of the genotype and not of the clinical phenotype.

A limitation in our study is that our Mexican mestizo population for ancestry has several genetic contributions, mainly Amerindians and Caucasians in different proportions.

Our result contributes to scientific knowledge, identifying candidate polymorphisms/genes in the development and progression of the HP. Nowadays we still require more assays to evaluate these variants like potential markers of clinical phenotypes for the disease, considering that HP is an inflammatory disease that in some people can develop chronic fibrosing disease, increasing morbidity and mortality.

5. Conclusions

Our findings demonstrate a subgroup of patients with hypersensitivity pneumonitis who develop autoantibodies without meeting the classification criteria for connective tissue disease. The presence of these antibodies contributes to a significant inflammatory response, possibly detonated by chronic exposure to a given environmental antigen.

Two polymorphisms in the *MMP1* and *MMP2* genes are associated with the risk of hypersensitivity pneumonitis in the Mexican mestizo population.

There are differences in the plasma levels of the MMP-2 protein among HP patients genotype-depending.

Our study suggests that polymorphisms and genes associated with metalloproteases influence the development of HP and worsening of lung function.

The identification of autoantibodies in patients with HP can have an impact on the course of the disease and the subsequent therapeutic management of interstitial lung diseases, since our results show, there are demographic and functional differences that probably influence prognosis.

6. Patents

None to declare.

Supplementary Materials: The following are available online at http://www.mdpi.com/2218-273X/9/10/574/s1.

Author Contributions: Conceptualization, I.B.-R., G.P.-R. and R.F.-V.; Data curation, E.A.-O. and R.F.-V.; Formal analysis, L.S.-R., I.B.-R, G.P.-R., M.M. (Martha Montaño) and R.F.-V.; Investigation, I.B.-R., G.P.-R., E.A.-O., M.M. (Mayra Mejía) and M.M. (Martha Montaño); Methodology, L.S.-R., E.A.-O., M.M. (Mayra Mejía) and M.M. (Martha Montaño); Project administration, R.F.-V.; Resources, M.M. (Mayra Mejía); Supervision, G.P.-R.; Validation, M.M. (Mayra Mejía); Visualization, R.F.-V.; Writing-original draft, L.S.-R., I.B.-R., G.P.-R. and R.F.-V.; Writing-review & editing, R.F.-V.

Funding: This research received no external funding.

Acknowledgments: To all participants who kindly accepted to contribute to this research.

Conflicts of Interest: The authors declare no conflict of interest.

References

1. Selman, M.; Buendía-Roldán, I. Immunopathology, diagnosis, and management of hypersensitivity pneumonitis. *Semin. Respir. Crit. Care Med.* **2012**, *33*, 543–554. [PubMed]
2. Spagnolo, P.; Rossi, G.; Cavazza, A.; Bonifazi, M.; Paladini, I.; Bonella, F.; Sverzellati, N.; Costabel, U. Hypersensitivity Pneumonitis: A Comprehensive Review. *J. Investig. Allergol. Clin. Immunol.* **2015**, *25*, 237–250. [PubMed]
3. García-de-Alba, C.; Becerril, C.; Ruiz, V.; González, Y.; Reyes, S.; García-Alvarez, J.; Selman, M.; Pardo, A. Expression of Matrix Metalloproteases by Fibrocytes. *Am. J. Respir. Crit. Care Med.* **2010**, *182*, 1144–1152. [CrossRef] [PubMed]
4. Rosas, I.O.; Richards, T.J.; Konishi, K.; Zhang, Y.; Gibson, K.; Lokshin, A.E.; Lindell, K.O.; Cisneros, J.; Macdonald, S.D.; Pardo, A.; et al. MMP1 and MMP7 as Potential Peripheral Blood Biomarkers in Idiopathic Pulmonary Fibrosis. *PLoS Med.* **2008**, *5*, e93. [CrossRef] [PubMed]

5. Adegunsoye, A.; Oldham, J.M.; Demchuk, C.; Montner, S.; Vij, R.; Strek, M.E. Predictors of survival in coexistent hypersensitivity pneumonitis with autoimmune features. *Respir. Med.* **2016**, *114*, 53–60. [CrossRef] [PubMed]
6. Nagase, H.; Visse, R.; Murphy, G. Structure and function of matrix metalloproteinases and TIMPs. *Cardiovasc. Res.* **2006**, *69*, 562–573. [CrossRef] [PubMed]
7. Visse, R.; Nagase, H. Matrix Metalloproteinases and Tissue Inhibitors of Metalloproteinases. *Circ. Res.* **2003**, *92*, 827–839. [CrossRef] [PubMed]
8. Herrera, I.; Cisneros, J.; Maldonado, M.; Ramírez, R.; Ortiz-Quintero, B.; Anso, E.; Chandel, N.S.; Selman, M.; Pardo, A. Matrix metalloproteinase (MMP)-1 induces lung alveolar epithelial cell migration and proliferation, protects from apoptosis, and represses mitochondrial oxygen consumption. *J. Biol. Chem.* **2013**, *288*, 25964–25975. [CrossRef] [PubMed]
9. Firszt, R.; Francisco, D.; Church, T.D.; Thomas, J.M.; Ingram, J.L.; Kraft, M. Interleukin-13 induces collagen type-1 expression through matrix metalloproteinase-2 and transforming growth factor-β1 in airway fibroblasts in asthma. *Eur. Respir. J.* **2014**, *43*, 464–473. [CrossRef] [PubMed]
10. Vasků, A.; Goldbergová, M.; Hollá, L.I.; Šišková, L.; Groch, L.; Beránek, M.; Tschöplová, S.; Znojil, V.; Vácha, J. A haplotype constituted of four MMP-2 promoter polymorphisms (-1575G/A, -1306C/T, -790T/G and -735C/T) is associated with coronary triple-vessel disease. *Matrix Biol.* **2004**, *22*, 585–591. [CrossRef] [PubMed]
11. Morgan, A.R.; Han, D.Y.; Thompson, J.M.; Mitchell, E.A.; Ferguson, L.R. Analysis of MMP2 promoter polymorphisms in childhood obesity. *BMC Res. Notes* **2011**, *4*, 253. [CrossRef] [PubMed]
12. Hua, Y.; Song, L.; Wu, N.; Xie, G.; Lu, X.; Fan, X.; Meng, X.; Gu, D.; Yang, Y. Polymorphisms of MMP-2 gene are associated with systolic heart failure prognosis. *Clin. Chim. Acta* **2009**, *404*, 119–123. [CrossRef] [PubMed]
13. Perotin, J.-M.; Adam, D.; Vella-Boucaud, J.; Delepine, G.; Sandu, S.; Jonvel, A.C.; Prevost, A.; Berthiot, G.; Pison, C.; Lebargy, F.; et al. Delay of airway epithelial wound repair in COPD is associated with airflow obstruction severity. *Respir. Res.* **2014**, *15*, 151. [CrossRef] [PubMed]
14. McQuibban, G.A.; Gong, J.H.; Tam, E.M.; McCulloch, C.A.; Clark-Lewis, I.; Overall, C.M. Inflammation dampened by gelatinase A cleavage of monocyte chemoattractant protein-3. *Science* **2000**, *289*, 1202–1206. [CrossRef] [PubMed]

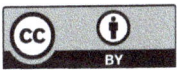

© 2019 by the authors. Licensee MDPI, Basel, Switzerland. This article is an open access article distributed under the terms and conditions of the Creative Commons Attribution (CC BY) license (http://creativecommons.org/licenses/by/4.0/).

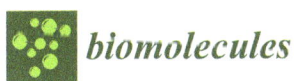

Article

Expression of MMP-2, MMP-9, and NGAL in Tissue and Serum of Patients with Vascular Aneurysms and Their Modulation by Statin Treatment: A Pilot Study

Erika Cione [1,†], Elena Piegari [2,†], Giuseppe Gallelli [3], Maria Cristina Caroleo [1], Elena Lamirata [4], Francesca Curcio [4], Federica Colosimo [5], Roberto Cannataro [1], Nicola Ielapi [6], Manuela Colosimo [7], Stefano de Franciscis [4] and Luca Gallelli [8,*]

1. Department of Pharmacy, Health and Nutritional Sciences, Department of Excellence 2018-2022, University of Calabria, 87036 Rende, Italy; erika.cione@unical.it (E.C.); mariacristinacaroleo@virgilio.it (M.C.C.); r.cannataro@gmail.com (R.C.)
2. Department of Experimental Medicine, Section of Pharmacology, University of Campania "Luigi Vanvitelli", 80138 Napoli, Italy; elena.piegari@unicampania.it
3. Unit of Vascular Surgery, Department of Surgery, "Pugliese Ciaccio" Hospital, 88100 Catanzaro, Italy; giuseppegallelli@hotmail.it
4. Department of Experimental Medicine, University of Catanzaro, and Vascular Surgery Unit, 88100 Mater Domini Hospital, 88100 Catanzaro, Italy; elena.lamirata@libero.it (E.L.); francesca.curcio@icloud.com (F.C.); defranci@unicz.it (S.d.F.)
5. National Institution of Social Insurance, Department of Medical Law, 88100 Catanzaro, Italy; federicacolosimo@virgilio.it
6. Department of Public Health and Infectious Disease, "Sapienza" University of Rome 5, 00185 Roma, Italy; infermierenicola@hotmail.it
7. Unit of Microbiology and Virology, "Pugliese Ciaccio" Hospital, 88100 Catanzaro, Italy; manuelacolosimo@hotmail.it
8. Department of Health Sciences, University of Catanzaro, and Clinical Pharmacology and Pharmacovigilance Unit, Mater Domini Hospital, 88100 Catanzaro, Italy
* Correspondence: gallelli@unicz.it; Tel.: +39-030961712322
† These authors contributed equally to this paper.

Received: 27 December 2019; Accepted: 23 February 2020; Published: 26 February 2020

Abstract: Background: Matrix metalloproteinases (MMPs) are involved in vascular wall degradation, and drugs able to modulate MMP activity can be used to prevent or treat aneurysmal disease. In this study, we evaluated the effects of statins on MMP-2, MMP-9, and neutrophil gelatinase-associated lipocalin (NGAL) in both plasma and tissue in patients with aneurysmal disease. Methods: We performed a prospective, single-blind, multicenter, control group clinical drug trial on 184 patients of both sexes >18 years old with a diagnosis of arterial aneurysmal disease. Enrolled patients were divided into two groups: Group I under statin treatment and Group II not taking statins. In addition, 122 patients without aneurysmal disease and under statin treatment were enrolled as a control group (Group III). The expression of MMPs and NGAL in plasma was evaluated using ELISA, while their expression in endothelial tissues was evaluated using Western blot. Results: The ELISA test revealed greater plasma levels ($p < 0.01$) of MMPs and NGAL in Groups I and II vs. Group III. Western blot analysis showed higher expression ($p < 0.01$) of MMPs and NGAL in Group II vs. Group I, and this increase was significantly higher ($p < 0.01$) in patients treated with low potency statins compared to high potency ones. Conclusions: MMPs and NGAL seem to play a major role in the development of aneurysms, and their modulation by statins suggests that these drugs could be used to prevent arterial aneurysmal disease.

Keywords: MMPs; NGAL; statins; arterial aneurysms; patients

1. Introduction

An aneurysm is the dilatation of the aorta induced by vascular wall degradation that can localize centrally or peripherally, affecting all portions of the aortic tube [1]. Several biochemical mediators are involved in the vascular wall degradation of the aorta, e.g., neutrophil elastase, serine proteases, and matrix metalloproteinases (MMPs) [2]. This latter class of enzymes is divided into collagenases (MMP-1, MMP-8, MMP-13, MMP-18), stromolysins (MMP-3 and MMP-10), matrilysins (MMP-7 and MMP-26), and gelatinases (MMP-2 and MMP-9), according to their protein degradation capabilities. In general, MMPs are able to degrade most components of the extracellular matrix (ECM) of the vessel wall, leading to an imbalance between ECM synthesis and degradation [3]. MMP-2 and MMP-9 are the most common MMPs involved in endothelial degradation [4–6]. Their activity chiefly depends on the balance between the formation of complexes containing MMP-9, neutrophil gelatinase-associated lipocalin (NGAL), and the expression of MMP tissue inhibitors (TIMPs) [7]. An imbalance between these factors results in uncontrolled changes in the ECM, which may lead to a widening of the aneurysm vessel with a future aortic aneurysm rupture [3,8–10]. Previously, we reported that plasma MMP-9 and NGAL levels were significantly elevated in patients with cerebral artery aneurysms [11]. Moreover, we also documented that several drugs/compounds can modulate the activity of MMPs, improving a patient's clinical outcomes [12,13]. It has been documented that HMG-CoA reductase inhibitors, also known as statins, inhibit the synthesis of cholesterol in the liver and can decrease arterial aneurysm growth rates by stabilizing endothelial function [14–16] and reducing inflammation and oxidative stress [17,18]. In this pilot clinical trial, we evaluated the effects of statins on MMP-2, MMP-9, and NGAL plasma levels in patients with aneurysmal disease.

2. Materials and Methods

2.1. Study Design

We performed a prospective, single-blind, multicenter, control group study from October 2017 to October 2019 in subjects admitted to the Department of Medical and Surgical Science at University Magna Graecia, Catanzaro and to the Unit of Vascular and Endovascular Surgery at the Regional Hospital "Pugliese Ciaccio", Catanzaro.

The study was approved by the Investigational Review Board, in accordance with the Declaration of Helsinki and the Guideline for Good Clinical Practice. Before the beginning of the study, all participants provided written informed consent.

2.2. Patients

In this prospective, pilot clinical drug trial, we enrolled patients of both sexes >18 years old with aneurysmal disease that had been diagnosed clinically and instrumentally. Patients who had not signed the informed consent form were excluded from the study. The diagnosis of aneurysmal disease was determined by assessing patient presentation and vascular examination, including an ankle–brachial index of <0.9 (in peripheral diseases) and duplex ultrasonography.

2.3. Experimental Study

Enrolled patients were divided into two groups: Group I (statin-treated): patients with a central or peripheral aneurysm under statin treatment; Group II (statin-free): patients with a central or peripheral aneurysm without a history of statin use. The cardiovascular risk factors that were analyzed included a history of smoking, diabetes mellitus, hypertension, hyperlipidemia, and coronary artery disease based on a presenting thallium nuclear stress test or transthoracic echocardiogram. Chronic renal failure was defined as serum creatinine level >1.5 mg/dL.

At the time of admission, each patient underwent a baseline contrast-enhanced computed tomography scan for diagnosis of the disease and for evaluation of the aneurysm length, maximum aneurysm diameter, diameter of the access vessels, and presence or absence of a wall thrombus at the level of the central or peripheral aneurysm. Follow-ups were performed at 1 (T1) and 3 (T2) months after surgery. Finally, patients >18 years old without aneurysmal disease, but treated with statins, were enrolled as **Group III** and were defined as a control group.

2.4. Endpoints

Primary endpoint: Statistically significant difference ($p < 0.05$) in the plasma levels of MMP-2, MMP-9, and NGAL between patients with central and peripheral aneurysms treated or not treated with HMG-CoA reductase inhibitors. In addition, the statistically significant difference ($p < 0.05$) of plasma levels of MMP-2, MMP-9, and NGAL among patients with aneurysmal disease taking statins at high and low doses/potencies.

Secondary endpoint: Correlation between the expression of MMP-2, MMP-9, and NGAL in plasma and tissue levels and the maximum diameter of the aneurysm.

Safety endpoint: Development of muscle pain in patients under statin treatment compared to the patients free of statins and correlation with plasma levels of MMP-2, MMP-9, and NGAL.

2.5. Enzyme-Linked Immunosorbent Assay (ELISA)

In patients enrolled in Groups I and II, to evaluate the plasma levels of MMP-2, MMP-9, and NGAL, blood samples collected at the time of admission (T0) and during the follow-ups (T1 and T2) were frozen at −80 °C for ELISA evaluation. In contrast, in patients enrolled in Group III, blood collected during the routine evaluation for lipid plasma levels (T0) was frozen at −80 °C for ELISA evaluation. The ELISA test was conducted according to our previous study [19–21]. Commercially available sandwich ELISA kits for the inactive form of MMP-2, MMP-9, and NGAL (Biotrak MMP-2 and MMP-9 Human ELISA System, Amersham Pharmacia Biotech, Buckinghamshire, UK; NGAL Human ELISA System, Bioporto Diagnostics, Gentofte, Denmark) were used, following the manufacturers' instructions. The absorbance of each well was measured with a microtiter plate reader (Synergy H1, BioTeck, Winooski, VT, USA).

2.6. Protein Extraction and Immunoblot Analysis

Western blot analysis was performed in agreement with our previous studies [22–24] and only on tissue derived from arterial aneurysms (Groups I and II). About 40 mg of arterial aneurysm obtained by removing the aneurysm wall during the surgical procedures was immediately washed in ice-cold physiological saline. In agreement with the instructions of the total protein extraction kit, the tissues were lysed in 2 mL of tissue protein extraction reagent (25 mmol/L bicine, 150 mmol/L sodium chloride pH 7.6 (Thermo Scientific, Waltham, MA, USA)) and then were placed in ice for homogenization by grinding. Tissue homogenates were centrifuged twice for 10 min at 12,000× g and 4 °C. Supernatants were collected and proteins were quantified according to the instructions of the Quant-iT™ Protein Assaykit (Thermo Fisher). They were then lyophilized and resuspended in 100 µL tissue protein extraction reagent, and an equal amount of protein extracts was then separated using 15% sodium dodecyl sulfate–polyacrylamide gel electrophoresis (SDS-PAGE) under constant voltage (about 150 V) and transferred to nitrocellulose membranes (Amersham Pharmacia, Little Chalfont, UK). Immunoblotting of protein was performed using anti-MMP-2, anti-MMP-9, and anti-NGAL (abcam #ab86607, #ab119906, and #ab23477, respectively) monoclonal primary antibodies (1:1000); each one was separately incubated for 1 h at room temperature in TBST 1x and 5% of milk under shake. Then, goat antimouse IgG-HRP (abcam #ab205719) secondary antibody (1:5000) was incubated for 2 h at room temperature in TBST 1x as described [7]. Loading conditions were determined with polyclonal GAPDH (Sigma-Aldrich) primary antibody (1:1000) after membrane stripping for 1 h at room temperature in TBST 1x and 5% of milk under shake. Then, goat antirabbit IgG-HRP (Santa Cruz #sc-2004) secondary antibody (1:10,000) was incubated for 2 h at room temperature in TBST 1x. Bands were visualized by enhanced chemiluminescence (ECL Plus, Amersham Pharmacia); the intensities of experimental bands were analyzed and normalized by loading control GAPDH by computer-assisted densitometry using Photoshop and then expressed as arbitrary units. All experiments were performed in triplicate.

2.7. Safety Evaluation

The development of adverse drug reactions (ADRs) (e.g., liver toxicity and myalgia) and drug–drug interactions were evaluated using the Naranjo scale and the drug interactions probability scales, respectively, in agreement with our previous studies [25–28].

2.8. Statistical Analysis

Patient characteristics data (Table 1) are expressed as absolute values or as mean ± standard deviation. MMP and NGAL expression data (Figures 1–4) are represented as mean values ± standard error of the mean (SEM). The Student's t-test was performed to analyze the difference between each group and the control. Analysis of variance was used to evaluate the difference between the groups. The threshold of statistical significance was set at * $p < 0.05$. SPSS (SPSS Inc., Chicago, IL, USA) software was used for statistical analyses. We defined and labeled this study as exploratory; therefore, we did not determine a power calculation.

Table 1. Enrolled patients in Group I (statin-treated), Group II (statin-free), and Group III (without aneurysm, taking statins, defined control group). Data are expressed as absolute values or as mean ± standard deviation.

Characteristics	Group I (n = 95)	Group II (n = 119)	Group III (n = 122)
Mean age (years)	71.5 ± 6.3	70.6 ± 6.4	69.3 ± 6.3
Male	65	78	68
Female	30	41	54
Aneurysm diameter	54.2 ± 15.2	49.3 ± 17.9	----
Cigarette smokers	42	63	59
Body mass index			
>30	12	10	22
25–29.9	70	94	83
18.5–24.9	13	15	17
<18.5	0	0	0
Glutamic oxaloacetic transaminase	33.3 ± 3.2	28.1 ± 4.9	26.7 ± 4.1
Glutamic pyruvic transaminase	32.5 ± 4.3	31.1 ± 3.6	29.3 ± 5.5
Platelet count	290.630 ± 21.315/µL	312.250 ± 28.530/µL	279.870 ± 53.210/µL
Comorbidity			
Blood hypertension	86	112	108
COPD	45	60	36
Hypercholesterolemia	95	----	68
Acute coronary syndrome	55	----	15
Diabetes type II	42	21	35
Diabetes type I	8	10	9
Pharmacological therapy			
Antihypertensive	86	112	108
Antiarrhythmic	32	----	2
Bronchodilators	45	60	36
Statins	95	----	68
Hypoglycemic drugs	39	16	35
Insulin	8	10	9
ADRs related to statins			
Myalgia	38		39
Gastrointestinal disturbance	12		16
Increase in transaminases	8		10

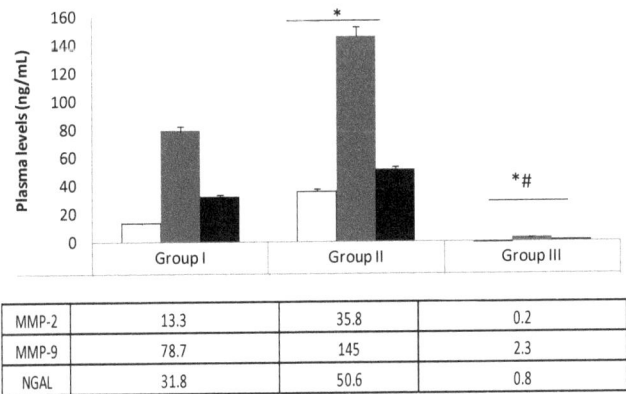

MMP-2	13.3	35.8	0.2
MMP-9	78.7	145	2.3
NGAL	31.8	50.6	0.8

Figure 1. Plasma levels of matrix metalloproteinase (MMP)-2, MMP-9, and neutrophil gelatinase-associated lipocalin (NGAL) in enrolled patients at the time of admission (T = 0). Group I: aneurysmal patients using statins; Group II: aneurysmal patients, statin-free; Group III: control patients. Group III vs. Group I, * $p < 0.01$; Group III vs. Group II, # $p < 0.01$.

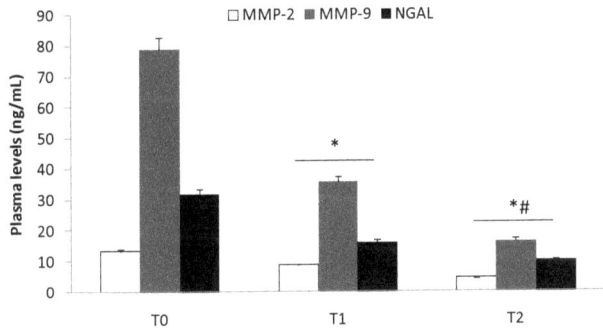

Figure 2. Plasma levels of MMP-2, MMP-9, and NGAL in aneurysmal patients under statin treatment (Group I) at the time of admission (T0) and 1 (T1) and 3 (T2) months later. T1 vs. T0, * $p < 0.01$; T2 vs. T1, # $p < 0.01$.

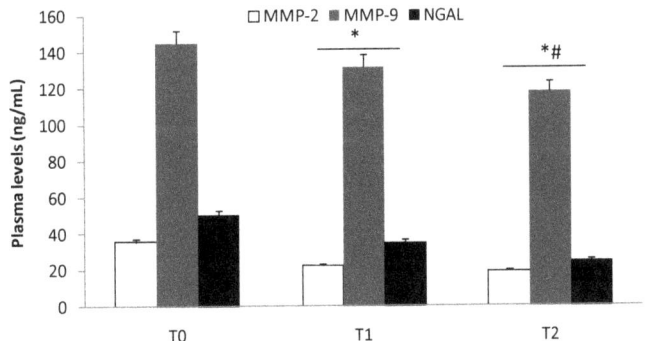

Figure 3. Plasma levels of MMP-2, MMP-9, and NGAL in aneurysmal patients free of statin treatment (Group II) at the time of admission (T0) and 1 (T1) and 3 (T2) months later. T1 vs. T0, * $p < 0.05$; T2 vs. T1, # $p < 0.05$.

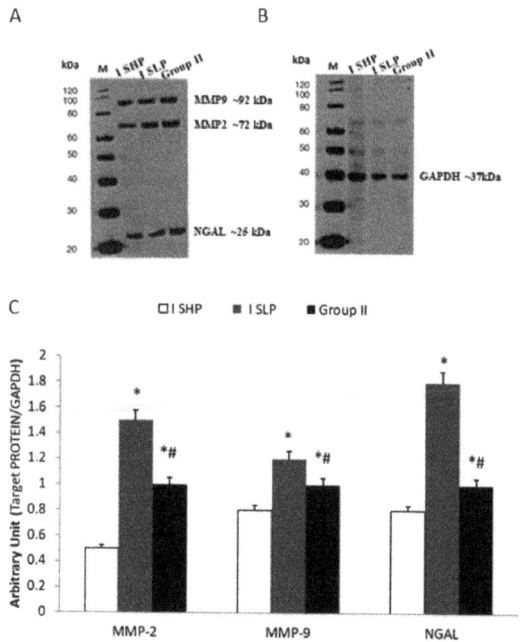

Figure 4. (**A**) Representative tissue levels of MMP-2, MMP-9, and NGAL in aneurysmal tissue. (**B**) GAPDH is used as loading control. (**C**) Tissue expression of MMP2, MMP-9, and NGAL in patients enrolled in Group I and treated with statin high potency (I SHP) (taking rosuvastatin 40 mg/day or atorvastatin 80 mg/day) or statin low potency (I SLP) (taking rosuvastatin <40 mg/day or atorvastatin <80 mg/day) and in patients enrolled in Group II (statin-free treatment). The results are expressed as mean ± standard error of the mean (SEM); * $p < 0.01$ vs. Group I SHP; # $p < 0.01$ vs. Group I SLP.

3. Results

3.1. Patients

In this study, we enrolled 184 patients—123 males (mean age 73.2 ± 8.6 years) and 61 females (mean age 68.7 ± 4.1 years)—with a diagnosis of central or peripheral aneurysmal disease: 15 in the popliteal artery (APA = 8.1%), 6 in the femoral artery (AFA = 3.3%), 28 in the iliac artery (AIA = 15.2%), and 135 in the abdominal aorta (AAA = 73.4%). Group I statin-treated: there were 65 patients—45 males (mean age 73.5 ± 8.4 years) and 20 females (mean age 69.4 ± 4.3 years)—taking rosuvastatin 10–40 mg/day or atorvastatin 20–80 mg/day. In this group, we designated further subgroups as statin high potency (SHP) (taking rosuvastatin 40 mg/day or atorvastatin 80 mg/day) and statin low potency (SLP) (taking rosuvastatin <40 mg/day or atorvastatin <80 mg/day). Group II statin-free: there were 119 patients—78 males (mean age 72.9 ± 8.8 years) and 41 females (mean age 68.3 ± 4.0 years)—who had never used statins as pharmacological treatment. Both groups had true aneurysms and had not received a vascular intervention or any other operative vascular interventions within the 3 years prior to inclusion in this study.

The control group was classified as Group III. In this group, there were 122 patients—68 males (median age 71 ± 7.3) and 54 females (median age 67.5 ± 5.2)—under statin treatment; they were screened with duplex ultrasonography to exclude the presence of asymptomatic central or peripheral aneurysms. Finally, in 58 patients of Group I (61%) and in 65 patients of Group III (53.3%), adverse drug reactions related to statin use were present. Despite this, statin treatment was not dismissed.

Patients' characteristics are shown in Table 1.

3.2. Elisa Test of MMP-2, MMP-9, and NGAL Plasma Levels

ELISA biochemical determination revealed greater plasma levels ($p < 0.01$) of MMP-2 and MMP-9 in patients with aneurysms (Groups I and II), compared to control patients (Group III); lower levels of MMP-2, MMP-9, and NGAL ($p < 0.01$) were found in patients treated with statins (Group I) compared with untreated patients (Group II) (Figure 1).

The same trend was evident in Groups I and II (Figures 2 and 3; $p < 0.05$). The reduction (T2) remained significantly higher ($p < 0.01$) compared to patients enrolled in Group III (Figure 4). Finally, we did not record any difference in the expression of MMP-2 and MMP-9 in patients who developed myalgia during statin treatment.

3.3. Protein Expression Levels of MMP-2, MMP-9, and NGAL in Aneurysmal Tissues

Western blot analysis showed increased protein expression ($p < 0.01$) of MMP-2, MMP-9, and NGAL in tissues of statin-untreated patients (Group II) compared to statin-treated patients (Group I). This increase was significantly higher ($p < 0.01$) in patients receiving low potency statins (Group I SLP) compared to patients treated with high potency statins (Group I SHP) (Figure 4A–C).

4. Discussion

In this study, we evaluated the expression of MMP-2, MMP-9, and NGAL in the plasma and tissue of patients with aneurysmal diseases. The modulation of these three biochemical indicators of aortic integrity in patients under statin treatment was also studied. Recently, in a preclinical experimental model, Krueger et al. [29] documented that vascular damage is associated with the upregulation of MMPs, which are involved in elastin degradation. An uncreated expression of MMPs causes loss of elastin and can induce compensatory fibrosis and inflammation with the destruction of all major matrix components, excessive distension, and vessel wall rupture [30–32]. In this view, recently, we documented that vascular damage induces an inflammatory response that can evoke a local reaction with the activation and recall of cytokines and inflammatory mediators [33] involved in aneurysmal diseases [32,34]. In an interesting pilot study, Yuwen et al. [35], investigating the expression of a plethora of cytokines in patients with aortic aneurysmal disease compared to healthy patients, described the role of several cytokines (i.e., CC chemokines, CXC chemokines, proinflammatory cytokines, growth factors, proteolytic proteins, and cell adhesion cytokines) in the pathogenesis of the aneurysms. In this study, several cytokines (e.g., IL-1α, IL-1β, IL-2, and IL-17) and growth factors (e.g., insulin-like growth factor-1, transforming growth factor-α, and tumor necrosis factor-α) were reported to activate NGAL, a marker of neutrophil activation [36] that is involved in tissue injury [37,38]. In our previous study, we documented an increase in plasma levels and tissue expression of both MMP-9 and NGAL in patients with central and peripheral aneurysms [7]. In the present study, we confirmed the involvement of MMP-2, MMP-9, and NGAL in aneurysmal lesions (Figure 1), and we also demonstrated their plasma decrease during the follow-ups (Figures 2 and 3). We also detected the protein expression levels of those biochemical mediators in aneurysmatic tissues, with no differences with respect to the location of the lesion. MMP-2 is derived from smooth muscle cells and fibroblasts and to a lesser extent macrophages [39], whereas MMP-9 is predominantly derived from macrophages and neutrophils [40]. Both are involved in the development of thoracic and aortic aneurysms [41,42]. On the other hand, NGAL levels reflect both inflammation and leukocyte activation in patients with arterial aneurysms and are correlated with aneurysm growth [43]. Of note, NGAL is released in the acute phase of inflammation by the secretory machinery of leukocytes and, in the glycosylated form, covalently binds to MMP-9 to make the MMP-9/NGAL complex. This complex, in turn, triggers an enhancement of the enzymatic activity of MMP-9 and protects MMP-9 from proteolytic degradation by TIMP1 and 2 proteins [37,44]. The crucial role of MMP-9 in the imbalance of the aortic wall drives the need to have pharmacological tools that can decrease its levels in the aneurysmal patient. In this view, we documented that several drugs/compounds are able to inhibit MMP expression [13,20].

Likewise, we reported that HMG-CoA reductase inhibitors (simvastatin and rosuvastatin) can block RAS prenylation, and thus are able to inhibit NF-κB signaling as well as decrease MMP-2 and MMP-9 protein expression in cell culture models [17,18]. In the present study, we reported that treatment with HMG-CoA reductase inhibitors at a high dose decreases the aneurysmal tissue levels of MMP-2, MMP-9, and NGAL (Figure 4). In an experimental study, Luan et al. [45] reported that statins inhibit in a dose-dependent manner the secretion of MMPs and decrease their collagenolytic, caseinolytic, and gelatinolytic activities. Moreover, other authors have documented that statins reduce the secretion of a broad spectrum of MMPs from macrophages and vascular endothelial cells, suggesting a beneficial effect of these drugs on these cells [46,47]. In our study, we documented that high potency statins compared to low potency ones have chemical characteristics that allow them to independently affect MMP-2, MMP-9, and NGAL in aneurysmal tissue levels, with no difference with respect to the site of the aneurysm. On the other hand, in the current study, we documented that 61% of patients in Group I and its relative subgroups, as well as 53.3% of patients in Group III, developed muscle pain as ADRs related to statin use. It is worth mentioning that the inhibition of HMG-CoA reductase blocks the synthesis of mevalonate, a precursor of farnesyl pyrophosphate that, in addition to being a substrate of cholesterol, is also the substrate for ubiquinone, also known as coenzyme Q synthesis [48]. Therefore, integrating coenzyme Q with supplements can be a strategy for reducing muscle pain mediated by statins [49,50]. Our study adds knowledge for clinical practice, but it also has some limitations. First, we measured the immune reactivity of MMP-2, MMP-9, and NGAL in the plasma of patients suffering from aneurysmal disease. These biochemical assays do not reflect the enzymatic activity of the protease. Second, the aneurysmal tissues were obtained from surgery patients in which the aneurysm had reached a specific size, so we do not know if the early stages of aneurysms have the same alterations described here. Third, more biochemical and mechanistic studies are required to determine the action of HMG-CoA reductase inhibitors, since NGAL decreased as well as MMP-9.

5. Conclusions

In conclusion, MMP-2, MMP-9, and NGAL levels seem to play a major role in the development of aneurysms, and their levels are modulated by statin treatment, suggesting that HMG-CoA reductase inhibitors have a role in the prevention of these clinical manifestations.

Author Contributions: Conceptualization, E.C., E.P., L.G., G.G., and S.d.F.; methodology, E.P., M.C.C., F.C. (Federica Colosimo), and M.C.; clinical study, G.G., S.d.F., E.L., F.C. (Francesca Curcio), and L.G.; statistical analysis, R.C. and N.I.; writing—original draft preparation, E.C., E.L., F.C. (Francesca Curcio) and F.C. (Federica Colosimo); writing—review and editing, E.P., M.C.C., and S.d.F.; supervision, L.G.; resources, S.d.F. All authors have read and agreed to the published version of the manuscript.

Funding: This research received no external funding.

Conflicts of Interest: The authors declare no conflict of interest.

References

1. Davies, M.J. Aortic aneurysm formation: Lessons from human studies and experimental models. *Circulation* **1998**, *98*, 193–195. [CrossRef] [PubMed]
2. Fontaine, V.; Jacob, M.P.; Houard, X.; Rossignol, P.; Plissonnier, D.; Angles-Cano, E.; Michel, J.B. Involvement of the mural thrombus as a site of protease release and activation in human aortic aneurysms. *Am. J. Pathol.* **2002**, *161*, 1701–1710. [CrossRef]
3. Petersen, E.; Wagberg, F.; Angquist, K.A. Proteolysis of the abdominal aortic aneurysm wall and the association with rupture. *Eur. J. Vasc. Endovasc. Surg.* **2002**, *23*, 153–157. [CrossRef] [PubMed]
4. Sakalihasan, N.; Delvenne, P.; Nusgens, B.V.; Limet, R.; Lapiere, C.M. Activated forms of mmp2 and mmp9 in abdominal aortic aneurysms. *J. Vasc. Surg.* **1996**, *24*, 127–133. [CrossRef]
5. Katsuda, S.; Okada, Y.; Imai, K.; Nakanishi, I. Matrix metalloproteinase-9 (92-kd gelatinase/type iv collagenase equals gelatinase b) can degrade arterial elastin. *Am. J. Pathol.* **1994**, *145*, 1208–1218.

6. Goodall, S.; Crowther, M.; Hemingway, D.M.; Bell, P.R.; Thompson, M.M. Ubiquitous elevation of matrix metalloproteinase-2 expression in the vasculature of patients with abdominal aneurysms. *Circulation* **2001**, *104*, 304–309. [CrossRef]
7. Serra, R.; Grande, R.; Montemurro, R.; Butrico, L.; Calio, F.G.; Mastrangelo, D.; Scarcello, E.; Gallelli, L.; Buffone, G.; de Franciscis, S. The role of matrix metalloproteinases and neutrophil gelatinase-associated lipocalin in central and peripheral arterial aneurysms. *Surgery* **2015**, *157*, 155–162. [CrossRef]
8. Ziora, D.; Dworniczak, S.; Kozielski, J. Induced sputum metalloproteinases and their inhibitors in relation to exhaled nitrogen oxide and sputum nitric oxides and other inflammatory cytokines in patients with chronic obstructive pulmonary disease. *J. Physiol. Pharmacol.* **2008**, *59* (Suppl. 6), 809–817.
9. De Franciscis, S.; Gallelli, L.; Amato, B.; Butrico, L.; Rossi, A.; Buffone, G.; Calio, F.G.; De Caridi, G.; Grande, R.; Serra, R. Plasma mmp and timp evaluation in patients with deep venous thrombosis: Could they have a predictive role in the development of post-thrombotic syndrome? *Int. Wound J.* **2016**, *13*, 1237–1245. [CrossRef]
10. Wilson, W.R.; Anderton, M.; Schwalbe, E.C.; Jones, J.L.; Furness, P.N.; Bell, P.R.; Thompson, M.M. Matrix metalloproteinase-8 and -9 are increased at the site of abdominal aortic aneurysm rupture. *Circulation* **2006**, *113*, 438–445. [CrossRef]
11. Serra, R.; Volpentesta, G.; Gallelli, L.; Grande, R.; Buffone, G.; Lavano, A.; de Franciscis, S. Metalloproteinase-9 and neutrophil gelatinase-associated lipocalin plasma and tissue levels evaluation in middle cerebral artery aneurysms. *Br. J. Neurosurg.* **2014**. [CrossRef] [PubMed]
12. Serra, R.; Gallelli, L.; Conti, A.; De Caridi, G.; Massara, M.; Spinelli, F.; Buffone, G.; Calio, F.G.; Amato, B.; Ceglia, S.; et al. The effects of sulodexide on both clinical and molecular parameters in patients with mixed arterial and venous ulcers of lower limbs. *Drug Des. Dev. Ther.* **2014**, *8*, 519–527. [CrossRef] [PubMed]
13. Serra, R.; Gallelli, L.; Buffone, G.; Molinari, V.; Stillitano, D.M.; Palmieri, C.; de Franciscis, S. Doxycycline speeds up healing of chronic venous ulcers. *Int. Wound J.* **2015**, *12*, 179–184. [CrossRef] [PubMed]
14. Piechota-Polanczyk, A.; Goraca, A.; Demyanets, S.; Mittlboeck, M.; Domenig, C.; Neumayer, C.; Wojta, J.; Nanobachvili, J.; Huk, I.; Klinger, M. Simvastatin decreases free radicals formation in the human abdominal aortic aneurysm wall via nf-kappab. *Eur. J. Vasc. Endovasc. Surg.* **2012**, *44*, 133–137. [CrossRef]
15. Piechota-Polanczyk, A.; Demyanets, S.; Nykonenko, O.; Huk, I.; Mittlboeck, M.; Domenig, C.M.; Neumayer, C.; Wojta, J.; Nanobachvili, J.; Klinger, M. Decreased tissue levels of cyclophilin a, a cyclosporine a target and phospho-erk1/2 in simvastatin patients with abdominal aortic aneurysm. *Eur. J. Vasc. Endovasc. Surg.* **2013**, *45*, 682–688. [CrossRef]
16. Liao, J.K. Effects of statins on 3-hydroxy-3-methylglutaryl coenzyme a reductase inhibition beyond low-density lipoprotein cholesterol. *Am. J. Cardiol.* **2005**, *96*, 24F–33F. [CrossRef]
17. Gallelli, L.; Falcone, D.; Scaramuzzino, M.; Pelaia, G.; D'Agostino, B.; Mesuraca, M.; Terracciano, R.; Spaziano, G.; Maselli, R.; Navarra, M.; et al. Effects of simvastatin on cell viability and proinflammatory pathways in lung adenocarcinoma cells exposed to hydrogen peroxide. *BMC Pharmacol. Toxicol.* **2014**, *15*, 67. [CrossRef]
18. Falcone, D.; Gallelli, L.; Di Virgilio, A.; Tucci, L.; Scaramuzzino, M.; Terracciano, R.; Pelaia, G.; Savino, R. Effects of simvastatin and rosuvastatin on ras protein, matrix metalloproteinases and nf-kappab in lung cancer and in normal pulmonary tissues. *Cell Prolif.* **2013**, *46*, 172–182. [CrossRef]
19. Pelaia, G.; Cuda, G.; Vatrella, A.; Gallelli, L.; Fratto, D.; Gioffre, V.; D'Agostino, B.; Caputi, M.; Maselli, R.; Rossi, F.; et al. Effects of hydrogen peroxide on mapk activation, il-8 production and cell viability in primary cultures of human bronchial epithelial cells. *J. Cell. Biochem.* **2004**, *93*, 142–152. [CrossRef]
20. Serra, R.; Grande, R.; Buffone, G.; Scarcello, E.; Tripodi, F.; Rende, P.; Gallelli, L.; de Franciscis, S. Effects of glucocorticoids and tumor necrosis factor-alpha inhibitors on both clinical and molecular parameters in patients with takayasu arteritis. *J. Pharmacol. Pharmacother.* **2014**, *5*, 193–196.
21. Singh, S.R.; Sullo, N.; Matteis, M.; Spaziano, G.; McDonald, J.; Saunders, R.; Woodman, L.; Urbanek, K.; De Angelis, A.; De Palma, R.; et al. Nociceptin/orphanin FQ (N/OFQ) modulates immunopathology and airway hyperresponsiveness representing a novel target for the treatment of asthma. *Br. J. Pharmacol.* **2016**, *8*, 1286–1301. [CrossRef] [PubMed]
22. Serra, R.; Gallelli, L.; Grande, R.; Amato, B.; De Caridi, G.; Sammarco, G.; Ferrari, F.; Butrico, L.; Gallo, G.; Rizzuto, A.; et al. Hemorrhoids and matrix metalloproteinases: A multicenter study on the predictive role of biomarkers. *Surgery* **2016**, *159*, 487–494. [CrossRef] [PubMed]

23. Pelaia, G.; Gallelli, L.; Renda, T.; Fratto, D.; Falcone, D.; Caraglia, M.; Busceti, M.T.; Terracciano, R.; Vatrella, A.; Maselli, R.; et al. Effects of statins and farnesyl transferase inhibitors on erk phosphorylation, apoptosis and cell viability in non-small lung cancer cells. *Cell Prolif.* **2012**, *45*, 557–565. [CrossRef] [PubMed]
24. Gallelli, L.; Pelaia, G.; Fratto, D.; Muto, V.; Falcone, D.; Vatrella, A.; Curto, L.S.; Renda, T.; Busceti, M.T.; Liberto, M.C.; et al. Effects of budesonide on p38 mapk activation, apoptosis and il-8 secretion, induced by tnf-alpha and haemophilus influenzae in human bronchial epithelial cells. *Int. J. Immunopathol. Pharmacol.* **2010**, *23*, 471–479. [CrossRef]
25. Rende, P.; Paletta, L.; Gallelli, G.; Raffaele, G.; Natale, V.; Brissa, N.; Costa, C.; Gratteri, S.; Giofre, C.; Gallelli, L. Retrospective evaluation of adverse drug reactions induced by antihypertensive treatment. *J. Pharmacol. Pharmacother.* **2013**, *4*, S47–S50.
26. Gallelli, L.; Galasso, O.; Urzino, A.; Sacca, S.; Falcone, D.; Palleria, C.; Longo, P.; Corigliano, A.; Terracciano, R.; Savino, R.; et al. Characteristics and clinical implications of the pharmacokinetic profile of ibuprofen in patients with knee osteoarthritis. *Clin. Drug Investig.* **2012**, *32*, 827–833. [CrossRef]
27. Gallelli, L.; Colosimo, M.; Tolotta, G.A.; Falcone, D.; Luberto, L.; Curto, L.S.; Rende, P.; Mazzei, F.; Marigliano, N.M.; De Sarro, G.; et al. Prospective randomized double-blind trial of racecadotril compared with loperamide in elderly people with gastroenteritis living in nursing homes. *Eur. J. Clin. Pharmacol.* **2010**, *66*, 137–144. [CrossRef]
28. Ciliberto, D.; Ierardi, A.; Caroleo, B.; Scalise, L.; Cimellaro, A.; Colangelo, L.; Spaziano, G.; Gallelli, L. Panitumumab induced forearm panniculitis in two women with metastatic colon cancer. *Curr. Drug Saf.* **2019**, *14*, 233–237.
29. Krueger, F.; Kappert, K.; Foryst-Ludwig, A.; Kramer, F.; Clemenz, M.; Grzesiak, A.; Sommerfeld, M.; Paul Frese, J.; Greiner, A.; Kintscher, U.; et al. At1-receptor blockade attenuates outward aortic remodeling associated with diet-induced obesity in mice. *Clin. Sci. (Lond)* **2017**, *131*, 1989–2005. [CrossRef]
30. Dorman, G.; Cseh, S.; Hajdu, I.; Barna, L.; Konya, D.; Kupai, K.; Kovacs, L.; Ferdinandy, P. Matrix metalloproteinase inhibitors: A critical appraisal of design principles and proposed therapeutic utility. *Drugs* **2010**, *70*, 949–964. [CrossRef]
31. Hu, J.; Van den Steen, P.E.; Sang, Q.X.; Opdenakker, G. Matrix metalloproteinase inhibitors as therapy for inflammatory and vascular diseases. *Nat. Rev. Drug Discov.* **2007**, *6*, 480–498. [CrossRef] [PubMed]
32. Maguire, E.M.; Pearce, S.W.A.; Xiao, R.; Oo, A.Y.; Xiao, Q. Matrix metalloproteinase in abdominal aortic aneurysm and aortic dissection. *Pharmaceuticals* **2019**, *12*, 118. [CrossRef] [PubMed]
33. Gallelli, L. Escin: A review of its anti-edematous, anti-inflammatory, and venotonic properties. *Drug Design Dev. Ther.* **2019**, *13*, 3425–3437. [CrossRef] [PubMed]
34. Serra, R.; Butrico, L.; Grande, R.; Placida, G.D.; Rubino, P.; Settimio, U.F.; Quarto, G.; Amato, M.; Furino, E.; Compagna, R.; et al. Venous aneurysm complicating arteriovenous fistula access and matrix metalloproteinases. *Open Med. (Wars)* **2015**, *10*, 519–522.
35. Yuwen, L.; Ciqiu, Y.; Yi, S.; Ruilei, L.; Yuanhui, L.; Bo, L.; Songqi, L.; Weiming, L.; Jie, L. A pilot study of protein microarray for simultaneous analysis of 274 cytokines between abdominal aortic aneurysm and normal aorta. *Angiology* **2019**, *70*, 830–837. [CrossRef]
36. De Franciscis, S.; Mastroroberto, P.; Gallelli, L.; Buffone, G.; Montemurro, R.; Serra, R. Increased plasma levels of metalloproteinase-9 and neutrophil gelatinase-associated lipocalin in a rare case of multiple artery aneurysm. *Ann. Vasc. Surg.* **2013**, *27*, 1185.e5–1185.e7. [CrossRef]
37. Yan, L.; Borregaard, N.; Kjeldsen, L.; Moses, M.A. The high molecular weight urinary matrix metalloproteinase (mmp) activity is a complex of gelatinase b/mmp-9 and neutrophil gelatinase-associated lipocalin (ngal). Modulation of mmp-9 activity by ngal. *J. Biol. Chem.* **2001**, *276*, 37258–37265. [CrossRef]
38. De Franciscis, S.; De Caridi, G.; Massara, M.; Spinelli, F.; Gallelli, L.; Buffone, G.; Calio, F.G.; Butrico, L.; Grande, R.; Serra, R. Biomarkers in post-reperfusion syndrome after acute lower limb ischaemia. *Int. Wound J.* **2016**, *13*, 854–859. [CrossRef]
39. Davis, V.; Persidskaia, R.; Baca-Regen, L.; Itoh, Y.; Nagase, H.; Persidsky, Y.; Ghorpade, A.; Baxter, B.T. Matrix metalloproteinase-2 production and its binding to the matrix are increased in abdominal aortic aneurysms. *Arterioscler. Thromb. Vasc. Biol.* **1998**, *18*, 1625–1633. [CrossRef]
40. Zhang, X.; Shen, Y.H.; LeMaire, S.A. Thoracic aortic dissection: Are matrix metalloproteinases involved? *Vascular* **2009**, *17*, 147–157. [CrossRef]

41. Jones, J.A.; Zavadzkas, J.A.; Chang, E.I.; Sheats, N.; Koval, C.; Stroud, R.E.; Spinale, F.G.; Ikonomidis, J.S. Cellular phenotype transformation occurs during thoracic aortic aneurysm development. *J. Thorac. Cardiovasc. Surg.* **2010**, *140*, 653–659. [CrossRef] [PubMed]
42. Jones, J.A.; Barbour, J.R.; Lowry, A.S.; Bouges, S.; Beck, C.; McClister, D.M., Jr.; Mukherjee, R.; Ikonomidis, J.S. Spatiotemporal expression and localization of matrix metalloproteinas-9 in a murine model of thoracic aortic aneurysm. *J. Vasc. Surg.* **2006**, *44*, 1314–1321. [CrossRef] [PubMed]
43. Ramos-Mozo, P.; Madrigal-Matute, J.; Vega de Ceniga, M.; Blanco-Colio, L.M.; Meilhac, O.; Feldman, L.; Michel, J.B.; Clancy, P.; Golledge, J.; Norman, P.E.; et al. Increased plasma levels of ngal, a marker of neutrophil activation, in patients with abdominal aortic aneurysm. *Atherosclerosis* **2012**, *220*, 552–556. [CrossRef] [PubMed]
44. Swedenborg, J.; Eriksson, P. The intraluminal thrombus as a source of proteolytic activity. *Ann. N. Y. Acad. Sci.* **2006**, *1085*, 133–138. [CrossRef]
45. Luan, Z.; Chase, A.J.; Newby, A.C. Statins inhibit secretion of metalloproteinases-1, -2, -3, and -9 from vascular smooth muscle cells and macrophages. *Arterioscler. Thromb. Vasc. Biol.* **2003**, *23*, 769–775. [CrossRef] [PubMed]
46. Bellosta, S.; Via, D.; Canavesi, M.; Pfister, P.; Fumagalli, R.; Paoletti, R.; Bernini, F. Hmg-coa reductase inhibitors reduce mmp-9 secretion by macrophages. *Arterioscler. Thromb. Vasc. Biol.* **1998**, *18*, 1671–1678. [CrossRef] [PubMed]
47. Wong, B.; Lumma, W.C.; Smith, A.M.; Sisko, J.T.; Wright, S.D.; Cai, T.Q. Statins suppress thp-1 cell migration and secretion of matrix metalloproteinase 9 by inhibiting geranylgeranylation. *J. Leukoc. Biol.* **2001**, *69*, 959–962.
48. Kawamukai, M. Biosynthesis of coenzyme q in eukaryotes. *Biosci. Biotechnol. Biochem.* **2016**, *80*, 23–33. [CrossRef]
49. Zlatohlavek, L.; Vrablik, M.; Grauova, B.; Motykova, E.; Ceska, R. The effect of coenzyme q10 in statin myopathy. *Neuro Endocrinol. Lett.* **2012**, *33* (Suppl. 2), 98–101.
50. Qu, H.; Guo, M.; Chai, H.; Wang, W.T.; Gao, Z.Y.; Shi, D.Z. Effects of coenzyme q10 on statin-induced myopathy: An updated meta-analysis of randomized controlled trials. *J. Am. Heart Assoc.* **2018**, *7*, e009835. [CrossRef]

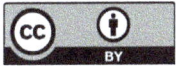 © 2020 by the authors. Licensee MDPI, Basel, Switzerland. This article is an open access article distributed under the terms and conditions of the Creative Commons Attribution (CC BY) license (http://creativecommons.org/licenses/by/4.0/).

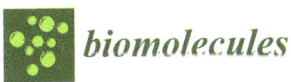

Article

An Oral Rinse Active Matrix Metalloproteinase-8 Point-of-Care Immunotest May Be Less Accurate in Patients with Crohn's Disease

Jaana Rautava [1,2,*], Ulvi K. Gürsoy [3], Adrian Kullström [1,3], Eija Könönen [3,4], Timo Sorsa [5,6], Taina Tervahartiala [5] and Mervi Gürsoy [3]

[1] Department of Oral Pathology and Oral Radiology, Institute of Dentistry, University of Turku, 20520 Turku, Finland; adrian.a.kullstrom@utu.fi
[2] Department of Pathology, Turku University Hospital, 20521 Turku, Finland
[3] Department of Periodontology, Institute of Dentistry, University of Turku, 20520 Turku, Finland; ulvi.gursoy@utu.fi (U.K.G.); eija.kononen@utu.fi (E.K.); mervi.gursoy@utu.fi (M.G.)
[4] Oral Health Care, Welfare Division, City of Turku, 20101 Turku, Finland
[5] Department of Oral and Maxillofacial Disease, Helsinki University Hospital, University of Helsinki, 00014 Helsinki, Finland; timo.sorsa@helsinki.fi (T.S.); taina.tervahartiala@helsinki.fi (T.T.)
[6] Department of Dental Medicine, Karolinska Institute, 14152 Huddinge, Sweden
* Correspondence: jaapoh@utu.fi; Tel.: +358-29-4505000

Received: 3 February 2020; Accepted: 26 February 2020; Published: 4 March 2020

Abstract: The diagnostic accuracy of point-of-care (PoC) applications may be compromised in individuals with additional inflammatory conditions. This cross-sectional study examined the performance of a commercial oral rinse active matrix metalloproteinase-8 (aMMP-8) PoC immunotest in individuals with ($n = 47$) and without Crohn's disease (CD) ($n = 41$). Oral rinse collected from the participants was analyzed by the PoC immunotest. Molecular forms and fragments of salivary MMP-8 were detected by western immunoblotting. The sensitivity of the immunotest for periodontitis was 60.0% in the CD group and 90.0% in the control group. The respective specificity was 75.0% and 80.0%. In both groups, clinical diagnosis of periodontitis exhibited a significant association with the immunotest results, however, the odds ratio (OR) was more than ten-fold in controls (OR 54.3, 95% CI: 3.1–953, $p = 0.006$) in comparison to CD patients (OR 5.2, 95% CI: 1.3–21.6, $p = 0.022$). According to Western immunoblot results, the immunotest MMP-8 positivity was not related to elevated levels of molecular forms and fragments of MMP-8 in the CD group, as in the control group. The diagnostic accuracy of the aMMP-8 PoC oral rinse immunotest is reduced in CD patients, which may be related to lower levels or undetectable complexes.

Keywords: collagenases; Crohn's disease; dental caries; mouth; periodontitis

1. Introduction

Crohn's disease (CD) is a chronic inflammatory disease of the gastrointestinal tract, involving a complex interplay between genetic risk, environmental exposures, the microbiota, and the immune system. Individuals suffering from CD seem to be prone to developing periodontitis, caries, and oral mucosal lesions [1–3]. CD patients have a higher decayed-missed-filled teeth (DMFT) index than healthy individuals, which could be due to differences in their diet [3]. Indeed, CD patients reportedly exhibit an increased sugar consumption and have insufficient oral hygiene [4]. The suggested link between CD and periodontitis may be explained by shared pathways in their pathogenesis related to altered gut/oral microbiota [5,6] and immune responsiveness [7]. Both CD and periodontitis have been linked to a disrupted immunological response to the local microbiota. The innate immune system, particularly neutrophils and their inadequate function, plays a major role in the pathogenesis of these diseases [8–10]. Of tissue-degrading matrix metalloproteinases (MMPs), MMP-8 is the key inflammatory mediator in their inter-relationship; elevated MMP-8 levels have been detected in CD patients both in the intestine and in the oral cavity [11,12].

Periodontitis is diagnosed based on clinical signs of gingival bleeding, loss of clinical attachment, deepened periodontal pockets, and the presence of radiographical alveolar bone loss [13,14]. Yet, the use of these parameters carries limitations, since they do not recognize the onset of inflammation or identify individuals who are at risk of disease initiation or progression in a given population [15]. Instead, biomarker-based diagnostic methods are less laborious, non-invasive, and do not require trained dentists, being especially useful in studies with large study populations [16].

In periodontology, point-of-care (PoC) tests aim to detect periodontal diseases by analyzing the levels of biomarkers in oral fluids (saliva, oral rinse, and/or gingival crevicular fluid) without need of a laboratory [17,18]. Among the tested biomarkers, salivary and oral rinse levels of MMP-8 are shown to be effective in distinguishing periodontitis patients from periodontally healthy individuals [19–21]. For instance, PoC tests using active MMP (aMMP)-8 as a diagnostic marker with a threshold of 20 ng/mL can successfully identify periodontitis with 64–95% sensitivity and 60–100% specificity [22–25]. Notably, the test sensitivity improves in line with disease severity [22,24].

To date, no data exist on the performance of the selected oral rinse aMMP-8 PoC immunotest in individuals with compromised immune responsiveness. In the present case-control study, we hypothesized that CD, a systemic condition with impaired immune function, leads to decreased sensitivity and specificity of the PoC immunotest. Our aim was to evaluate the utility of the immunotest for chair-side diagnostics of periodontal disease in subjects with and without CD. As a main conclusion, we state that the accuracy of the immunotest was impaired in individuals with CD.

2. Materials and Methods

2.1. Study Design and Enrolment of Participants

This was a case-control study conducted at the Institute of Dentistry, University of Turku, from January 2017 to May 2018. The CD group, consisting of 47 CD patients between the ages of 22 and 77 years, was recruited from a Crohn and Colitis patient organization (IBD Association of Finland). Their diagnosis of CD had previously been confirmed by endoscopy and histopathological analysis of intestinal biopsy specimens. The control group, including 41 age- and gender-matched individuals without CD or other immune-related diseases, was recruited using advertisements placed at the Institute of Dentistry, University of Turku. Exclusion criteria for both groups included diabetes mellitus, smoking, excessive use of alcohol, less than 24 teeth, and the use of antimicrobial medication in the preceding six months prior to the clinical examination. In addition, individuals with periodontitis as a manifestation of systemic disease [26] as well as pregnant or lactating women were excluded.

The research protocol was approved by the Ethical Committee of the Hospital District of Southwest Finland (114/1801/2016), and the study was conducted according to the guidelines of the World Medical Association Declaration of Helsinki. Each participant was informed of the purpose, potential side effects and benefits of the study and gave their written consent. A structured questionnaire was collected from all participants regarding their demographic data (such as age, sex, and residence), general health, medications, and previous dental care. Additionally, the short Crohn's disease activity index (CDAI) was used to assess the disease activity of the CD patients [27].

2.2. Clinical Oral Examination

The full-mouth clinical examination included registrations of oral mucosal status performed by a specialist in oral pathology (JR) together with cariological and periodontal measurements generated by a periodontist (MG). Before this study, the intra-examiner (MG) agreement was tested in double measurements of 10 patients and discovered to be very good.

The oral mucosal examination included visual inspection of the lips, mucous membranes of the oral cavity, and oropharynx while pressing the tongue down as well as manual palpation of the neck. All mucosal findings were described by clinical appearance and the site of the lesion. CD-associated mucosal lesions (sulcular ulceration, aphthous stomatitis, mucosal cobblestone appearance, lip swelling, angular cheilitis, mucogingivitis) were registered separately [28,29].

Cariological status was assessed based on visual inspection, fiber-optic transillumination and tactile examination on the five surfaces of each tooth. Additionally, initial caries lesions together with other hard tissue defects on tooth surfaces, such as erosion and attrition, were determined. Caries prevalence in the whole dentition (excluding the third molars) was expressed using the decayed-missed-filled surface (DMFS) index. The participants were classified as having caries when they had at least one tooth surface with a carious lesion.

Periodontal status was obtained from six sites per each natural tooth and dental implant using a WHO probe (LM-Instruments Oy, Parainen, Finland) with a ball-tip end diameter of 0.5 mm. A full-mouth dichotomous visible plaque index (VPI) score was recorded as percentage. Gingival recession (REC) was detected as the distance between the cemento-enamel junction and free gingival margin, while probing pocket depth (PPD) was measured from the free gingival margin to the most apical penetration point of the probe. Loss of clinical attachment level (CAL) was determined as the sum of REC and PPD. A full-mouth dichotomous gingival bleeding score was obtained upon bleeding on probing (BOP) and presented as percentage. In addition, furcation defects and tooth mobility scores were recorded.

Individuals with BOP < 15%, PPD < 4 mm, and no loss of CAL were regarded as periodontally healthy, whereas gingivitis was diagnosed in the presence of BOP ≥15% without periodontal pockets and loss of CAL [30]. The diagnostic criteria for periodontitis included PPD ≥ 4 mm and/or loss of CAL on ≥ 2 non-adjacent teeth together with BOP [31]. The severity of the disease was classified based on PPD and loss of CAL as follows: initial periodontitis (PPD 4 mm, CAL loss 1–2 mm), moderate periodontitis (PPD 5–6 mm, CAL loss 3–4 mm), and severe periodontitis (PPD ≥ 7 mm, CAL loss ≥ 5 mm). After the clinical examination, the patient was informed both orally and in written form of the findings. The patients with need for treatment were advised to contact their own dentist.

2.3. Application of an Oral Rinse aMMP-8 PoC Immunotest

The study participants were instructed to avoid tooth brushing, eating, and chewing gum 30 min prior to the visit. Oral rinse sampling was performed before the clinical oral examination. First, each participant pre-rinsed the mouth with tap water for 30 s and then spitted out or swallowed the fluid. After 60 s of waiting, they re-rinsed vigorously the mouth with 5 mL of rinsing fluid‡ for 30 s and then poured the entire sample into a measuring cup, from which the sample was drawn up into a syringe and used for the aMMP-8 PoC analysis.

The immunotest (PerioSafe® PRO, Dentognostics GmbH, Jena, Germany) was used according to the manufacturer's instructions. A single examiner (UKG) ran all tests, and the result was interpreted by visual estimation 5 min after testing. The outcome was defined as positive (+) when a double line (i.e., both test and control line) was visible on the test window or negative (−) when only a single line was observed [22].

2.4. MMP-8 Western Immunoblot

Stimulated saliva samples were collected for 5 min from the patients, separately from the immunotest. A modified enhanced chemiluminescence (ECL) western blotting kit (GE Healthcare, Amersham, UK) was used to detect the molecular forms of MMP-8 from the stimulated saliva as described earlier [32,33]. Salivary flow levels were measured to minimize the variations in sample collection and sample loading during immunoblottings. Briefly, the saliva samples were mixed with Laemmli's buffer without any reducing reagents. The samples were heated for 5 min, followed by protein separation with 11% sodium dodecyl sulphate (SDS)-polyacrylamide gels. The proteins were then electro-transferred onto nitrocellulose membranes (Protran, Whatman GmbH, Dassel, Germany). Milk powder (5%; Valio Ltd., Helsinki, Finland) was used to block non-specific binding in TBST buffer (10 mM Tris-HCl, pH 7.5, containing 22 mM NaCl and 0.05% Triton-X) for 1 h. The membranes were incubated with polyclonal primary antibodies anti-MMP-8 [34] overnight and followed by the horseradish peroxidase-linked secondary antibody (GE Healthcare, Buckinghamshire, UK) for 1 h. The target proteins were visualized using the ECL system, and scanned and converted into arbitrary units (relative levels of mean intensity) using GS-700 Imaging Densitometer Scanner (BioRad, Hercules, CA, USA) and Bio-Rad Quantity One program. Purified human activated MMP-8 (BioTeZ, Berlin, Germany) was used as positive control and low range prestained SDS-PAGE Standards (BioRad) served as a molecular weight marker.

2.5. Statistical Analyses

All statistical analyses were performed using the SPSS statistical program (version 24.0; IBM Inc., Armonk, NY, USA). The Chi square test was used for comparing demographic and clinical data (with the exception of age and number of teeth) between the CD and control groups. Age, salivary flow rate, and number of teeth were compared between the groups with one-way ANOVA test. Multinomial regression analyses were performed to describe the associations between periodontal diseases and the immunotest result, after adjusting for furcation and attrition defects. Statistical significance was defined as $p < 0.05$.

3. Results

3.1. Crohn's Disease Status

Of the 47 CD patients, 89.4% received medication for CD and 34.0% had undergone surgical treatment for CD. According to the short CDAI score, 53.2% of the subjects were in remission (short CDAI < 150 points), 31.9% had mild disease (short CDAI 150–219 points), 14.9% had moderate disease (short CDAI 220–450 points), and none had severe disease (CDAI > 450 points).

3.2. Oral Health Status

Characterization of the CD and control groups on the basis of periodontal findings is presented in Table 1.

Table 1. Characterization of the study groups (patients with Crohn's disease and their age- and gender-matched healthy controls) according to periodontal health status and stimulated salivary flow. PPD = probing pocket depth; BOP = bleeding on probing.

Findings	Crohn's Disease Group (N = 47)	Control Group (N = 41)	Difference P-Value
Gender (male %)	23.4	29.3	0.629
Age, years (mean, st.dev)	46.4 (13.9)	47.4 (13.2)	0.734
No. of teeth (mean, st.dev)	27 (2.3)	27.6 (2.4)	0.192
VPI % (mean, st.dev)	23.8 (20.8)	22.9 (18.7)	0.828
BOP % (mean, st.dev)	32.7 (23.3)	33.9 (28.6)	0.820
Individuals with PPD 4 mm (n, %)	22 (46.8)	13 (31.7)	0.192
Individuals with PPD 5–6 mm (n, %)	1 (2.1)	8 (19.5)	**0.011**
Individuals with PPD ≥ 7 mm (n, %)	0	5 (12.2)	**0.019**
Individuals with REC ≥ 1 mm (n, %)	33 (70.2)	28 (68.3)	1.000
Individuals with REC ≥ 3 mm (n, %)	14 (29.8)	12 (29.3)	0.073
Periodontal diagnosis			**0.021**
Periodontally healthy (n, %)	12 (25)	15 (36.6)	
Gingivitis (n, %)	20 (42.6)	15 (36.6)	
Initial periodontitis (n, %)	14 (29.8)	4 (9.8)	
Moderate periodontitis (n, %)	1 (2.1)	2 (4.9)	
Severe periodontitis (n, %)	0 (0)	5 (12.2)	
Stimulated salivary flow, ml/min (mean, st.dev)	1.42 (0.72)	1.59 (0.90)	0.313

The DMFS index was 35.8 for the CD patients and 23.9 for the controls ($p = 0.015$). At least one dentin caries lesion was found in 31.9% of the CD patients and 12.2% of the controls ($p = 0.028$). The mean stimulated salivary flow was 1.42 mL/min and 1.59 mL/min, respectively. CD-associated mucosal lesions were detected in 10.6% of the CD patients. Mucosal lesions not associated with CD were found in 34.0% of the CD patients and 36.6% of the controls.

3.3. Oral Rinse aMMP-8 PoC Immunotest

The outcomes of the aMMP-8 PoC immunotest were tested against various clinical outcomes and diagnoses in terms of its sensitivity and specificity as presented in Table 2. Sensitivity and specificity values of the aMMP-8 PoC immunotest for detecting periodontitis were 60.0% and 75.0% in the CD patients, 90.9% and 80.0% in the controls, and 73.1% and 77.4% in the whole population, respectively.

Table 2. Sensitivity and specificity of the oral rinse active matrix metalloproteinase-8 oral rinse point-of-care immunotest in relation to the presence of probing pocket depth (PPD), bleeding on probing (BOP), furcation defects, attrition, periodontal diseases (gingivitis or periodontitis), and periodontitis. (- = no individuals with PPD ≥ 7 mm)

Periodontal Findings	Sensitivity/Spesificity	Crohn's Disease Group (N = 47)	Control Group (N = 41)	Whole Population (N = 88)
PPD 4 mm	Sensitivity	54.5	84.6	65.7
	Specificity	80	82.1	81.1
PPD 5–6 mm	Sensitivity	100	87.5	88.9
	Specificity	65.2	72.7	68.4
PPD ≥ 7 mm	Sensitivity	-	100	100
	Specificity	-	69.4	66.3
BOP ≥ 15%	Sensitivity	37.1	57.7	45.9
	Specificity	66.7	93.3	81.5
Furcation defect	Sensitivity	40	66.7	54.5
	Specificity	64.9	72.4	68.2
Attrition	Sensitivity	52.4	38.9	46.2
	Specificity	76.9	60.9	69.4
Periodontal diseases	Sensitivity	35.3	57.7	45
	Specificity	61.5	93.3	78.6
Periodontitis	Sensitivity	60	90.9	73.1
	Specificity	75	80	77.4

The results of the aMMP-8 PoC immunotest were significantly associated with the diagnosis of periodontitis in the CD patients (OR: 5.2, 95% CI: 1.26–21.6, $p = 0.022$), in the controls (OR: 54.3, 95% CI: 3.09–953, $p = 0.006$), and in the whole population (OR: 8.5, 95% CI: 2.88–25.3, $p < 0.001$), as shown in Table 3.

Table 3. Unadjusted and adjusted (furcation defects and attrition) associations of the selected oral rinse active matrix metalloproteinase 8 point-of-care immunotest with periodontal diseases (gingivitis or periodontitis) or with periodontitis. Data are given as odds ratio (95% confident intervals), and p-value.

Group	Periodontal Diseases		Periodontitis	
	Unadjusted	Adjusted	Unadjusted	Adjusted
Crohn's disease group (N = 47)	0.9 (0.23–3.26), 0.84	1.3 (0.29–5.58), 0.752	4.5 (1.22–16.6), 0.024	5.2 (1.26–21.6), 0.022
Control group (N = 41)	19.1 (2.17–167), 0.08	20.4 (1.92–216), 0.012	40 (4.25–376), 0.001	54.3 (3.09–953), 0.006
Whole population (N = 88)	3.0 (1.06–8.45), 0.038	4.16 (1.34–12.9), 0.014	9.3 (3.25–26.6), <0.001	8.5 (2.88–25.3), <0.001

3.4. MMP-8 Immunoblot

Figure 1 presents the relative levels of molecular forms, activations, and fragments of MMP-8 in saliva.

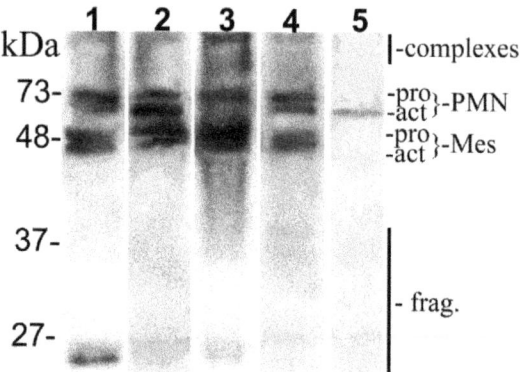

Figure 1. Western immunoblot analysis of salivary samples studied for molecular forms, degree of activation and related fragmentation of matrix metalloproteinase (MMP)-8. "PMN" indicates neutrophil-type collagenase (70–80 kDa) and "Mes" fibroblast-type MMP-8 collagenase (50–65 kDa) together with their pro and active forms. "Complexes" indicate multiple forms of MMP-8 (>110 kDa) and "fragments" the fragmented MMP-8 species (20–30 kDa). Lanes 1 and 2 illustrate the Crohn's disease group, and lanes 3 and 4 the control group. All laboratory conditions (incl. time of exposure) and image analyses were standardized. Purified human activated MMP-8## was used as positive control (lane 5). Mobilities of the molecular weight markers (low range prestained SDS-PADE Standards (Bio-Rad Laboratories, Inc, Richmond, CA, USA) are indicated on the left.

According to the immunoblot results, in the control group the PoC immunotest positivity is related to elevated levels of different forms and fragments of MMP-8 in saliva (Table 4). In CD patients, however, no difference in the levels of salivary forms of MMP-8 was observed between the PoC immunotest positive and negative individuals.

Table 4. Relative levels of mean intensity (median, min-max) of molecular forms and fragments of salivary MMP-8 as regards to oral rinse point-of care immunotest positivity (+) and negativity (−). p values indicating a significant difference (<0.05) are bolded.

Group		Complexes of MMP-8	PMN		Mesenchymal		Fragments of MMP-8	Total MMP-8
			Pro MMP-8	aMMP-8	Pro MMP-8	aMMP-8		
Crohn's disease Group	+ (N = 17)	1.8 (0.6–4.1)	0.4 (0.1–2.1)	0.0 (0.0–1.2)	0.6 (0.0–1.5)	0.5 (0.0–1.6)	0.1 (0.0–1.4)	3.8 (1.0–9.5)
	− (N = 30)	1.5 (0.2–4.2)	0.4 (0.0–1.1)	0.1 (0.0–1.3)	0.8 (0.0–1.6)	0.8 (0.0–1.7)	0.6 (0.0–0.5)	3.7 (1.5–8.2)
	p	0.330	0.877	0.708	0.303	0.061	0.192	0.982
Control Group	+ (N = 16)	1.4 (0.1–4.7)	0.6 (0.0–1.5)	0.4 (0.0–1.4)	1.0 (0.1–1.8)	0.9 (0.0–1.9)	0.1 (0.0–2.4)	4.9 (0.4–11.8)
	− (N = 25)	0.5 (0.0–3.7)	0.2 (0.0–1.8)	0.0 (0.0–1.0)	0.6 (0.0–1.6)	0.7 (0.0–1.7)	0.0 (0.0–0.5)	2.2 (0.2–7.6)
	p	**0.022**	**0.037**	**0.015**	0.121	0.209	**0.046**	**0.015**
Whole Population	+ (N = 33)	1.6 (0.1–4.7)	0.4 (0.0–2.1)	0.1 (0.0–1.4)	0.8 (0.0–1.8)	0.2 (0.0–1.9)	0.1 (0.0–2.4)	3.9 (0.4–11.8)
	− (N = 55)	1.0 (0.0–4.2)	0.3 (0.0–1.8)	0.5 (0.0–1.3)	0.7 (0.0–1.6)	0.7 (0.0–1.7)	0.1 (0.0–0.5)	3.1 (0.2–8.2)
	p	**0.032**	0.174	0.140	0.670	0.689	**0.020**	0.062

4. Discussion

To our knowledge, this is the first study to investigate the sensitivity and specificity of a chairside diagnostic kit in detection of periodontitis in patients with disrupted immune responsiveness. Our findings demonstrate that both the sensitivity and specificity of the aMMP-8 oral rinse PoC immunotest are significantly impaired in CD patients.

A comprehensive examination of periodontal, cariological, and oral mucosal health is the strength of the present study. Although there was no significant decrease in salivary flow in the CD group, the DMFS index was significantly higher in CD patients than in controls. Only 25% of the CD patients were periodontally healthy compared to 37% of the control group. In addition, CD patients presented more gingivitis and initial periodontitis than their generally healthy controls. These clinical findings are in line with several previous studies indicating differences in caries and periodontal states of CD patients in comparison to systemically healthy individuals [1–3]. On one hand, a higher DMF index may be attributed to nutritional and behavioral changes, such as an increased intake of carbohydrates and alterations in bacterial conditions in the oral cavity favoring mutans streptococci and lactobacilli [4,34,35], although these factors were not examined in the present study. On the other hand, the association between CD and periodontitis has been attributed to common predisposing factors, including age, genetic predisposition, and lifestyle factors, but perhaps more importantly to defects in the mucosal barrier, disrupted immune responses, and the exuberant host-response to bacteria leading to chronic inflammation [36]. Moreover, CD patients seem to exhibit a higher prevalence and more generalized and more severe periodontitis than non-CD individuals [2,3,37,38]. Contrarily, in the present study, severe periodontitis (12%) was diagnosed only in the control group. The small group size may have an impact on the results, but it was not possible to expand the present study sample size due to the low prevalence of Crohn's disease. The cross-sectional study design is another limitation of the present study, and thus, we cannot infer any temporal association between CD and oral disease. Moreover, the recruitment of the control group was in part undertaken at a dental clinic, which may result in a selection bias. However, this does not weaken the associations between the outcomes of the chairside test and periodontitis diagnosis after adjusting for clinical parameters.

The PoC oral rinse and salivary tests can be used as noninvasive and economic methods for screening and diagnosing disease. Various inflammatory proteins present in saliva have been tested as candidate biomarkers for periodontitis [39–43]. For example, salivary MMP-8 can be detected in different isoforms based on its origin (neutrophilic or mesenchymal type) or molecular forms (active, pro-, fragmented, complex) [32,33]. Moreover, neutrophils, fibroblasts, and endothelial cells are the main sources of MMP-8 in the oral cavity [44,45]. Some studies have indicated that dental caries has an impact on oral MMP-8 levels, and thereby, caries lesions may affect the outcome of oral rinse aMMP-8 PoC immunotests [22,46]. The causal relationship between caries and salivary MMP-8 has not been established, but the association between the number of cariotic lesions and MMP-8 levels suggests a role for the collagenase in the dentin caries process [46]. In our study, the sensitivity and specificity of the kit for caries detection in the whole population were low, 55.0% and 67.6%, respectively. One explanation for this could be the activity of the cariotic process. In comparison to chronic or stable caries lesions, active lesions seem to correlate more with MMP activity [47]. In addition, open caries lesions may more likely cause leakage of MMPs into the saliva in comparison to non-cavitated small caries lesions [47].

Recent research has shown promising results regarding the use of aMMP-8 as a diagnostic biomarker in PoC oral rinse tests for periodontitis [22–25,43,48]. The oral rinse aMMP-8 PoC immunotest, also used in the present study, applies lateral flow chromatography and detects the active form of MMP-8 with targeted antibodies [43,48]. A positive result of the test is based on a cutoff of 20 ng/mL for aMMP-8, and it can identify periodontitis with 64–95% sensitivity and 60–100% specificity [22–25]. In comparison to salivary MMP-8 analyses, the oral rinse aMMP-8 PoC immunotest has demonstrated a higher accuracy when differentiating periodontal health from the disease [43,48]. However, little information is still available regarding the limitations of this test.

There are common and discordant elements in the pathogenesis of CD and periodontitis. Indeed, both disorders lead to a substantial defect in the mucosal barrier and exuberant host response to bacteria, resulting in inflammation and tissue destruction. It is reasonable to speculate that the dysregulation of the immune system in CD may have an effect on MMP-8 levels in the oral cavity. It has been shown in a mouse model simulating inflammatory bowel disease that inflammation in the colon changes the microbiota not only in the colon but also in the oral cavity [9]. In the current study, the sensitivity and specificity estimates of the aMMP-8 PoC immunotest for detecting periodontitis were found to be poorer in CD patients (60.0% and 75.0%) than in systemically healthy controls (90.9% and 80.0%). The reasons for this are most likely multifactorial. Firstly, it can be argued that the prescribed immunomodulatory or anti-inflammatory medications affect the test accuracy. However, these medications act as suppressors of inflammatory response, which means that both clinical and sub-clinical indices of periodontitis (i.e., bleeding on probing as well as MMP-8 expression and activation, respectively) can be restrained. Thus, the use of medications does not fully explain the low sensitivity and specificity values of aMMP-8 PoC test in periodontitis patients with Crohn's disease. Secondly, impaired neutrophil MMP-8 function might be another explanation for the low sensitivity of the test in CD patients. Our western immunoblot experiment of salivary MMP-8 indicated that the aMMP-8 PoC oral rinse immunotest positivity in the CD group does not reflect the changes in the levels of molecular forms and fragments of MMP-8, varying from that observed in the control group. The difference may be explained, at least in part, by genetics. Indeed, a mutation in the nucleotide-binding oligomerization domain 2/caspase recruitment domain 15 (NOD2/CARD15) gene, which impairs the ability to recognize bacterial components and thus triggers an inadequate immune response, has been reported in patients with CD [49]. Interestingly, when patients suffering from rheumatoid arthritis - another example of a disease with dysregulated immune system - were compared to systemically healthy periodontitis patients, they exhibited increased aMMP-8 levels in gingival crevicular fluid [50]. Additionally, in presence of vascular leakage components in saliva samples, alpha 2-macroglobulin may form complexes with proteases, which in turn may partly explain the high-molecular weight complexes [51]. Formation of these complexes, however, may not totally explain the current results, since all samples were free of blood contamination. Finally, all these observations indicate that patients with a systemic disease manifested with impaired immune responsiveness need to be evaluated in a disease-specific manner before any diagnostic test can be reliably utilized. The reasons why (1) MMP-8 is not a functioning biomarker in CD patients or (2) aMMP-8 PoC immunotest seem to produce less accurate results in CD patients remain unsolved. Therefore, further studies are still required.

5. Conclusions

In conclusion, the performance of the oral rinse aMMP-8 PoC immunotest for recognizing periodontitis seem to be less reliable in CD patients than in systemically healthy individuals.

6. Patents

Professor Timo Sorsa is an inventor of US patents 5652223, 5736341, 5866932, 6143476, 20145192, 15/121801 and US 10,488,415 B2.

Author Contributions: Conceptualization, J.R., U.K.G. and M.G.; Data curation, U.K.G.; Formal analysis, J.R., U.K.G., A.K., T.T. and M.G.; Funding acquisition, J.R. and T.S.; Investigation, J.R., U.K.G., A.K., T.T. and M.G.; Methodology, J.R., U.K.G., A.K., E.K., T.S., T.T. and M.G.; Project administration, E.K.; Resources, E.K. and T.S.; Supervision, E.K. and T.S.; Visualization, T.T. and M.G.; Writing—original draft, J.R., U.K.G., A.K. and T.T.; Writing—review & editing, E.K., T.S. and M.G. All authors have read and agreed to the published version of the manuscript.

Conflicts of Interest: The authors declare no conflicts of interests related to this study.

Abbreviations

PoC = point-of-care; MMP = matrix metalloproteinase; aMMP-8 = active matrix metalloproteinase-8; CD = Crohn's disease; OR = odds ratio; DMFT index = decayed-missed-filled teeth index; CDAI = Crohn's disease activity index; VPI = visible plaque index; REC = gingival recession; PPD = probing pocket depth; CAL = loss of clinical attachment level; BOP = bleeding on probing; ECL = enhanced chemiluminescence.

References

1. Papageorgiou, S.N.; Hagner, M.; Nogueira, A.V.B.; Franke, A.; Jäger, A.; Deschner, J. Inflammatory bowel disease and oral health: Systematic review and a meta-analysis. *J. Clin. Periodontol.* **2017**, *44*, 382–393. [CrossRef] [PubMed]
2. Habashneh, R.A.; Khader, Y.S.; Alhumouz, M.K.; Jadallah, K.; Ajlouni, Y. The association between inflammatory bowel disease and periodontitis among Jordanians: A case-control study. *J. Periodontal. Res.* **2012**, *47*, 293–298. [CrossRef] [PubMed]
3. Brito, F.; de Barros, F.C.; Zaltman, C.; Carvalho, A.T.; Carneiro, A.J.; Fischer, R.G.; Gustafsson, A.; Figueredo, C.M. Prevalence of periodontitis and dmft index in patients with Crohn's disease and ulcerative colitis. *J. Clin. Periodontol.* **2008**, *35*, 555–560. [CrossRef]
4. Schütz, T.; Drude, C.; Paulisch, E.; Lange, K.P.; Lochs, H. Sugar intake, taste changes and dental health in Crohn's disease. *Dig. Dis.* **2003**, *21*, 252–257. [CrossRef] [PubMed]
5. Said, H.S.; Suda, W.; Nakagome, S.; Chinen, H.; Oshima, K.; Kim, S.; Kimura, R.; Iraha, A.; Ishida, H.; Fujita, J.; et al. Dysbiosis of salivary microbiota in inflammatory bowel disease and its association with oral immunological biomarkers. *DNA Res.* **2014**, *21*, 15–25. [CrossRef] [PubMed]
6. Rautava, J.; Pinnell, L.J.; Vong, L.; Akseer, N.; Assa, A.; Sherman, P.M. Oral microbiome composition changes in mouse models of colitis. *J. Gastroenterol. Hepatol.* **2015**, *30*, 521–527. [CrossRef]
7. Keskin, M.; Zeidán-Chuliá, F.; Gürsoy, M.; Könönen, E.; Rautava, J.; Gürsoy, U.K. Two cheers for Crohn's disease and periodontitis: Beta-defensin-2 as an actionable target to intervene on two clinically distinct diseases. *OMICS* **2015**, *19*, 443–450. [CrossRef]
8. Goethel, A.; Croitoru, K.; Philpott, D.J. The interplay between microbes and the immune response in inflammatory bowel disease. *J. Physiol.* **2018**, *596*, 3869–3882. [CrossRef]
9. Somasundaram, R.; Nuij, V.J.; van der Woude, C.J.; Kuipers, E.J.; Peppelenbosch, M.P.; Fuhler, G.M. Peripheral neutrophil functions and cell signalling in Crohn's disease. *PLoS ONE* **2013**, *8*, e84521. [CrossRef]
10. Levine, A.P.; Segal, A.W. What is wrong with granulocytes in inflammatory bowel diseases? *Dig. Dis.* **2013**, *31*, 321–327. [CrossRef]
11. Schmidt, J.; Weigert, M.; Leuschner, C.; Hartmann, H.; Raddatz, D.; Haak, R.; Mausberg, R.F.; Kottmann, T.; Schmalz, G.; Ziebolz, D. Active matrix metalloproteinase-8 and periodontal bacteria-interlink between periodontitis and inflammatory bowel disease? *J. Periodontol.* **2018**, *89*, 699–707. [CrossRef] [PubMed]
12. Koelink, P.J.; Overbeek, S.A.; Braber, S.; Morgan, M.E.; Henrkicks, P.A.J.; Roda, M.A.; Verspaget, H.W.; Wolfkamp, S.C.; te Velde, A.A.; Jones, C.W.; et al. Collagen degradation and neutrophilic infiltration: A vicious circle in inflammatory bowel disease. *Gut* **2014**, *63*, 578–587. [CrossRef] [PubMed]
13. Papapanou, P.N.; Sanz, M.; Buduneli, N.; Dietrich, T.; Feres, M.; Fine, D.H.; Flemmig, T.F.; Garcia, R.; Giannobile, W.V.; Graziani, F.; et al. Periodontitis: Consensus report of workgroup 2 of the 2017 World Workshop on the classification of periodontal and peri-implant diseases and conditions. *J. Periodontol.* **2018**, *89*, S173–S182. [CrossRef] [PubMed]
14. Tonetti, M.S.; Greenwell, H.; Kornman, K.S. Staging and grading of periodontitis: Framework and proposal of a new classification and case definition. *J. Periodontol.* **2018**, *89*, S159–S172. [CrossRef]
15. Ramseier, C.A.; Kinney, J.S.; Herr, A.E.; Braun, T.; Sugai, J.V.; Shelburne, C.A.; Rayburn, L.A.; Tran, H.M.; Singh, A.K.; Giannobile, W.V. Identification of pathogen and host-response markers correlated with periodontal disease. *J. Periodontol.* **2009**, *80*, 436–446. [CrossRef]
16. Gürsoy, U.K.; Pussinen, P.J.; Salomaa, V.; Syrjäläinen, S.; Könönen, E. Cumulative use of salivary markers with an adaptive design improves detection of periodontal disease over fixed biomarker thresholds. *Acta Odontol. Scand.* **2018**, *76*, 493–496. [CrossRef]
17. Sorsa, T.; Gürsoy, U.K.; Nwhator, S.; Hernandez, M.; Tervahartiala, T.; Leppilahti, J.; Gürsoy, M.; Könönen, E.; Emingil, G.; Pussinen, P.J.; et al. Analysis of matrix metalloproteinases, especially MMP-8, in gingival crevicular fluid, mouthrinse and saliva for monitoring periodontal diseases. *Periodontol. 2000* **2016**, *70*, 142–163. [CrossRef]
18. Ji, S.; Choi, Y. Point-of-care diagnosis of periodontitis using saliva: Technically feasible but still a challenge. *Front. Cell Infect. Microbiol.* **2015**, *5*, 65. [CrossRef]
19. Mauramo, M.; Ramseier, A.M.; Mauramo, E.; Buser, A.; Tervahartiala, T.; Sorsa, T.; Waltimo, T. Associations of oral fluid MMP-8 with periodontitis in Swiss adult subjects. *Oral Dis.* **2018**, *24*, 449–455. [CrossRef]

20. Zhang, L.; Li, X.; Yan, H.; Huang, L. Salivary matrix metalloproteinase (MMP)-8 as a biomarker for periodontitis: A PRISMA-compliant systematic review and meta-analysis. *Medicine (Baltimore)* **2018**, *97*, e9642. [CrossRef]
21. Sorsa, T.; Alassiri, S.; Grigoriadis, A.; Räisänen, I.T.; Pärnänen, P.; Nwhator, S.O.; Gieselmann, D.-R.; Sakellari, D. Active MMP-8 (aMMP-8) as a grading and staging biomarker in the periodontitis classification. *Diagnostics* **2020**, *10*, 61, in press. [CrossRef] [PubMed]
22. Heikkinen, A.M.; Nwhator, S.O.; Rathnayake, N.; Mäntylä, P.; Vatanen, P.; Sorsa, T. Pilot study on oral health status as assessed by an active matrix metalloproteinase-8 chairside mouthrinse test in adolescents. *J. Periodontol.* **2016**, *87*, 36–40. [CrossRef] [PubMed]
23. Johnson, N.; Ebersole, J.L.; Kryscio, R.J.; Danaher, R.J.; Dawson, D., 3rd; Al-Sabbagh, M.; Miller, C.S. Rapid assessment of salivary MMP-8 and periodontal disease using lateral flow immunoassay. *Oral Dis.* **2016**, *22*, 681–687. [CrossRef] [PubMed]
24. Räisänen, I.T.; Heikkinen, A.M.; Siren, E.; Tervahartiala, T.; Gieselmann, D.R.; van der School, G.J.; van der Schoor, P.; Sorsa, T. Point-of-care/chairside aMMP-8 analytics of periodontal diseases activity and episodic progression. *Diagnostics* **2018**, *8*, 74. [CrossRef]
25. Nwhator, S.O.; Ayanbadejo, P.O.; Umeizudike, K.A.; Opeodu, O.I.; Agbelusi, G.A.; Olamijulo, J.A.; Arowojolu, M.O.; Sorsa, T.; Babajide, B.S.; Opedun, D.O. Clinical correlates of a lateral-flow immunoassay rinse risk indicator. *J. Periodontol.* **2014**, *85*, 188–194. [CrossRef]
26. Jepsen, S.; Caton, J.G.; Albandar, J.M.; Bissada, N.F.; Bouchard, P.; Cortellini, P.; Demirel, K.; de Sanctis, M.; Ercoli, C.; Fan, J.; et al. Periodontal manifestations of systemic diseases and developmental and acquired conditions: Consensus report of workgroup of the 2017 World Workshop on the classification of periodontal and peri-implant diseases and conditions. *J. Periodontol.* **2018**, *89*, S237–S248. [CrossRef]
27. Thia, K.; Faubion, W.A., Jr.; Loftus, E.V., Jr.; Persson, T.; Persson, A.; Sandborn, W.J. Short CDAI: Development and validation of a shortened and simplified Crohn's disease activity index. *Inflamm. Bowel Dis.* **2011**, *17*, 105–111. [CrossRef]
28. Lankarani, K.B.; Sivandzadeh, G.R.; Hassanpour, S. Oral manifestation in inflammatory bowel disease: A review. *World J. Gastroenterol.* **2013**, *19*, 8571–8579. [CrossRef]
29. Harty, S.; Fleming, P.; Rowland, M.; Crushell, E.; McDermott, M.; Drumm, B.; Bourke, B. A prospective study of the oral manifestations of Crohn's disease. *Clin. Gastroenterol. Hepatol.* **2005**, *3*, 886–891. [CrossRef]
30. Sanz, M.; Bäumer, A.; Buduneli, N.; Dommisch, H.; Farina, R.; Könönen, E.; Linden, G.; Meyle, J.; Preshaw, P.M.; Quirynen, M.; et al. Effect of professional mechanical plaque removal on secondary prevention of periodontitis and the complications of gingival and periodontal preventive measures: Consensus report of group 4 of the 11th European Workshop on Periodontology on effective prevention of periodontal and peri-implant diseases. *J. Clin. Periodontol.* **2015**, *42*, S214–S220.
31. American Academy of Periodontology task force report on the update to the 1999 classification of periodontal diseases and conditions. *J. Periodontol.* **2015**, *86*, 835–838. [CrossRef] [PubMed]
32. Buduneli, E.; Mäntylä, P.; Emingil, G.; Tervahartiala, T.; Pussinen, P.; Barış, N.; Akıllı, A.; Atilla, G.; Sorsa, T. Acute myocardial infarction is reflected in salivary matrix metalloproteinase-8 activation level. *J. Periodontol.* **2011**, *82*, 716–725. [CrossRef] [PubMed]
33. Gürsoy, U.K.; Könönen, E.; Tervahartiala, T.; Gürsoy, M.; Pitkänen, J.; Torvi, P.; Suominen, A.L.; Pussinen, P.; Sorsa, T. Molecular forms and fragments of salivary MMP-8 in relation to periodontitis. *J. Clin. Periodontol.* **2018**, *45*, 1421–1428. [CrossRef] [PubMed]
34. Grössner-Schreiber, B.; Fetter, T.; Hedderich, J.; Kocher, T.; Schreiber, S.; Jepsen, S. Prevalence of dental caries and periodontal disease in patients with inflammatory bowel disease: A case-control study. *J. Clin. Periodontol.* **2006**, *33*, 478–484. [CrossRef] [PubMed]
35. Järnerot, G.; Järnmark, I.; Nilsson, K. Consumption of refined sugar by patients with Crohn's disease, ulcerative colitis, or irritable bowel syndrome. *Scand. J. Gastroenterol.* **1983**, *18*, 999–1002. [CrossRef] [PubMed]
36. Indriolo, A.; Greco, S.; Ravelli, P.; Fagiuoli, S. What can we learn about biofilm/host interactions from the study of inflammatory bowel disease. *J. Clin. Periodontol.* **2011**, *38*, 36–43. [CrossRef]
37. Stein, J.M.; Lammert, F.; Zimmer, V.; Granzow, M.; Reichert, S.; Schulz, S.; Ocklenburg, C.; Conrads, G. Clinical periodontal and microbiologic parameters in patients with Crohn's disease with consideration of the CARD 15 genotype. *J. Periodontol.* **2010**, *81*, 535–545. [CrossRef]

38. Flemmig, T.F.; Shanahan, F.; Miyasaki, K.T. Prevalence and severity of periodontal disease in patients with inflammatory bowel disease. *J. Clin. Periodontol.* **1991**, *18*, 690–697. [CrossRef]
39. Rathnayake, N.; Akerman, S.; Klinge, B.; Lundegren, N.; Jansson, H.; Tryselius, Y.; Sorsa, T.; Gustafsson, A. Salivary biomarkers of oral health: A cross-sectional study. *J. Clin. Periodontol.* **2013**, *40*, 140–147. [CrossRef]
40. Miller, C.S.; King, C.P., Jr.; Langub, M.C.; Kryscio, R.J.; Thomas, M.V. Salivary biomarkers of existing periodontal disease: A cross-sectional study. *J. Am. Dent. Assoc.* **2006**, *137*, 322–329. [CrossRef]
41. Sexton, W.M.; Lin, Y.; Kryscio, R.J.; Dawson, D.R., 3rd; Ebersole, J.L.; Miller, C.S. Salivary biomarkers of periodontal disease in response to treatment. *J. Clin. Periodontol.* **2011**, *38*, 434–441. [CrossRef] [PubMed]
42. Gürsoy, U.K.; Könönen, E.; Pradhan-Palikhe, P.; Tervahartiala, T.; Pussinen, P.J.; Suominen-Taipale, L.; Sorsa, T. Salivary MMP-8, TIMP-1, and ICTP as markers of advanced periodontitis. *J. Clin. Periodontol.* **2010**, *37*, 487–493. [CrossRef] [PubMed]
43. Räisänen, I.T.; Sorsa, T.; van der Schoor, G.J.; Tervahartiala, T.; van der Schoor, P.; Gieselmann, D.R.; Heikkinen, A.M. Active matrix metalloproteinase-8 point-of-care (PoC)/chairside mouthrinse test vs. bleeding on probing in diagnosing subclinical periodontitis in adolescents. *Diagnostics* **2019**, *23*, 9. [CrossRef] [PubMed]
44. Hanemaaijer, R.; Sorsa, T.; Konttinen, Y.T.; Ding, Y.; Sutinen, M.; Visser, H.; van Hinsbergh, V.W.; Helaakoski, T.; Kainulainen, T.; Rönkä, H.; et al. Matrix metalloproteinase-8 is expressed in rheumatoid synovial fibroblasts and endothelial cells. Regulation by tumor necrosis factor-alpha and doxycycline. *J. Biol. Chem.* **1997**, *272*, 31504–31509. [CrossRef] [PubMed]
45. Herman, M.P.; Sukhova, G.K.; Libby, P.; Gerdes, N.; Tang, N.; Horton, D.B.; Kilbride, M.; Breitbart, R.E.; Chun, M.; Schönbeck, U. Expression of neutrophil collagenase (matrix metalloproteinase-8) in human atheroma: A novel collagenolytic pathway suggested by transcriptional profiling. *Circulation* **2001**, *104*, 1899–1904. [CrossRef]
46. Hedenbjörk-Lager, A.; Bjørndal, L.; Gustafsson, A.; Sorsa, T.; Tjäderhane, L.; Åkerman, S.; Ericson, D. Caries correlates strongly to salivary levels of matrix metalloproteinase-8. *Caries Res.* **2015**, *49*, 1–8. [CrossRef]
47. Nascimento, F.D.; Minciotti, C.L.; Feraldeli, S.; Carrilho, M.R.; Pashely, D.F.; Tay, F.R.; Nader, H.B.; Salo, T.; Tjäderhane, L.; Tersariol, I.L. Cysteine cathepsins in human carious dentin. *J. Dent. Res.* **2011**, *90*, 506–511. [CrossRef]
48. Räisänen, I.T.; Heikkinen, A.M.; Nwhator, S.O.; Umeizudike, K.A.; Tervahartiala, T.; Sorsa, T. On the diagnostic discrimination ability of mouthrinse and salivary aMMP-8 point-of-care testing regarding periodontal health and disease. *Diagn. Microbiol. Infect. Dis.* **2019**, *95*, 114871. [CrossRef]
49. Hugot, J.P.; Chamaillard, M.; Zouali, H.; Lesage, S.; Cezard, J.P.; Belaiche, J.; Almer, S.; Tysk, C.; O'Morain, C.A.; Gassull, M.; et al. Association of NOD2 leucine-rich repeat variants with susceptibility to Crohn's disease. *Nature* **2001**, *411*, 599–603. [CrossRef]
50. Kirchner, A.; Jäger, J.; Krohn-Grimberghe, B.; Patschan, S.; Kottmann, T.; Schmalz, G.; Mausberg, R.F.; Haak, R.; Ziebolz, D. Active matrix metalloproteinase-8 and periodontal bacteria depending on periodontal status in patients with rheumatoid arthritis. *J. Periodontal Res.* **2017**, *52*, 745–754. [CrossRef]
51. Serifova, X.; Ugarte-Berzal, E.; Opdenakker, G.; Vandooren, J. Homotrimeric MMP-9 is an active hitchhiker on alpha-2-macroglobulin partially escaping protease inhibition and internalization through LRP-1. *Cell Mol. Life Sci.* **2019**. Oct 23, Epub ahead of print. [CrossRef] [PubMed]

 © 2020 by the authors. Licensee MDPI, Basel, Switzerland. This article is an open access article distributed under the terms and conditions of the Creative Commons Attribution (CC BY) license (http://creativecommons.org/licenses/by/4.0/).

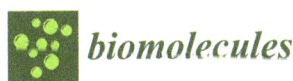

Article

Variations in Circulating Active MMP-9 Levels during Renal Replacement Therapy

Elena Rodríguez-Sánchez [1,†], José Alberto Navarro-García [1,†], Jennifer Aceves-Ripoll [1], Judith Abarca-Zabalía [1], Andrea Susmozas-Sánchez [1], Teresa Bada-Bosch [2], Eduardo Hernández [2], Evangelina Mérida-Herrero [2], Amado Andrés [2], Manuel Praga [2], Mario Fernández-Ruiz [3], José María Aguado [3], Julián Segura [1], Luis Miguel Ruilope [1,4,5] and Gema Ruiz-Hurtado [1,5,*]

1. Cardiorenal Translational Laboratory, Institute of Research i+12 (imas12), Hospital Universitario 12 de Octubre, 28041 Madrid, Spain; elena.rodsanchez@gmail.com (E.R.-S.); jalbertong@gmail.com (J.A.N.-G.); jen.ace.rip@hotmail.com (J.A.-R.); judithrit@hotmail.com (J.A.-Z.); andreasusmozas@gmail.com (A.S.-S.); hta@juliansegura.com (J.S.); ruilope@icloud.com (L.M.R.)
2. Service of Nephrology, Hospital Universitario 12 de Octubre, 28041 Madrid, Spain; teresa_bada@hotmail.com (T.B.-B.); ehm3871@yahoo.es (E.H.); evameridaherrero@hotmail.com (E.M.-H.); amado.andres@salud.madrid.org (A.A.); mpragat@senefro.com (M.P.)
3. Unit of Infectious Diseases, Hospital Universitario 12 de Octubre, 28041 Madrid, Spain; mario_fdezruiz@yahoo.com (M.F.-R.); jaguadog1@gmail.com (J.M.A.)
4. School of Doctoral Studies and Research, European University of Madrid, 28670 Madrid, Spain
5. CIBER-CV, Hospital Universitario 12 de Octubre, 28041 Madrid, Spain
* Correspondence: gemaruiz@h12o.es; Tel.: +34-91-390-8001
† Both authors contributed equally and are first authors.

Received: 27 February 2020; Accepted: 23 March 2020; Published: 26 March 2020

Abstract: Renal replacement therapy (RRT) is complicated by a chronic state of inflammation and a high mortality risk. However, different RRT modalities can have a selective impact on markers of inflammation and oxidative stress. We evaluated the levels of active matrix metalloproteinase (MMP)-9 in patients undergoing two types of dialysis (high-flux dialysis (HFD) and on-line hemodiafiltration (OL-HDF)) and in kidney transplantation (KT) recipients. Active MMP-9 was measured by zymography and ELISA before (pre-) and after (post-) one dialysis session, and at baseline and follow-up (7 and 14 days, and 1, 3, 6, and 12 months) after KT. Active MMP-9 decreased post-dialysis only in HFD patients, while the levels in OL-HDF patients were already lower before dialysis. Active MMP-9 increased at 7 and 14 days post-KT and was restored to baseline levels three months post-KT, coinciding with an improvement in renal function and plasma creatinine. Active MMP-9 correlated with pulse pressure as an indicator of arterial stiffness both in dialysis patients and KT recipients. In conclusion, active MMP-9 is better controlled in OL-HDF than in HFD and is restored to baseline levels along with stabilization of renal parameters after KT. Active MMP-9 might act as a biomarker of arterial stiffness in RRT.

Keywords: matrix metalloproteinase-9; dialysis; on-line hemodiafiltration; high-flux dialysis; renal replacement therapy; kidney transplantation

---

1. Introduction

Chronic kidney disease (CKD) is defined as abnormalities of kidney structure and/or function for a period of at least three months, with implications for health [1]. CKD is an irreversible disorder and often progresses to end-stage renal disease (ESRD), which is life-threatening and requires some form of renal replacement therapy (RRT) such as dialysis or kidney transplantation (KT). Since KT is limited by organ availability, dialysis is the most common form of RRT to remove uremic toxins in ESRD.

There are two types of dialysis treatments that can be applied to the ESRD patient: peritoneal dialysis and hemodialysis. Hemodialysis can be further classified depending on the membrane modality (convective vs. diffusive). For example, high-flux dialysis (HFD) is based on the use of high diffusion and low convection, whereas on-line hemodiafiltration (OL-HDF) is based on lower diffusion and higher convection, enabling the removal of middle- and larger-molecular weight substances. However, whatever the dialysis strategy used, it is only a temporary solution until the patient can undergo KT.

Patients with CKD, especially ESRD, are regarded as being at high risk of fatal and non-fatal cardiovascular events because cardiovascular and renal disease often have similar origins and risk factors [2]. Cardiovascular risk is particularly high for patients undergoing dialysis [3] because of CKD-associated complications such as atherosclerosis and systemic inflammation [4]. Indeed, this enhanced risk of atherosclerotic cardiovascular events begins from the earliest stages of CKD. Moreover, dialysis-specific risk factors such as mineral bone disorders and excess fluid load induce vascular calcification and hypertension, which in turn induce arterial stiffness [5], a process characterized by a thickening of the arterial wall and a loss of elastin fiber integrity leading to a decrease in elasticity [6]. Arterial stiffness is a predictor of cardiovascular disease in dialysis and KT recipients [7,8], and is associated with graft dysfunction and rejection [9]. Interestingly, vascular thickening tends to diminish after KT [10] and, in fact, KT improves the longevity and quality of life of patients as compared with long-term dialysis treatment [11], although cardiovascular risk remains higher than in the general population [12].

The anomalous turnover of extracellular matrix components favors deleterious vascular remodeling, which is a major mechanism underlying arterial stiffness. Matrix metalloproteinases (MMPs) play a central role in the regulation of both physiological and pathological connective tissue turnover. In particular, the inducible MMP-9, degrades laminin, elastin, and type IV collagen [13], which are the main components of the glomerular basement membrane of the kidney. In fact, the exaggerated activation of MMP-9 has been associated with an abnormal glomerular basement membrane structure and consequent albuminuria escape in treated hypertension [14]. MMP-9 activation is triggered under stress conditions including inflammation and oxidative stress [13] and is consequently upregulated in inflammation-dependent conditions such as hypertension and associated with cardiovascular risk in patients undergoing hemodialysis [15].

Although the use of MMP-9 as a marker of cardiovascular risk has been widely described, there is a paucity of studies examining how RRT affects its activity [16]. MMP-9 can be assessed as total MMP-9 or active MMP-9 levels measured by the MMP-9/tissue inhibitor of MMP (TIMP)-1 ratio, zymography, or solid-phase immunoassays. Total MMP-9 abundance is, however, not a direct measure of its activity, as both active and inactive MMP-9 are considered. Likewise, the indirect measure of active MMP-9 using the MMP-9/TIMP-1 ratio might be inadequate because it considers that TIMP-1, the endogenous inhibitor of MMP-9, interacts completely with MMP-9 in a 1:1 stoichiometry [17]. It is known that reactive oxygen and nitrogen species can interact with both TIMP-1 and MMP-9, blocking endogenous MMP-9 inhibition and activating MMP-9 constitutively [13] and, therefore, assessment of the MMP-9/TIMP-1 ratio as an indicator of MMP-9 activation is not recommended [18], especially in conditions of oxidative stress such as CKD or ESRD.

Given the heterogeneity in MMP-9 measurements and the gap in our knowledge on MMP-9 activity in RRT, the aim of this study was to assess the effect of different types of RRT (HFD, OL-HDF, and KT) on active MMP-9 measured in a direct manner by zymography and enzyme-linked immunosorbent assay (ELISA), as well as by the direct protein interaction between MMP-9 and TIMP-1 using AlphaLISA® technology (PerkinElmer, Waltham, MA, USA).

2. Materials and Methods

2.1. Study Population

The study included two independent cohorts of patients receiving RRT: 32 dialysis-dependent patients recruited for a cross-sectional analysis between November 2016 and March 2017 [19], and 46 KT recipients recruited for a longitudinal study between November 2014 and June 2016 [20,21]. The exclusion criterion for KT recipients was development of acute rejection in the first year post-KT. Both cohorts of patients were recruited at the Nephrology Unit of the Hospital Universitario 12 de Octubre (Madrid, Spain). Dialysis-dependent patients underwent clinical examination before dialysis, and KT patients underwent clinical examination before transplant. Pulse pressure (PP) was determined as the difference between systolic blood pressure (SBP) and diastolic (DBP) blood pressure [9]. Blood samples were drawn before (pre-) and after (post-) one dialysis session, or in the case of KT at baseline and 7 days, 14 days, 1 month, 3 months, 6 months, and 12 months post-KT. Blood samples were collected in heparin tubes and immediately centrifuged at 2000 rpm for 10 min. Plasma samples were stored at −80 °C until use.

All patients signed informed consent. The study was approved by the local ethics committee in compliance with the guidelines of the Declaration of Helsinki.

2.2. Assessment of Active MMP-9

Active MMP-9 was assessed by zymography and ELISA. Zymography was performed under non-reducing conditions using 10% SDS/PAGE containing 0.1% gelatin. Following electrophoresis, gels were incubated in 500 mM Tris, 6 mM CaCl2, and stained with Coomassie Brilliant Blue R-250 (Bio-Rad, Hercules, CA, USA). Digitalized gel images were analyzed with ImageJ software (NIH, Bethesda, MD, USA). Quantification of active MMP-9 was performed with a commercially available ELISA kit (QuickZyme BioSciences, Leiden, The Netherlands). Given the consistency between zymography and ELISA, follow-up of KT patients was exclusively assessed by ELISA at 7 days, 3 months, and 12 months post-KT. In the case of dialysis-dependent patients, active MMP-9 post-dialysis was corrected according to the weight loss during dialysis using the following equation:

$$Cc = \frac{Cpost}{1 + \frac{BWpre - BWpost}{0.2 * BWpost}}, \qquad (1)$$

where Cc is the corrected concentration post-dialysis, $Cpost$ is the concentration post-dialysis, $BWpre$ is the body weight pre-dialysis, and $BWpost$ is the body weight post-dialysis [22].

2.3. Assessment of Total MMP-9, Total TIMP-1, and MMP-9/TIMP-1 Interaction

Quantification of total MMP-9 and TIMP-1 was performed in KT patients at baseline, 7 days, 3 months, and 12 months post-KT using commercial ELISA Quantikine kits (R&D Systems, Minneapolis, MN, USA). MMP-9/TIMP-1 was calculated by dividing the levels of total MMP-9 by the levels of TIMP-1.

AlphaLISA® technology was used to detect the interaction between MMP-9 and TIMP-1 following a published protocol [18]. Briefly, AlphaLISA® acceptor beads (PerkinElmer, Waltham, MA, USA) were conjugated with an anti-MMP-9 antibody (ThermoFisher Scientific, Waltham, MA, USA) and then incubated with plasma samples from KT recipients and a biotinylated anti-TIMP-1 antibody (ThermoFisher Scientific). Streptavidin-coated donor beads were then added to bind the biotinylated anti-TIMP-1 antibody and detect the MMP-9/TIMP-1 interactions. Plates were read on an EnSpire Multimode Microplate Reader (PerkinElmer) using an excitation wavelength of 680 nm and an emission wavelength of 615 nm.

2.4. Statistical Analysis

Normality of data was determined with the Kolmogorov–Smirnov test. HFD and OL-HDF groups were compared using unpaired Student's t-test or the Mann–Whitney U test. Categorical variables were compared with Fisher's exact test. Pre- and post-dialysis groups were compared using the Wilcoxon signed-rank test, and KT follow-up groups were compared using the Friedman test. Spearman's rank-order correlation was used to analyze correlations. Results are expressed as mean ± SEM unless otherwise stated, and p-values < 0.05 were considered significant. Analyses were performed using GraphPad Prism 6 (GraphPad Software Inc., San Diego, CA, USA) and SPSS Statistics v22 (IBM, Armonk, NY, USA).

3. Results

3.1. Clinical Characteristics

Baseline characteristics of all hemodialysis patients stratified according to the type of dialysis applied (HDF or OL-HDF) are shown in Table 1. No differences were found in the mean age between the two groups. Likewise, there were no differences between the HFD and OL-HDF groups for hypertension, SBP, PP, diabetes mellitus, or N-terminal pro-brain natriuretic peptides. Dialysis-related parameters were also the same between the groups except for the duration of dialysis. Patients in the OL-HDF group were significantly longer on dialysis (31.4 vs. 98.4 months for HFD and OL-HDF, respectively). There were no differences between the groups for the cause of CKD or the medication used. The proportion of men was significantly higher in the OL-HFD group (65%) than in the HFD group (11%). Baseline characteristics of the KT recipients are shown in Table 2.

Table 1. Baseline characteristics of dialysis patients.

	All Patients (n = 32)	HFD Patients (n = 9)	OL-HDF Patients (n = 23)	p-Value
Age (years)	60.0 ± 16,4	64.7 ± 22.0	58.2 ± 13.8	0.322
Male sex (n, %)	16 (50)	1 (11)	15 (65)	0.016
Hypertension (n, %)	25 (78)	7 (78)	18 (78)	0.999
SBP (mmHg)	128.4 ± 23.0	126.2 ± 23.2	129.3 ± 23.4	0.739
PP (mmHg)	55.5 ± 17.5	58.4 ± 14.6	54.3 ± 18.7	0.556
Diabetes mellitus (n, %)	7 (22)	2 (22)	5 (22)	0.999
NT-proBNP (pg/mL)	2565 ± 1735	2753 ± 1245	2509 ± 1881	0.769
Dialysis-related parameters				
Serum creatinine (mg/dL)	7.61 ± 2.22	7.16 ± 2.22	7.78 ± 2.25	0.486
Serum albumin (g/dL)	4.05 ± 0.43	3.91 ± 0.24	4.10 ± 0.48	0.259
Potassium (mEq/L)	5.15 ± 0.90	5.06 ± 0.78	5.19 ± 0.95	0.725
Bicarbonate (mEq/L)	21.3 ± 2.9	21.2 ± 3.8	21.3 ± 2.6	0.974
Dialysis vintage (months)	79.5 ± 74.3	31.4 ± 24.5	98.4 ± 79.1	0.020
Kt/V	1.63 ± 0.24	1.68 ± 0.25	1.61 ± 0.24	0.463
eGFR (ml/min/1.73 m^2)	6.92 ± 3.00	6.48 ± 2.92	7.09 ± 3.08	0.614
Residual diuresis (n, %)	15 (52)	5 (56)	10 (43)	0.699
Interdialytic urine volume (mL)	375 (163–875)	250 (100–500)	500 (175–1000)	0.518
Cause of CKD				0.547
Glomerulonephritis (n, %)	7 (22)	2 (22)	5 (22)	
Diabetic nephropathy (n, %)	5 (16)	1 (11)	4 (17)	
Polycystic kidney disease (n, %)	4 (12)	0 (0)	4 (17)	
Hypertensive nephropathy (n, %)	2 (6)	0 (0)	2 (9)	
Other or undetermined (n, %)	14 (44)	6 (67)	8 (35)	
Medication				
ACEi/ARB (n, %)	8 (25)	2 (22)	6 (26)	0.999
Diuretics (n, %)	3 (9)	0 (0)	3 (13)	0.541
β-blockers (n, %)	13 (41)	5 (56)	8 (35)	0.427
Cinacalcet (n, %)	3 (9)	0 (0)	3 (13)	0.541
Paricalcitol (n, %)	12 (38)	5 (56)	7 (30)	0.253

SBP: systolic blood pressure; PP: pulse pressure; NT-proBNP: N-terminal (NT)-pro B-type natriuretic peptide; Kt/V: where K is the dialyzer urea clearance, t is the total treatment time, and V is the total volume within the body that urea is distributed; eGFR: estimated glomerular filtration rate; CKD: chronic kidney disease; ACEi: angiotensin converting enzyme inhibitor; ARB: angiotensin receptor blocker.

Table 2. Baseline characteristics of kidney transplant recipients.

	All Patients (n = 46)
Age of the recipient (years)	54.6 ± 15.8
Male sex (n, %)	27 (59)
Previous kidney transplant (n, %)	4 (9)
Pretransplant dialysis (n, %)	41 (89)
Dialysis vintage (months)	21.0 ± 19.0
SBP (mmHg)	134.5 ± 14.8
PP (mmHg)	49.9 ± 12.9
Serum creatinine (mg/dL)	6.27 ± 2.56
Serum albumin (g/dL)	4.23 ± 0.52
eGFR (mL/min/1.73 m^2)	9.82 ± 4.28
Donor	
Male sex (n, %)	25 (54)
Age (years)	52.6 ± 14.6
Living donor (n, %)	5 (11)
Number of HLA-mismatches	5 (4–5)
Cause of CKD	
IgA nephropathy	9 (20)
Glomerulonephritis	2 (4)
Diabetic nephropathy	7 (15)
Polycystic kidney disease	8 (17)
Hypertensive nephropathy	3 (7)
Other or undetermined	17 (37)
Induction therapy	38 (83)
Maintenance immunosuppression	
Steroids	46 (100)
Tacrolimus	46 (100)
Mycophenolate mofetil/mycophenolic acid	42 (91)
Cyclosporine A	0 (0)

SBP: systolic blood pressure; PP: pulse pressure; eGFR: estimated glomerular filtration rate; CKD: chronic kidney disease; HLA: human leukocyte antigen.

3.2. Dialysis Reduces Active MMP-9 Levels

We first compared the plasma levels of active MMP-9 in all dialysis patients pre- and post-dialysis. Active MMP-9 estimated by zymography (Figure 1A) or quantified by ELISA (Figure 1B) was lower post-dialysis than pre-dialysis, and this was significant for the ELISA analysis. Baseline plasma levels of active MMP-9 were significantly lower in the OL-HDF group than in the HFD group, both by zymography (Figure 1C) and ELISA (Figure 1D), and active MMP-9 levels were reduced by dialysis only in the HFD group while OL-HDF patients' active MMP-9 levels remained at the same level after the dialysis process. Active MMP-9 negatively correlated with the interdialytic urine volume (Figure 1E), in the sense that less urine volume was associated with higher MMP-9 activity.

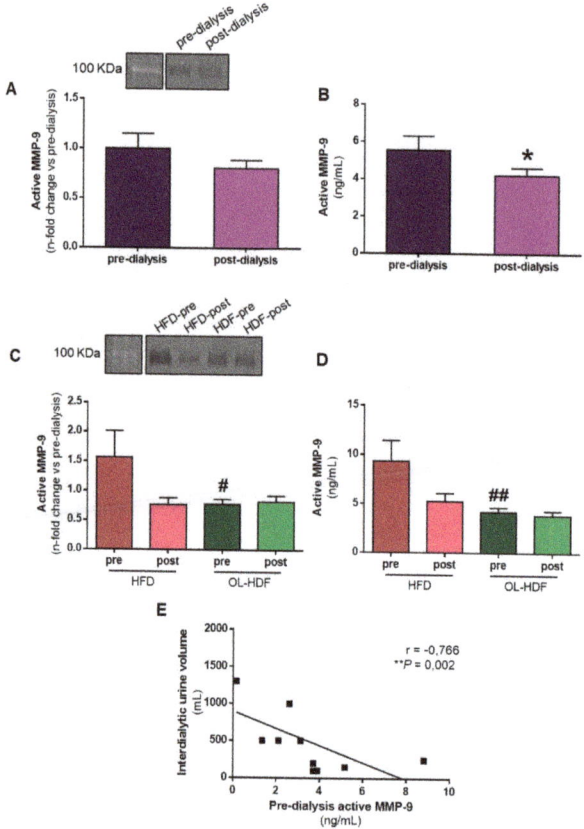

Figure 1. Matrix metalloproteinase (MMP)-9 activity in pre- and post-dialysis according to the type of dialysis applied. (**A**) Representative zymography gel showing plasma gelatinase MMP-9 activity (upper panel) and quantification (bottom panel). (**B**) Quantification of active MMP-9 by ELISA in plasma of dialysis patients before (pre-dialysis) and after (post-dialysis) one session of dialysis. (**C**) Representative zymography gel showing plasma gelatinase MMP-9 activity (upper panel) and quantification (bottom panel). (**D**) Quantification of active MMP-9 formed by ELISA in plasma of dialysis patients stratified as those on high-flux dialysis (HFD) (pre- and post-dialysis) and on-line hemodiafiltration (OL-HDF) (pre- and post-dialysis). (**E**) Negative correlation between interdialytic urine volume and pre-dialysis active MMP-9 in dialysis patients with residual urine volume. Correlation was performed using Spearman's test and a linear regression of the data is displayed. * $p < 0.05$ vs. pre-dialysis; # $p < 0.05$ and ## $p < 0.01$ vs. HFD pre-dialysis.

3.3. Kidney Transplantation Increases Total and Active MMP-9 and Total TIMP-1 Levels, but Not MMP-9:TIMP-1 Protein Interactions

Representative gel zymography of active MMP-9 in KT recipients before KT and at follow-up is shown in Figure 2A. Active MMP-9, measured by gel zymography (Figure 2B) or quantified by ELISA (Figure 2C), increased significantly 7 days after KT. Active MMP-9 levels remained high 14 days after KT (Figure 2A,B), but thereafter decreased significantly at one month after KT, reaching levels not significantly different to baseline at 3 and 12 months after KT (Figure 2A–C). Active MMP-9 levels were related to renal function, decreasing as estimated glomerular filtration rate (eGFR) increased and plasma creatinine decreased (Figure 2D).

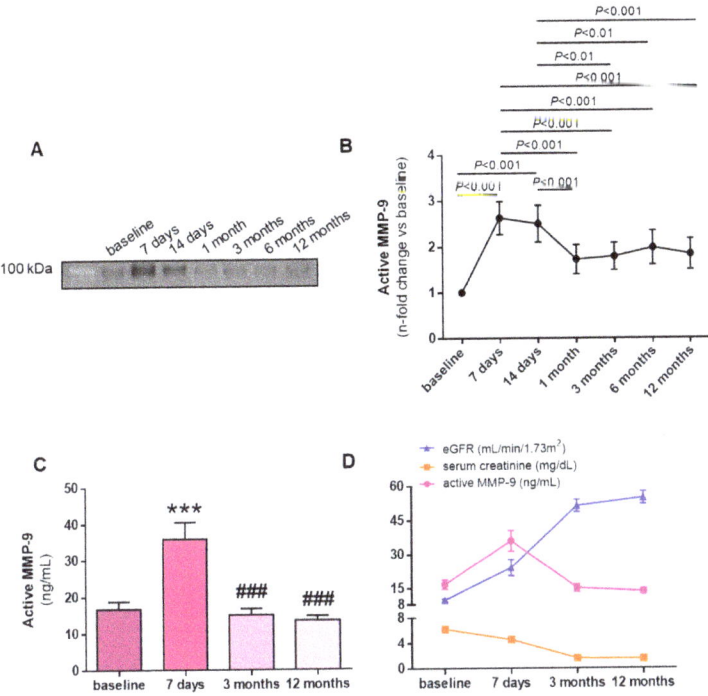

Figure 2. MMP-9 activity profile before and after kidney transplantation. (**A**) Representative zymography gel showing plasma gelatinase MMP-9 activity. (**B**) Quantification of active MMP-9 by zymography in plasma of kidney transplantation (KT) patients at baseline (before KT) and after 7 and 14 days, and 1, 3, 6, and 12 months. (**C**) Quantification of active MMP-9 by ELISA in plasma of KT patients at baseline and after 7 days, 3 months, and 12 months. (**D**) Evolution of eGFR, plasma creatinine, and active MMP-9 at baseline and 7 days, 3 months, and 12 months after KT. *** $p < 0.001$ vs. baseline and ### $p < 0.001$ vs. 7 days after KT.

To evaluate whether the changes in active MMP-9 abundance were due to changes in its expression or, alternatively, to its endogenous inhibition by TIMP-1, we measured total MMP-9 and TIMP-1 levels in KT recipients. Total MMP-9 levels increased significantly at 7 days after KT relative to baseline levels, but significantly decreased at 3 and 12 months after KT (Figure 3A). A similar pattern was observed for TIMP-1 levels, with a significant increase at 7 days after KT and a return to baseline levels at 3 months (Figure 3B). However, TIMP-1 levels continued to decrease at 12 months after KT and were significantly lower than baseline levels at this time (Figure 3B). To indirectly estimate MMP-9 activity and following the line of the majority of clinical studies, we calculated the MMP-9/TIMP-1 ratio, which revealed a significant increase in the MMP-9/TIMP-1 ratio over baseline levels at 7 days after KT (Figure 3C). The ratio decreased to baseline levels 3 months after KT but increased 12 months after KT, reaching an intermediate level (Figure 3C). To confirm the interaction between both molecules, we used the AlphaLISA protocol to measure MMP-9:TIMP-1 protein interactions [18]. No changes in MMP-9:TIMP-1 interactions were found until 12 months after KT, when the interaction was significantly higher than at baseline (Figure 3D).

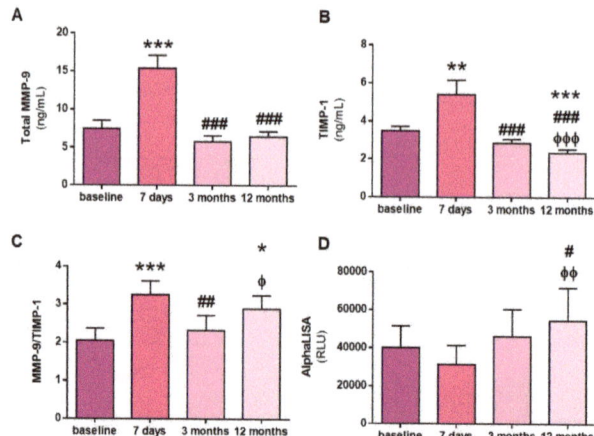

Figure 3. Total protein MMP-9 and tissue inhibitor of MMP (TIMP)-1 levels, MMP-9/TIMP-1 ratio, and MMP-9:TIMP-1 interactions before and after KT. (**A**) Total MMP-9 protein levels (**B**) and total TIMP-1 protein levels quantified by ELISA at baseline and at 7 days, 3 months, and 12 months after KT. (**C**) MMP-9/TIMP-1 ratio estimation. (**D**) AlphaLISA® MMP-9:TIMP-1 interaction immunoassay expressed as binding relative luminescence units (RLUs). * $p < 0.05$, ** $p < 0.01$, *** $p < 0.001$ vs. baseline; # $p < 0.05$, ## $p < 0.01$ and ### $p < 0.001$ vs. 7 days after KT; and φ $p < 0.05$, $\varphi\varphi$ $p < 0.01$, $\varphi\varphi\varphi$ $p < 0.001$ vs. 3 months after KT.

3.4. Active MMP-9 Positively Correlates with Arterial Stiffness in RRT Patients, but Not with Systolic Blood Pressure

We examined for correlations between active MMP-9 levels, SBP, and the arterial stiffness PP parameters in patients undergoing RRT. No correlation was found between active MMP-9 and SBP in the dialysis or KT cohorts (Figure 4A,B). However, we found a positive significant correlation between active MMP-9 levels and PP in both dialysis and KT cohorts (Figure 4A,B).

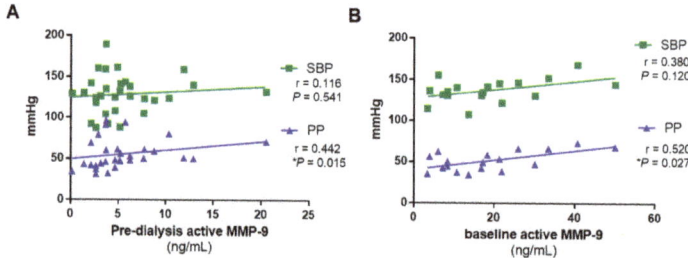

Figure 4. Correlation between MMP-9 activity and systolic blood pressure (SBP) and pulse pressure (PP) at pre-dialysis and before KT. (**A**) No association of MMP-9 activity with SBP (in green) and a positive significant correlation with PP (in blue) in dialysis patients in pre-dialysis. (**B**) No association of MMP-9 activity with SBP (in green) and a positive significant correlation with PP (in blue) in KT recipients before KT (baseline). Correlation was performed using Spearman's test and a linear regression of the data is displayed.

4. Discussion

Our study shows that: (i) patients undergoing OL-HDF have lower levels of active MMP-9 compared with those undergoing HFD; (ii) active MMP-9 increases early post-KT at 7 and 14 days and stabilizes in parallel with renal markers at 3 months after KT; and (iii) active MMP-9 is associated with arterial stiffness measured by PP in RRT (pre-dialysis and before KT).

Renal dysfunction is characterized by a uremic state that aggravates as renal function declines, reaching its maximum in ESRD. This state is intimately associated with all-cause mortality and especially with cardiovascular morbidity and mortality. Undoubtedly, RRT improves the lifespan and the quality of life of patients with ESRD. Among RRT patients, KT significantly improves the quality of life compared with dialysis, but the access to renal transplants is limited and not all ESRD patients can undergo a surgical procedure. Although dialysis is the cornerstone of RRT, it is also associated with a state of chronic inflammation and oxidative stress [23]. Dialysis *per se* triggers an increase in oxidative stress and inflammation because of incompatibilities with the dialysis membrane, which activates circulating leukocytes, and also because low-molecular weight antioxidant systems are filtered and therefore eliminated during the procedure. In addition, the type of dialysis used directly influences the oxidative status of the patients. Indeed, recent studies demonstrate that patients under OL-HDF have less inflammation, endothelial damage, and oxidative stress [19,24,25], which could be associated with the improved prognosis in this group [26,27]. The reduction in middle-molecules is associated with the preservation of residual renal function [28], which decreases the mortality risk in dialysis [29] and is improved in OL-HDF [30]. The systemic activation of MMP-9 is a marker of a lasting inflammatory state that is inherent to renal disease, as has been demonstrated even with adequate pharmacological treatment in patients with CKD [14,31]. In the case of ESRD, and especially dialysis, there are conflicting results on the levels of MMP-9 in the pre- and post-dialysis states [32,33]. This could be due to the different types of dialysis membranes [34,35], or to the type of dialysis itself [19,25]. We demonstrate herein that active MMP-9 is cleared during dialysis when the type of dialysis is not considered, but a decrease in active MMP-9 is only seen in HFD. Other authors have described a decrease in total MMP-9 during OL-HDF, but not during other hemodialysis [36]. Nevertheless, total MMP-9 does not necessarily correlate with active MMP-9, and the measurement of active MMP-9 is a more direct assessment of its pathophysiological activity [14]. The fact that only HFD effectively clears active MMP-9 might suggest that HFD is more efficient than OL-HDF; however, pre-dialysis active MMP-9 was significantly lower in the OL-HDF group than in HFD patients, indicating that the levels of active MMP-9 are better controlled in patients under OL-HDF. Moreover, residual renal function is associated with lower inflammation in OL-HDF [37,38]. Supporting this, we also observed that active MMP-9 is lower in patients with greater interdialytic urine volume, which is superior to eGFR as an estimate of residual renal function in dialysis [28].

KT is the only curative treatment for ESRD and long-term survival is significantly greater after KT than after dialysis. Despite its benefits, however, KT is not without risks, such as the inevitable ischemia and reperfusion (I/R) injury, which triggers several processes such as immune system activation, endothelial dysfunction, and cell death. Likewise, I/R induces morphological changes in the kidney that lead to fibrosis, as shown by the elevation of fibrosis-related biomarkers in the kidney of patients with chronic allograft nephropathy [39]. By contrast, a well-known benefit of KT is the normalization of inflammatory and oxidative stress markers [40]. For example, the C-terminal agrin fragment, a biomarker for kidney function and a breakdown product of agrin, the major proteoglycan of the glomerular basement membrane, strongly correlates with creatinine and eGFR and is stabilized at 1–3 months after KT [41]. In the same line, interleukin 6, a well-known precursor of MMP-9 activation, shows a burst of activity one week after KT before stabilizing [42]. In the present study, we demonstrate that systemic active MMP-9 levels increase one week after KT, but rapidly and significantly decrease from the second week after surgery. We speculate that the increase in active MMP-9 evident one week after KT likely originates from neutrophils in response to leukocyte activation inherent to I/R processes. This is supported by experimental studies demonstrating that MMP-9 promotes mononuclear cell infiltration in a rat model of early allograft nephropathy [43].

The peak in active MMP-9 observed early post-KT (after 7 and 14 days) might be due to an increase in total MMP-9 or an enhancement in the enzyme activation by the inflammatory environment.

MMP-9 is synthesized as a zymogen with a covered zinc-containing active site. Other MMPs and MMP-9 itself cleave the peptide chain that covers the active site in physiological conditions. However, reactive oxygen and nitrogen species can pathologically expose the active site by binding to the zinc ion. Reactive oxygen and nitrogen species can also bind to TIMP-1 and hamper the physiological inhibition of MMP-9. Indeed, MMP-9:TIMP-1 interactions are reduced under conditions of increased oxidative stress and can therefore mask the results obtained from the surrogate marker of MMP-9 activity, the MMP-9/TIMP-1 ratio [18]. Given the increase in oxidative stress associated with I/R, we aimed to investigate whether the peak in active MMP-9 was due to the pathological activation of MMP-9 or to an increase in MMP-9 protein levels. Our results indicate that the peak in active MMP-9 was in fact due to an increase in total MMP-9 expression, and the results of the MMP-9/TIMP-1 ratio indicate the same. However, the reduction in TIMP-1 levels at 12 months post-KT leads to an increase in the MMP-9/TIMP-1 ratio, erroneously suggesting increased MMP-9 activity. Indeed, active MMP-9 is unaltered 12 months post-KT because the MMP-9:TIMP-1 interaction is increased, supporting the importance of measuring active MMP-9 rather than the MMP-9/TIMP-1 ratio. The suggested increase in active MMP-9 by the MMP-9/TIMP-1 ratio indicates an increase in mortality risk [44]. However, total and real active MMP-9 do not vary, and TIMP-1, which is also associated with mortality [45], is reduced. Therefore, the patients might actually have a reduced risk of mortality as the KT becomes more stable.

Finally, arterial stiffness increases SBP by wave reflection and decreases DBP, which increases PP, a marker of large artery stiffness [46]. Arterial stiffness is attenuated after KT as compared with hemodialysis [9,47–50], and is subject to donor age, living kidney donation, and mean blood pressure [5]. Our study shows for the first time, to our knowledge, that active MMP-9 correlates with PP in patients treated with RRT. We found that, independently of the type of dialysis, PP is lower as the levels of active MMP-9 decline. A decrease in active MMP-9 suggests that arterial stiffness might be reduced in patients undergoing OL-HDF. However, we failed to find differences in PP between groups of patients on the different types of dialysis, in accord with results from other groups describing that arterial stiffness is not different between hemodialysis and HDF [5]. We also found that baseline active MMP-9 correlates with PP before KT, supporting the idea that a reduction in active MMP-9 levels in ESRD patients is needed to ameliorate arterial stiffness.

The main limitation of the present study was the small population of dialysis patients. More studies are needed in order to confirm our results, but this pilot study is the first step in assessing the insights of arterial stiffness in different types of dialysis.

5. Conclusions

Active MMP-9 is lower in OL-HDF than in HFD and shows a peak in KT recipients after I/R in the early post-KT stages (7 and 14 days). However, the peak in active MMP-9 is resolved in parallel with the restoration of renal function, indicating that MMP-9 activity is likely a surrogate of I/R injury. In both contexts—dialysis and KT—active MMP-9 is associated with PP in pre-dialysis and just before KT, indicating that MMP-9 is a marker of vascular dysfunction in patients undergoing RRT.

Author Contributions: E.R.-S., J.A.N.-G., J.A.-R., J.A.-Z. and A.S.-S. performed the experiments and the data analysis; T.B.-B., E.H., E.M.-H. and M.P. collected samples and followed dialysis patients; A.A., M.F.-R. and J.M.Á. recruited and followed KT patients. L.M.R., J.S., J.M.A. and G.R.-H. contributed to the funding acquisition. J.A.N.-G., E.R.-S. and G.R.-H. wrote the manuscript; G.R.-H. conceived the idea and designed the study. All authors reviewed and edited the manuscript. All authors have read and agreed to the published version of the manuscript.

Funding: This work was mainly supported by projects from the Instituto de Salud Carlos III (PIE13/00045, PI17/01093, PI17/01193, ayuda confinanciada por el Fondo Europeo de Desarrollo (FEDER) and CP15/00129, CP18/00073, FI18/00261 ayuda cofinanciada por el Fondo Social Europeo (FSE)) and partially supported by Sociedad Española de Nefrología/Fundación SENEFRO and Fundación Renal Íñigo Álvarez de Toledo (FRIAT), and co-funded by the European Regional Development Fund.

Acknowledgments: The authors thank Tamara Ruiz and Patricia Parra Aragón from Hospital Universitario 12 de Octubre.

Conflicts of Interest: The authors declare no conflict of interest.

References

1. Lamb, E.J.; Levey, A.S.; Stevens, P.E. The Kidney Disease Improving Global Outcomes (KDIGO) guideline update for chronic kidney disease: Evolution not revolution. *Clin. Chem.* **2013**, *59*, 462–465. [CrossRef] [PubMed]
2. Ruiz-Hurtado, G.; Ruilope, L.M. Does cardiovascular protection translate into renal protection? *Nat. Rev. Cardiol.* **2014**, *11*, 742–746. [CrossRef] [PubMed]
3. Wanner, C.; Amann, K.; Shoji, T. The heart and vascular system in dialysis. *Lancet* **2016**, *388*, 276–284. [CrossRef]
4. Valdivielso, J.M.; Rodríguez-Puyol, D.; Pascual, J.; Barrios, C.; Bermúdez-López, M.; Sánchez-Niño, M.D.; Pérez-Fernández, M.; Ortiz, A. Atherosclerosis in Chronic Kidney Disease: More, Less, or Just Different? *Arter. Thromb. Vasc. Biol.* **2019**, *39*, 1938–1966. [CrossRef] [PubMed]
5. Lioufas, N.; Hawley, C.M.; Cameron, J.D.; Toussaint, N.D. Chronic Kidney Disease and Pulse Wave Velocity: A Narrative Review. *Int. J. Hypertens* **2019**, *2019*, 9189362. [CrossRef]
6. Paloian, N.J.; Giachelli, C.M. A current understanding of vascular calcification in CKD. *Am. J. Physiol. Ren. Physiol.* **2014**, *307*, F891–F900. [CrossRef]
7. Verbeke, F.; Van Biesen, W.; Honkanen, E.; Wikström, B.; Jensen, P.B.; Krzesinski, J.M.; Rasmussen, M.; Vanholder, R.; Rensma, P.L.; Investigators, C.S. Prognostic value of aortic stiffness and calcification for cardiovascular events and mortality in dialysis patients: Outcome of the calcification outcome in renal disease (CORD) study. *Clin. J. Am. Soc. Nephrol.* **2011**, *6*, 153–159. [CrossRef]
8. Safar, M.E.; Blacher, J.; Pannier, B.; Guerin, A.P.; Marchais, S.J.; Guyonvarc'h, P.M.; London, G.M. Central pulse pressure and mortality in end-stage renal disease. *Hypertension* **2002**, *39*, 735–738. [CrossRef]
9. Korogiannou, M.; Xagas, E.; Marinaki, S.; Sarafidis, P.; Boletis, J.N. Arterial Stiffness in Patients With Renal Transplantation; Associations With Co-morbid Conditions, Evolution, and Prognostic Importance for Cardiovascular and Renal Outcomes. *Front. Cardiovasc. Med.* **2019**, *6*, 67. [CrossRef]
10. Litwin, M.; Wühl, E.; Jourdan, C.; Trelewicz, J.; Niemirska, A.; Fahr, K.; Jobs, K.; Grenda, R.; Wawer, Z.T.; Rajszys, P.; et al. Altered morphologic properties of large arteries in children with chronic renal failure and after renal transplantation. *J. Am. Soc. Nephrol.* **2005**, *16*, 1494–1500. [CrossRef]
11. Wolfe, R.A.; Ashby, V.B.; Milford, E.L.; Ojo, A.O.; Ettenger, R.E.; Agodoa, L.Y.; Held, P.J.; Port, F.K. Comparison of mortality in all patients on dialysis, patients on dialysis awaiting transplantation, and recipients of a first cadaveric transplant. *N Engl. J. Med.* **1999**, *341*, 1725–1730. [CrossRef] [PubMed]
12. Aakhus, S.; Dahl, K.; Widerøe, T.E. Cardiovascular morbidity and risk factors in renal transplant patients. *Nephrol. Dial. Transpl.* **1999**, *14*, 648–654. [CrossRef]
13. Newby, A.C. Dual role of matrix metalloproteinases (matrixins) in intimal thickening and atherosclerotic plaque rupture. *Physiol. Rev.* **2005**, *85*, 1–31. [CrossRef] [PubMed]
14. Pulido-Olmo, H.; García-Prieto, C.F.; Álvarez-Llamas, G.; Barderas, M.G.; Vivanco, F.; Aranguez, I.; Somoza, B.; Segura, J.; Kreutz, R.; Fernández-Alfonso, M.S.; et al. Role of matrix metalloproteinase-9 in chronic kidney disease: A new biomarker of resistant albuminuria. *Clin. Sci. (Lond)* **2016**, *130*, 525–538. [CrossRef]
15. Miljković, M.; Stefanović, A.; Bogavac-Stanojević, N.; Simić-Ogrizović, S.; Dumić, J.; Černe, D.; Jelić-Ivanović, Z.; Kotur-Stevuljević, J. Association of Pentraxin-3, Galectin-3 and Matrix Metalloproteinase-9/Timp-1 with Cardiovascular Risk in Renal Disease Patients. *Acta Clin. Croat.* **2017**, *56*, 673–680. [CrossRef] [PubMed]
16. Kousios, A.; Kouis, P.; Panayiotou, A.G. Matrix Metalloproteinases and Subclinical Atherosclerosis in Chronic Kidney Disease: A Systematic Review. *Int. J. Nephrol* **2016**, *2016*, 9498013. [CrossRef] [PubMed]
17. Nagase, H.; Visse, R.; Murphy, G. Structure and function of matrix metalloproteinases and TIMPs. *Cardiovasc. Res.* **2006**, *69*, 562–573. [CrossRef]
18. Pulido-Olmo, H.; Rodríguez-Sánchez, E.; Navarro-García, J.A.; Barderas, M.G.; Álvarez-Llamas, G.; Segura, J.; Fernández-Alfonso, M.; Ruilope, L.M.; Ruiz-Hurtado, G. Rapid, Automated, and Specific Immunoassay to Directly Measure Matrix Metalloproteinase-9-Tissue Inhibitor of Metalloproteinase-1 Interactions in Human Plasma Using AlphaLISA Technology: A New Alternative to Classical ELISA. *Front. Immunol.* **2017**, *8*, 853. [CrossRef]

19. Navarro-García, J.A.; Rodríguez-Sánchez, E.; Aceves-Ripoll, J.; Abarca-Zabalía, J.; Susmozas-Sánchez, A.; González Lafuente, L.; Bada-Bosch, T.; Hernández, E.; Mérida-Herrero, E.; Praga, M.; et al. Oxidative Status before and after Renal Replacement Therapy: Differences between Conventional High Flux Hemodialysis and on-Line Hemodiafiltration. *Nutrients* **2019**, *11*, 2809. [CrossRef]
20. Fernández-Ruiz, M.; Albert, E.; Giménez, E.; Ruiz-Merlo, T.; Parra, P.; López-Medrano, F.; San Juan, R.; Polanco, N.; Andrés, A.; Navarro, D.; et al. Monitoring of alphatorquevirus DNA levels for the prediction of immunosuppression-related complications after kidney transplantation. *Am. J. Transpl.* **2019**, *19*, 1139–1149. [CrossRef]
21. Utrero-Rico, A.; Laguna-Goya, R.; Cano-Romero, F.; Chivite-Lacaba, M.; Gonzalez-Cuadrado, C.; Rodríguez-Sánchez, E.; Ruiz-Hurtado, G.; Serrano, A.; Fernández-Ruiz, M.; Justo, I.; et al. Early Posttransplant Mobilization of M-MDSC Correlates with Increase in Soluble Immunosuppressive Factors and Predicts Cancer in Kidney Recipients. *Transplantation* **2020**. [CrossRef] [PubMed]
22. Patrier, L.; Dupuy, A.M.; Granger Vallée, A.; Chalabi, L.; Morena, M.; Canaud, B.; Cristol, J.P. FGF-23 removal is improved by on-line high-efficiency hemodiafiltration compared to conventional high flux hemodialysis. *J. Nephrol.* **2013**, *26*, 342–349. [CrossRef] [PubMed]
23. Cozzolino, M.; Mangano, M.; Stucchi, A.; Ciceri, P.; Conte, F.; Galassi, A. Cardiovascular disease in dialysis patients. *Nephrol Dial. Transpl.* **2018**, *33*, iii28–iii34. [CrossRef]
24. Morad, A.A.; Bazaraa, H.M.; Abdel Aziz, R.E.; Abdel Halim, D.A.; Shoman, M.G.; Saleh, M.E. Role of online hemodiafiltration in improvement of inflammatory status in pediatric patients with end-stage renal disease. *Iran. J. Kidney Dis.* **2014**, *8*, 481–485. [PubMed]
25. Ağbaş, A.; Canpolat, N.; Çalışkan, S.; Yılmaz, A.; Ekmekçi, H.; Mayes, M.; Aitkenhead, H.; Schaefer, F.; Sever, L.; Shroff, R. Hemodiafiltration is associated with reduced inflammation, oxidative stress and improved endothelial risk profile compared to high-flux hemodialysis in children. *PLoS ONE* **2018**, *13*, e0198320. [CrossRef] [PubMed]
26. Peters, S.A.; Bots, M.L.; Canaud, B.; Davenport, A.; Grooteman, M.P.; Kircelli, F.; Locatelli, F.; Maduell, F.; Morena, M.; Nubé, M.J.; et al. Haemodiafiltration and mortality in end-stage kidney disease patients: A pooled individual participant data analysis from four randomized controlled trials. *Nephrol. Dial. Transpl.* **2016**, *31*, 978–984. [CrossRef]
27. Nubé, M.J.; Peters, S.A.E.; Blankestijn, P.J.; Canaud, B.; Davenport, A.; Grooteman, M.P.C.; Asci, G.; Locatelli, F.; Maduell, F.; Morena, M.; et al. Mortality reduction by post-dilution online-haemodiafiltration: A cause-specific analysis. *Nephrol. Dial. Transpl.* **2017**, *32*, 548–555. [CrossRef]
28. Lee, M.J.; Park, J.T.; Park, K.S.; Kwon, Y.E.; Oh, H.J.; Yoo, T.H.; Kim, Y.L.; Kim, Y.S.; Yang, C.W.; Kim, N.H.; et al. Prognostic Value of Residual Urine Volume, GFR by 24-h Urine Collection, and eGFR in Patients Receiving Dialysis. *Clin. J. Am. Soc. Nephrol.* **2017**, *12*, 426–434. [CrossRef]
29. van der Wal, W.M.; Noordzij, M.; Dekker, F.W.; Boeschoten, E.W.; Krediet, R.T.; Korevaar, J.C.; Geskus, R.B.; (NECOSAD), N.C.S.o.t.A.o.D.S.G. Full loss of residual renal function causes higher mortality in dialysis patients; findings from a marginal structural model. *Nephrol. Dial. Transpl.* **2011**, *26*, 2978–2983. [CrossRef]
30. Hyodo, T.; Koutoku, N. Preservation of residual renal function with HDF. *Contrib. Nephrol.* **2011**, *168*, 204–212. [CrossRef]
31. Rodríguez-Sánchez, E.; Navarro-García, J.A.; Aceves-Ripoll, J.; Álvarez-Llamas, G.; Segura, J.; Barderas, M.G.; Ruilope, L.M.; Ruiz-Hurtado, G. Association between renal dysfunction and metalloproteinase (MMP)-9 activity in hypertensive patients. *Nefrologia* **2019**, *39*, 184–191. [CrossRef] [PubMed]
32. Lu, L.C.; Yang, C.W.; Hsieh, W.Y.; Chuang, W.H.; Lin, Y.C.; Lin, C.S. Decreases in plasma MMP-2/TIMP-2 and MMP-9/TIMP-1 ratios in uremic patients during hemodialysis. *Clin. Exp. Nephrol.* **2016**, *20*, 934–942. [CrossRef]
33. Pawlak, K.; Mysliwiec, M.; Pawlak, D. Peripheral blood level alterations of MMP-2 and MMP-9 in patients with chronic kidney disease on conservative treatment and on hemodialysis. *Clin. Biochem.* **2011**, *44*, 838–843. [CrossRef] [PubMed]
34. Chou, F.P.; Chu, S.C.; Cheng, M.C.; Yang, S.F.; Cheung, W.N.; Chiou, H.L.; Hsieh, Y.S. Effect of hemodialysis on the plasma level of type IV collagenases and their inhibitors. *Clin. Biochem.* **2002**, *35*, 383–388. [CrossRef]
35. Musiał, K.; Zwolińska, D.; Polak-Jonkisz, D.; Berny, U.; Szprynger, K.; Szczepańska, M. Soluble adhesion molecules in children and young adults on chronic hemodialysis. *Pediatr. Nephrol.* **2004**, *19*, 332–336. [CrossRef] [PubMed]

36. Derosa, G.; Libetta, C.; Esposito, P.; Borettaz, I.; Tinelli, C.; D'angelo, A.; Maffioli, P. Effects of two different dialytic treatments on inflammatory markers in people with end-stage renal disease with and without type 2 diabetes mellitus. *Cytokine* **2017**, *92*, 75–79. [CrossRef]
37. Raikou, V.D.; Kardalinos, V.; Kyriaki, D. The Relationship of Residual Renal Function with Cardiovascular Morbidity in Hemodialysis Patients and the Potential Role of Monocyte Chemoattractant Protein-1. *Kidney Dis. (Basel)* **2018**, *4*, 20–28. [CrossRef] [PubMed]
38. Malyszko, J.; Malyszko, J.S.; Koc-Zorawska, E.; Kozminski, P.; Mysliwiec, M. Neutrophil gelatinase-associated lipocalin in dialyzed patients is related to residual renal function, type of renal replacement therapy and inflammation. *Kidney Blood Press Res.* **2009**, *32*, 464–469. [CrossRef] [PubMed]
39. Mas, V.; Maluf, D.; Archer, K.; Yanek, K.; Mas, L.; King, A.; Gibney, E.; Massey, D.; Cotterell, A.; Fisher, R.; et al. Establishing the molecular pathways involved in chronic allograft nephropathy for testing new noninvasive diagnostic markers. *Transplantation* **2007**, *83*, 448–457. [CrossRef] [PubMed]
40. Cerrillos-Gutiérrez, J.I.; Miranda-Díaz, A.G.; Preciado-Rojas, P.; Gómez-Navarro, B.; Sifuentes-Franco, S.; Carrillo-Ibarra, S.; Andrade-Sierra, J.; Rojas-Campos, E.; Cueto-Manzano, A.M. The Beneficial Effects of Renal Transplantation on Altered Oxidative Status of ESRD Patients. *Oxid Med. Cell Longev.* **2016**, *2016*, 5757645. [CrossRef]
41. Steubl, D.; Hettwer, S.; Vrijbloed, W.; Dahinden, P.; Wolf, P.; Luppa, P.; Wagner, C.A.; Renders, L.; Heemann, U.; Roos, M. C-terminal agrin fragment–a new fast biomarker for kidney function in renal transplant recipients. *Am. J. Nephrol.* **2013**, *38*, 501–508. [CrossRef]
42. Simmons, E.M.; Langone, A.; Sezer, M.T.; Vella, J.P.; Recupero, P.; Morrow, J.D.; Ikizler, T.A.; Himmelfarb, J. Effect of renal transplantation on biomarkers of inflammation and oxidative stress in end-stage renal disease patients. *Transplantation* **2005**, *79*, 914–919. [CrossRef] [PubMed]
43. Gu, D.; Shi, Y.; Ding, Y.; Liu, X.; Zou, H. Dramatic early event in chronic allograft nephropathy: Increased but not decreased expression of MMP-9 gene. *Diagn. Pathol.* **2013**, *8*, 13. [CrossRef] [PubMed]
44. Provenzano, M.; Andreucci, M.; Garofalo, C.; Faga, T.; Michael, A.; Ielapi, N.; Grande, R.; Sapienza, P.; Franciscis, S.; Mastroroberto, P.; et al. The Association of Matrix Metalloproteinases with Chronic Kidney Disease and Peripheral Vascular Disease: A Light at the End of the Tunnel? *Biomolecules* **2020**, *10*, 154. [CrossRef] [PubMed]
45. LaRocca, G.; Aspelund, T.; Greve, A.M.; Eiriksdottir, G.; Acharya, T.; Thorgeirsson, G.; Harris, T.B.; Launer, L.J.; Gudnason, V.; Arai, A.E. Fibrosis as measured by the biomarker, tissue inhibitor metalloproteinase-1, predicts mortality in Age Gene Environment Susceptibility-Reykjavik (AGES-Reykjavik) Study. *Eur. Heart J.* **2017**, *38*, 3423–3430. [CrossRef] [PubMed]
46. Dao, H.H.; Essalihi, R.; Bouvet, C.; Moreau, P. Evolution and modulation of age-related medial elastocalcinosis: Impact on large artery stiffness and isolated systolic hypertension. *Cardiovasc. Res.* **2005**, *66*, 307–317. [CrossRef]
47. Feng, S.; Wang, H.; Yang, J.; Hu, X.; Wang, W.; Liu, H.; Li, H.; Zhang, X. Kidney transplantation improves arterial stiffness in patients with end-stage renal disease. *Int. Urol. Nephrol.* **2020**. [CrossRef]
48. Hornum, M.; Clausen, P.; Idorn, T.; Hansen, J.M.; Mathiesen, E.R.; Feldt-Rasmussen, B. Kidney transplantation improves arterial function measured by pulse wave analysis and endothelium-independent dilatation in uraemic patients despite deterioration of glucose metabolism. *Nephrol. Dial. Transpl.* **2011**, *26*, 2370–2377. [CrossRef]
49. Rodriguez, R.A.; Hae, R.; Spence, M.; Shea, B.; Agharazii, M.; Burns, K.D. A Systematic Review and Meta-analysis of Nonpharmacologic-based Interventions for Aortic Stiffness in End-Stage Renal Disease. *Kidney Int. Rep.* **2019**, *4*, 1109–1121. [CrossRef]
50. Sidibé, A.; Fortier, C.; Desjardins, M.P.; Zomahoun, H.T.V.; Boutin, A.; Mac-Way, F.; De Serres, S.; Agharazii, M. Reduction of Arterial Stiffness After Kidney Transplantation: A Systematic Review and Meta-Analysis. *J. Am. Heart Assoc.* **2017**, *6*. [CrossRef]

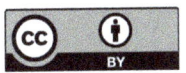

© 2020 by the authors. Licensee MDPI, Basel, Switzerland. This article is an open access article distributed under the terms and conditions of the Creative Commons Attribution (CC BY) license (http://creativecommons.org/licenses/by/4.0/).

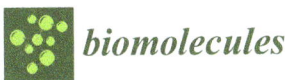

Article

CD147 is a Novel Interaction Partner of Integrin αMβ2 Mediating Leukocyte and Platelet Adhesion

David Heinzmann [1,*,†], Moritz Noethel [1,†], Saskia von Ungern-Sternberg [1], Ioannis Mitroulis [2], Meinrad Gawaz [1], Triantafyllos Chavakis [2], Andreas E. May [3] and Peter Seizer [1]

1. Medizinische Klinik III, Kardiologie und Kreislauferkrankungen, Eberhard-Karls Universität Tübingen, 72076 Tübingen, Germany
2. Institute for Clinical Chemistry and Laboratory Medicine, University Clinic and Faculty of Medicine Carl-Gustav-Carus, TU Dresden, 01397 Dresden, Germany
3. Department of Cardiology, Innere Medizin I, Klinikum Memmingen, 87700 Memmingen, Germany
* Correspondence: david.heinzmann@med.uni-tuebingen.de
† D.H. and M.N. contributed equally to this work.

Received: 23 February 2020; Accepted: 31 March 2020; Published: 2 April 2020

Abstract: Surface receptor-mediated adhesion is a fundamental step in the recruitment of leukocytes and platelets, as well as platelet–leukocyte interactions. The surface receptor CD147 is crucially involved in host defense against self-derived and invading targets, as well as in thrombosis. In the current study, we describe the previously unknown interaction of CD147 with integrin αMβ2 (Mac-1) in this context. Using binding assays, we were able to show a stable interaction of CD147 with Mac-1 in vitro. Leukocytes from Mac-1$^{-/-}$ and CD147$^{+/-}$ mice showed a markedly reduced static adhesion to CD147- and Mac-1-coated surfaces, respectively, compared to wild-type mice. Similarly, we observed reduced rolling and adhesion of monocytes under flow conditions when cells were pre-treated with antibodies against Mac-1 or CD147. Additionally, as assessed by antibody inhibition experiments, CD147 mediated the dynamic adhesion of platelets to Mac-1-coated surfaces. The interaction of CD147 with Mac-1 is a previously undescribed mechanism facilitating the adhesion of leukocytes and platelets.

Keywords: Mac-1; CD147; leukocytes; platelets; adhesion; integrin αMβ2

---

1. Introduction

The recruitment of leukocytes and platelets to activated endothelium as well as platelet-leukocyte interactions are of fundamental significance for innate and adaptive immunity, as well as thrombosis [1]. The surface receptor CD147 (basigin, extracellular matrix-metalloproteinase inducer; EMMPRIN) has been shown to be important in the host defense from self-derived as well as invading targets and is a major factor regulating the expression of matrix metalloproteinases (MMPs). CD147 is a pathophysiologically important multi-ligand receptor of the immunoglobulin superfamily. It is expressed in various tissues and cell types, including leukocytes, endothelial cells, and platelets. A range of different proteins, including cyclophilins, monocarboxylate transporters (MCTs) 1-4, CD43, CD44, CD98, NOD2, galectin-3, γ-catenin, apolipoprotein-D, members of the S100 protein family, and integrins, such as $α_3β_1$ and $α_6β_1$, have been reported to interact with CD147 [2–6].

In the context of thromboinflammation, CD147 acts as a pro-inflammatory and pro-thrombotic receptor, eliciting leukocyte chemotaxis and adhesion, as well as platelet activation and subsequent thrombus formation through the binding of various interaction partners [4,7–12]. Notably, its interaction with cyclophilin A (CyPA) contributes significantly to various inflammatory diseases. In the context of cardiovascular diseases, CyPA induces leukocyte chemotaxis and adhesion, and myocardial MMP expression, facilitating subsequent myocardial remodeling. Inhibition of extracellular

CyPA significantly decreases platelet activation and thrombus formation as well as the formation of monocyte–platelet aggregates [4,7,8,13,14]. Furthermore, our group identified glycoprotein VI (GPVI) to be an adhesion-mediating partner for CD147 on the platelet surface, which is the first time it has been demonstrated that CD147 plays a direct role in cell adhesive events, apart from mediating adhesion via intracellular signaling, leading to the expression of adhesion molecules [11].

Mac-1 (integrin αMβ2, complement receptor 3, CD11b/CD18) is a well-characterized heterodimeric integrin, mostly found on polymorphonuclear leukocytes [15]. As a member of the β2-integrin family, it is known to be involved in the leukocyte adhesion cascade. After the initial contact of the leukocyte with endothelial cells lining the vessel wall, a complex signaling cascade is initiated, leading to a selectin-dependent rolling motion of the leukocyte [16]. To establish a firm contact on the luminal side of the endothelium necessary for extravasation, chemokine-induced inside-out activation of integrins on the surface is necessary [17]. Especially on neutrophils, Mac-1 plays an important role in adhesion to the endothelium upon activation [18–20]. In this context, Mac-1-dependent adhesive interactions enable the cells to crawl on the surface of endothelial cells prior to extravasation [16,21]. Numerous cell surface receptors have been identified to interact with Mac-1 in its high-affinity state, including ICAM1-4, JAM-C, Thy-1, RAGE, DC-SIGN, and CD40L [15,22,23]. A plethora of soluble ligands for Mac-1 have been identified, amongst which are fibrin, fibrinogen, plasminogen, factor Xa, heparin, polysaccharides, ssDNA, and dsRNA [15,24]. Mac-1 can also interact with matrix proteins, including vitronectin, collagen, Cyr61, and fibronectin [15]. Mac-1 is also involved in complement-mediated immune responses by recognizing complement C3-opsonized pathogens as well as immune complexes [25].

In this study, we describe for the first time the interaction of integrin Mac-1 with CD147. We provide evidence that CD147 is a novel and relevant binding partner for Mac-1 on leukocytes and platelets.

2. Materials and Methods

2.1. Mac-1-CD147 Binding ELISA

Binding between Mac-1 and CD147 was evaluated using a modified enzyme-linked immunosorbent assay (ELISA). In a 96-well plate, wells were coated with recombinant Mac-1 (R&D Systems, Minneapolis, MN, USA) or bovine serum albumin (BSA) as the control. Recombinant CD147 was added in increasing concentrations (0–20 µg/mL) for 1 h. After removing CD147 and gentle washing, the wells were incubated with an anti-CD147 antibody (mouse-anti CD147, Abcam, Cambridge, UK) followed by a biotinylated secondary antibody (polyclonal rabbit anti mouse, Dako, Glostrup, Denmark) and a streptavidin/HRP complex (Life technologies, Carlsbad, CA, USA). The binding was detected using 3,3′,5,5′-tetramethylbenzidine (Serva, Heidelberg, Germany). The reaction was stopped using 1 M H_2SO_4. The absorption was measured using an ELISA plate reader at 450 nm with a reference value of 570 nm. Measurements from 6 independent experiments were analyzed.

2.2. Murine Leukocyte Isolation and Static Adhesion

Murine leukocytes were isolated from bone marrow. $CD11b^{-/-}$ mice were from Jackson Laboratories, and $CD147^{+/-}$ mice were a kind gift from Professor R. A. Nowak (Urbana, IL, USA). The femur and tibia were removed from sacrificed $CD11b^{+/+}$ and $CD11b^{-/-}$ (hereafter designated $Mac-1^{+/+}$ and $Mac-1^{-/-}$, respectively, n = 5), as well as from $CD147^{+/-}$ and $CD147^{+/+}$ (n = 12, respectively) mice (with a C57Bl/6 background). Throughout this, all efforts were made to minimize animal suffering. The bone marrow was washed out of the bones using RPMI 1640 medium (Life technologies, Carlsbad, CA, USA) supplemented with 10% FCS (Life technologies, Carlsbad, CA, USA), 1% Pen/Strep (Sigma-Aldrich, St. Louis, MO, USA), 1% HEPES (Sigma-Aldrich, St. Louis, MO, USA), and β-mercaptoethanol. The harvested cells were strained through a 70-µm strainer and were centrifuged (300× g for 5 min) and resuspended in ammonium chloride to lyse erythrocytes. For the leukocyte culture, cells were washed and resuspended in RPMI 1640 medium supplemented with 0.0001% GMCSF.

For the static adhesion assay, a 96-well plate was coated overnight with Mac-1 (10 μg/mL), CD147 (20 μg/mL), or BSA (1%). Hereafter, the coated wells were blocked with 4% BSA for 1 h. Then, 2×10^4 isolated leukocytes from Mac-1$^{+/+}$, Mac-1$^{-/-}$, CD147$^{+/+}$, or CD147$^{+/-}$ mice were added into each well. After allowing the cells to adhere to the coating for one hour, the plate was washed twice with medium to remove non-adherent cells. The number of adherent cells was analyzed using photo documentation.

2.3. Isolation of Human Monocytes

Human monocytes were isolated as described before [26]. Briefly, mononuclear cells were isolated form venous blood drawn from the antecubital vein of healthy volunteers. The blood was collected in citrate-phosphate-dextrose-adenine (CPDA) buffer and was centrifuged over a Ficoll gradient at $920 \times g$ for 20 min. Leukocytes were cultured overnight in RPMI 1640 (Life technologies, Carlsbad, CA, USA) supplemented with 10% FCS (Life technologies, Carlsbad, CA, USA) and 1% Pen/Strep (Sigma-Aldrich, St. Louis, MO, USA) in plastic dishes. Non-adherent cells were removed by gentle washing. The adherent cells were detached using trypsin (Life technologies, Carlsbad, CA, USA) and were resuspended in RPMI 1640 supplemented with 10% FCS and 1% Pen/Strep for further use.

2.4. Isolation of Human Platelets

Human platelets were isolated as described before [27]. In brief, venous blood was drawn from the antecubital vein of healthy volunteers in adenosine citrate dextrose (ACD) buffer. The blood was centrifuged at $210 \times g$ for 20 min. Hereafter, the platelet-rich plasma (PRP) was collected and Tyrodes-HEPES buffer (HEPES 2.5 mM; NaCl, 150 mM; KCl, 1 mM; NaHCO$_3$, 2.5 mM; glucose, 6 mM; BSA, 1 mg/mL; pH 7.4) was added and centrifuged at $836 \times g$ for 10 min. The pellet was resuspended in Tyrodes-HEPES buffer supplemented with 1 mM CaCl$_2$ and 1 mM MgCl$_2$ for further use.

2.5. Cell Adhesion under Flow Conditions

Using a flow chamber assay, human monocytes (2×10^5/mL, stimulated with 1 μg/mL LPS (Sigma-Aldrich, St. Louis, MO, USA) for 2 h (n ≥ 7) or platelets (1×10^8/mL, n = 7) were pre-incubated with anti-Mac-1 (clone #2LPM19c, monoclonal mouse-anti-Mac-1 Santa Cruz, Dallas, TX, USA), anti-CD147 antibody (clone #UM-8D6, monoclonal mouse-anti-CD147, Ancell, Bayport, MN, USA), or IgG control (all 20 μg/mL) for 2 h (monocytes) or 30 min (platelets). The cells were then perfused over Mac-1-, CD147-, or BSA-coated coverslips with arterial shear rates (2000 s^{-1}). All experiments were recorded in real time and were analyzed for adherent and rolling monocytes/platelets, respectively.

2.6. Ethics Statement

All experiments were conducted in accordance with the German animal protection law and according to the Declaration of Helsinki. All protocols were conducted according to current animal protection laws and were approved by Regierungspräsidium Tübingen and the local ethics committee (Anzeige nach §8a TierSchG).

2.7. Statistical Analysis

Data are shown as mean ± SEM. Differences between groups with cardinal values were evaluated using Student's *t*-test for two groups or ANOVA with subsequent post hoc analyses. Differences were considered statistically significant if $p < 0.05$. Analysis was performed using Prism 8 (GraphPad Software, La Jolla, CA, USA).

3. Results

3.1. Mac-1 Interaction with CD147

We used a binding ELISA to assess whether Mac-1 and CD147 can interact in a stable manner. As a negative control, coating with bovine serum albumin showed no significant interaction. When Mac-1 was used for coating the respective capture signal of CD147 was significantly enhanced, demonstrating a direct and stable interaction between the two molecules (Figure 1).

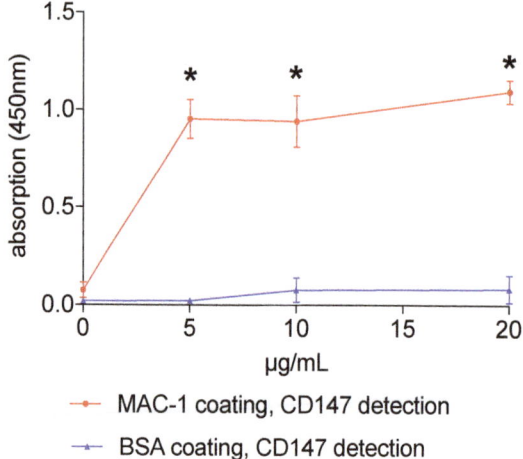

Figure 1. Mac-1 and CD147 interaction. Mac-1/CD147 interaction was assessed using an ELISA with recombinant Mac-1 or BSA (control) coating. Recombinant CD147 was added in ascending concentrations for 1 h. Evaluation was facilitated using a biotinylated secondary anti-CD147 antibody with a streptavidin/HRP complex. Changes in absorption of 3,3′,5,5′-tetramethylbenzidine were measured at 450 nm. Measurements from 6 independent experiments were analyzed, * indicates $p < 0.05$.

3.2. Mac-1/CD147 Interaction under Static Conditions

Based on the initial interaction study, we hypothesized that the interaction of these molecules could play a role in leukocyte adhesive events, as both have been described in this context separately. To this end, we performed a static adhesion assay with leukocytes from Mac-1-deficient and -sufficient mice. Mac-1$^{-/-}$ leukocytes showed a markedly reduced adhesion to immobilized CD147 compared to wild-type mice, indicating a relevant binding strength. With heterozygous leukocytes from CD147$^{+/-}$ mice, the effect was expected to be less pronounced. CD147$^{+/-}$ cells showed a higher adhesion under basal conditions with a slight non-significant increase of adhesion to the Mac-1-coated surface (Figure 2).

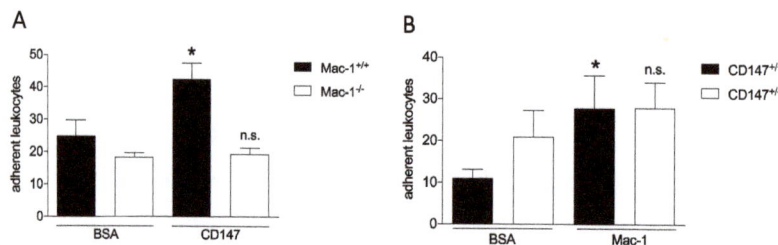

Figure 2. Mac-1/CD147 interaction in static leukocyte adhesion. A static adhesion assay with leukocytes form wild-type, Mac$^{-/-}$ (n = 5) (**A**), and CD147$^{+/-}$ (n = 12) (**B**) mice was used. Leukocytes were allowed to adhere to CD147- or BSA-coated surfaces (**A**) or to Mac-1- or BSA-coated surfaces (**B**) for 1 h. * indicates $p < 0.05$, n.s. indicates $p > 0.05$ compared to BSA control, respectively.

3.3. Mac-1/CD147 Interaction under Dynamic Conditions

After establishing a possibly relevant interaction strength for pathophysiological mechanisms, we studied LPS-stimulated human monocytes, as prototypical members of innate immunity under dynamic flow conditions. LPS-stimulated leukocytes were perfused over coated surfaces to evaluate the relative ability of the Mac-1/CD147 interaction to induce adhesion. Using a flow chamber assay, we observed a stable number of rolling and adherent cells on CD147- as well as on Mac-1-coated surfaces, compared to BSA under arterial shear rates (n = 9). In both cases, the effect could be reduced by the addition of either anti-CD147 or anti-Mac-1 antibody to the setup. The number of adherent monocytes over CD147 failed to reach statistical significance when treated with anti-Mac-1 ($p = 0.06$) (Figure 3).

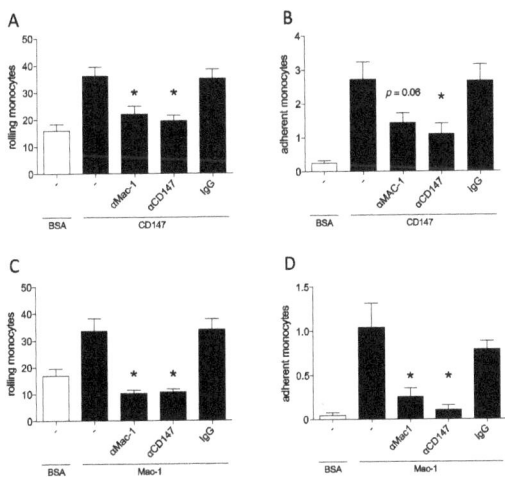

Figure 3. Mac-1/CD147 interaction facilitates leukocyte adhesion under dynamic flow conditions. To evaluate the relevance of the Mac-1/CD147 interaction for adhesion under arterial shear conditions, a flow chamber assay was used. LPS-stimulated human monocytes were perfused over BSA- or CD147-coated surfaces (**A** rolling cells, **B** adherent cells), or over BSA- or Mac-1-coated surfaces (**C** rolling cells, **D** adherent cells). Inhibitory antibodies against CD147 or Mac-1, as well as IgG control were added to determine the relevance of the respective protein for adhesion to its proposed counterpart. Results of ≥7 independent experiments are shown, * indicates $p < 0.05$ compared to uninhibited control.

3.4. Mac-1/CD147 Interaction in Platelets

To establish whether this mechanism is specific to leukocytes, we decided to perform a similar dynamic adhesion assay using isolated human platelets. When isolated platelets were perfused over immobilized Mac-1, adhesion was greatly induced compared to perfusion over BSA, which was used as a control. When anti-Mac-1 or anti-CD147 antibody was added, adhesion to Mac-1 was significantly reduced, almost reaching control levels (n = 7). The addition of IgG antibody had no modifying effect (Figure 4).

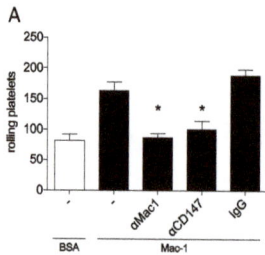 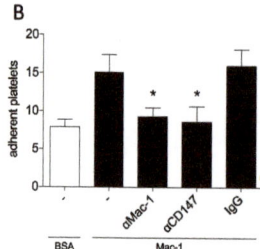

Figure 4. Mac-1/CD147 interaction facilitates platelet adhesion under dynamic flow conditions. The adhesion of platelets was studied in a similar flow chamber assay with arterial shear conditions. Isolated human platelets were perfused over Mac-1- or BSA-coated surfaces. Inhibiting antibodies against CD147 or Mac-1, as well as IgG control were added to determine the relevance of the protein for adhesion. Video analysis was performed to assess rolling (**A**) and adherent cells (**B**). Results of 7 independent experiment are shown, * indicates $p < 0.05$ compared to uninhibited control.

4. Discussion

The recruitment of leukocytes is a vital mechanism for innate and adaptive immunological response. Especially, integrins have been found to play a central role for the adhesion of activated leukocytes to the endothelium [28].

CD147 is a promiscuous surface receptor expressed on a variety of cell types. Ligand binding to CD147 has been shown to elicit many pro-inflammatory and pro-fibrotic aspects, such as induction of matrix-metalloproteinases, induction of leukocyte chemotaxis, platelet activation, and adhesion [4,7,8,29].

Thus far, especially, homodimeric signaling of CD147 and the interaction with extracellular cyclophilin A has been characterized in the inflammatory and pro-fibrotic context [30,31]. In this study, we proposed Mac-1 as a previously unknown binding partner for CD147 on leukocytes and platelets.

Initial interaction studies showed a stable binding of the two molecules, making detection via an ELISA-based interaction assay feasible. As both molecules have been found to be involved in leukocyte recruitment, we used static and dynamic adhesion assays to establish whether the stability of the interaction could be of pathophysiological significance. We found that inhibition of either binding partner strongly reduced the ability of leukocytes and especially monocytes to adhere to CD147- or Mac-1-coated surfaces under static and dynamic conditions.

With this in mind, we were interested in identifying the mechanism by using leukocytes from Mac-1 knock-out mice and CD147 heterozygous mice. Both genotypes showed little adhesion to the immobilized binding partner, whereas leukocytes from wild-type mice showed strong adhesion. Interestingly, this interaction also seems to be of importance for the adhesion of platelets. While platelets play a role in inflammation by releasing pro-inflammatory and pro-fibrotic chemokines, in clinical practice, their pro-thrombotic properties are especially of great interest, as the initial contact of the platelets with the activated endothelium and associated factors triggers a wide range of responses, including degranulation, activation by the presentation of adhesion molecules, and shape changes. Under flow conditions, platelet adhesion to Mac-1 was abolished by the addition of anti-Mac-1 or anti-CD147 antibodies. This finding suggests that the binding between Mac-1 and CD147 may mediate platelet–leukocyte interactions as well.

CD147 has been identified to play a prominent role in the induction of pro-inflammatory and pro-thrombotic effects in various disease models and across species. Our group has previously described platelet glycoprotein VI (GPVI) as a novel receptor for CD147, mediating platelet rolling and monocyte–platelet aggregates [11]. Furthermore, the interaction of CD147 with cyclophilin A (CyPA) has been intensively investigated in the context of thromboinflammation. CyPA can be released from the cytoplasm by various pro-inflammatory stimuli. The binding of CyPA to CD147 on the surface of platelets induces rapid degranulation and activation, leading to shape changes and the release of pro-inflammatory chemokines [4]. Furthermore, the CD147–CyPA interaction induces leukocyte chemotaxis and activation, expression of matrix-metalloproteinases, promotes atherosclerotic plaque formation, and plays critical roles in several inflammatory and cardiovascular diseases [14,31–33]. CD147 has also been associated with other integrins, including $\alpha_3\beta_1$ and $\alpha_6\beta_1$ [2]. S100A9, belonging to the S100 family of proteins, has been identified to induce leukocyte migration, thrombosis, and cytokine release via CD147 [5,34]. Mac-1, predominantly expressed on myeloid cells, has also been extensively implicated in various thromboinflammatory mechanisms, including leukocyte migration, phagocytosis, and the facilitation of monocyte–platelet aggregates [15,35].

The presented data therefore links two molecules, both deeply embedded in thromboinflammatory mechanisms, complimenting the existing literature. However, the pathophysiological importance in vivo remains to be elucidated. This study was primarily designed to establish a plausible link between CD147 and Mac-1 in the context of thromboinflammation using in vitro experiments. Further investigations are necessary to characterize the underlying signaling mechanisms and to subsequently evaluate its pathophysiological relevance.

5. Conclusions

In this study, we described for the first time the interaction of integrin Mac-1 with CD147. We furthermore provide evidence that CD147 is a novel and relevant binding partner for Mac-1 on leukocytes and platelets.

Author Contributions: Conceptualization, P.S., A.E.M., M.G., D.H., I.M., and T.C., Methodology, P.S., M.G., D.H., I.M., M.N., and S.v.U.-S.; Investigation, D.H., M.N., S.v.U.-S.; Resources, D.H., P.S., M.G.; Writing—Original Draft Preparation, D.H., and P.S.; Writing—Review and Editing, D.H., M.N., S.v.U.-S., I.M., M.G., A.E.M., T.C., P.S.; Visualization, D.H., M.N., S.v.U.-S.; Supervision, P.S., A.E.M., M.G., and P.S.; Funding Acquisition, M.G., P.S., and D.H. All authors have read and agreed to the published version of the manuscript.

Funding: This work was supported by grants from the German Research Foundation (Deutsche Forschungsgemeinschaft, DFG #374031971-TRR 240-CRU-240), and the German Heart Foundation (Deutsche Herzstiftung).

Acknowledgments: The authors thank K. Posavec for providing outstanding technical assistance.

Conflicts of Interest: The authors declare no conflict of interest. The funders had no role in the design of the study; in the collection, analyses, or interpretation of data; in the writing of the manuscript, or in the decision to publish the results.

References

1. Pircher, J.; Engelmann, B.; Massberg, S.; Schulz, C. Platelet-neutrophil crosstalk in atherothrombosis. *Thromb. Haemost.* **2019**, *119*, 1274–1282. [CrossRef] [PubMed]
2. Berditchevski, F.; Chang, S.; Bodorova, J.; Hemler, M.E. Generation of monoclonal antibodies to integrin-associated proteins. Evidence that alpha3beta1 complexes with EMMPRIN/basigin/OX47/M6. *J. Biol. Chem.* **1997**, *272*, 29174–29180. [CrossRef]
3. Dai, J.Y.; Dou, K.F.; Wang, C.H.; Zhao, P.; Lau, W.B.; Tao, L.; Wu, Y.M.; Tang, J.; Jiang, J.L.; Chen, Z.N. The interaction of HAb18G/CD147 with integrin alpha6beta1 and its implications for the invasion potential of human hepatoma cells. *BMC Cancer* **2009**, *9*, 337. [CrossRef] [PubMed]
4. Seizer, P.; Ungern-Sternberg, S.N.; Schonberger, T.; Borst, O.; Munzer, P.; Schmidt, E.M.; Mack, A.F.; Heinzmann, D.; Chatterjee, M.; Langer, H.; et al. Extracellular cyclophilin A activates platelets via EMMPRIN (CD147) and PI3K/Akt signaling, which promotes platelet adhesion and thrombus formation in vitro and in vivo. *Arterioscler. Thromb. Vasc. Biol.* **2015**, *35*, 655–663. [CrossRef]
5. Hibino, T.; Sakaguchi, M.; Miyamoto, S.; Yamamoto, M.; Motoyama, A.; Hosoi, J.; Shimokata, T.; Ito, T.; Tsuboi, R.; Huh, N.-H. S100A9 is a novel ligand of EMMPRIN that promotes melanoma metastasis. *Cancer Res.* **2013**, *73*, 172–183. [CrossRef] [PubMed]
6. Muramatsu, T. Basigin (CD147), a multifunctional transmembrane glycoprotein with various binding partners. *J Biochem.* **2016**, *159*, 481–490. [CrossRef] [PubMed]

7. Seizer, P.; Ochmann, C.; Schonberger, T.; Zach, S.; Rose, M.; Borst, O.; Klingel, K.; Kandolf, R.; MacDonald, H.R.; Nowak, R.A.; et al. Disrupting the EMMPRIN (CD147)-cyclophilin A interaction reduces infarct size and preserves systolic function after myocardial ischemia and reperfusion. *Arterioscler. Thromb. Vasc. Biol.* **2011**, *31*, 1377–1386. [CrossRef] [PubMed]
8. Seizer, P.; Schonberger, T.; Schott, M.; Lang, M.R.; Langer, H.F.; Bigalke, B.; Kramer, B.F.; Borst, O.; Daub, K.; Heidenreich, O.; et al. EMMPRIN and its ligand cyclophilin A regulate MT1-MMP, MMP-9 and M-CSF during foam cell formation. *Atherosclerosis* **2010**, *209*, 51–57. [CrossRef] [PubMed]
9. Elvers, M.; Herrmann, A.; Seizer, P.; Munzer, P.; Beck, S.; Schonberger, T.; Borst, O.; Martin-Romero, F.J.; Lang, F.; May, A.E.; et al. Intracellular cyclophilin A is an important Ca^{2+} regulator in platelets and critically involved in arterial thrombus formation. *Blood* **2012**, *120*, 1317–1326. [CrossRef]
10. Seizer, P.; Geisler, T.; Bigalke, B.; Schneider, M.; Klingel, K.; Kandolf, R.; Stellos, K.; Schreieck, J.; Gawaz, M.; May, A.E. EMMPRIN and its ligand Cyclophilin A as novel diagnostic markers in inflammatory cardiomyopathy. *Int. J. Cardiol.* **2013**, *163*, 299–304. [CrossRef]
11. Seizer, P.; Borst, O.; Langer, H.F.; Bultmann, A.; Munch, G.; Herouy, Y.; Stellos, K.; Kramer, B.; Bigalke, B.; Buchele, B.; et al. EMMPRIN (CD147) is a novel receptor for platelet GPVI and mediates platelet rolling via GPVI-EMMPRIN interaction. *Thromb. Haemost.* **2009**, *101*, 682–686. [CrossRef] [PubMed]
12. Flora, G.K.; Anderton, R.S.; Meloni, B.P.; Guillemin, G.J.; Knuckey, N.W.; MacDougall, G.; Matthews, V.; Boulos, S. Microglia are both a source and target of extracellular cyclophilin A. *Heliyon* **2019**, *5*, e02390. [CrossRef]
13. von Ungern-Sternberg, S.N.I.; Vogel, S.; Walker-Allgaier, B.; Geue, S.; Maurer, A.; Wild, A.M.; Munzer, P.; Chatterjee, M.; Heinzmann, D.; Kremmer, E.; et al. Extracellular cyclophilin A augments platelet-dependent thrombosis and thromboinflammation. *Thromb. Haemost.* **2017**, *117*, 2063–2078. [CrossRef] [PubMed]
14. von Ungern-Sternberg, S.N.I.; Zernecke, A.; Seizer, P. Extracellular matrix metalloproteinase inducer EMMPRIN (CD147) in cardiovascular disease. *Int. J. Mol. Sci.* **2018**, *19*, 507. [CrossRef] [PubMed]
15. Bednarczyk, M.; Stege, H.; Grabbe, S.; Bros, M. β2 Integrins-multi-functional leukocyte receptors in health and disease. *Int. J. Mol. Sci.* **2020**, *21*, 1402. [CrossRef] [PubMed]
16. Futosi, K.; Fodor, S.; Mocsai, A. Neutrophil cell surface receptors and their intracellular signal transduction pathways. *Int. Immunopharmacol.* **2013**, *17*, 638–650. [CrossRef]
17. Mitroulis, I.; Alexaki, V.I.; Kourtzelis, I.; Ziogas, A.; Hajishengallis, G.; Chavakis, T. Leukocyte integrins: Role in leukocyte recruitment and as therapeutic targets in inflammatory disease. *Pharmacol. Ther.* **2015**, *147*, 123–135. [CrossRef]
18. Keiper, T.; Al-Fakhri, N.; Chavakis, E.; Athanasopoulos, A.N.; Isermann, B.; Herzog, S.; Bohle, R.M.; Haendeler, J.; Preissner, K.T.; Santoso, S.; et al. The role of junctional adhesion molecule-C (JAM-C) in oxidized LDL-mediated leukocyte recruitment. *FASEB J. Off. Publ. Fed. Am. Soc. Exp. Biol.* **2005**, *19*, 2078–2080. [CrossRef]
19. Chavakis, T.; Athanasopoulos, A.; Rhee, J.S.; Orlova, V.; Schmidt-Woll, T.; Bierhaus, A.; May, A.E.; Celik, I.; Nawroth, P.P.; Preissner, K.T. Angiostatin is a novel anti-inflammatory factor by inhibiting leukocyte recruitment. *Blood* **2005**, *105*, 1036–1043. [CrossRef]
20. Hajishengallis, G.; Chavakis, T. Endogenous modulators of inflammatory cell recruitment. *Trends Immunol.* **2013**, *34*, 1–6. [CrossRef]
21. Li, N.; Yang, H.; Wang, M.; Lu, S.; Zhang, Y.; Long, M. Ligand-specific binding forces of LFA-1 and Mac-1 in neutrophil adhesion and crawling. *Mol. Biol. Cell* **2018**, *29*, 408–418. [CrossRef] [PubMed]
22. Chavakis, T.; Santoso, S.; Clemetson, K.J.; Sachs, U.J.; Isordia-Salas, I.; Pixley, R.A.; Nawroth, P.P.; Colman, R.W.; Preissner, K.T. High molecular weight kininogen regulates platelet-leukocyte interactions by bridging Mac-1 and glycoprotein Ib. *J. Biol. Chem.* **2003**, *278*, 45375–45381. [CrossRef] [PubMed]
23. Santoso, S.; Sachs, U.J.; Kroll, H.; Linder, M.; Ruf, A.; Preissner, K.T.; Chavakis, T. The junctional adhesion molecule 3 (JAM-3) on human platelets is a counterreceptor for the leukocyte integrin Mac-1. *J. Exp. Med.* **2002**, *196*, 679–691. [CrossRef]
24. Lishko, V.K.; Podolnikova, N.P.; Yakubenko, V.P.; Yakovlev, S.; Medved, L.; Yadav, S.P.; Ugarova, T.P. Multiple binding sites in fibrinogen for integrin alphaMbeta2 (Mac-1). *J. Biol. Chem.* **2004**, *279*, 44897–44906. [CrossRef] [PubMed]
25. Vorup-Jensen, T.; Jensen, R.K. Structural immunology of complement receptors 3 and 4. *Front. Immunol.* **2018**, *9*, 2716. [CrossRef]

26. Schmidt, R.; Bultmann, A.; Ungerer, M.; Joghetaei, N.; Bulbul, O.; Thieme, S.; Chavakis, T.; Toole, B.P.; Gawaz, M.; Schömig, A.; et al. Extracellular matrix metalloproteinase inducer regulates matrix metalloproteinase activity in cardiovascular cells: Implications in acute myocardial infarction. *Circulation* **2006**, *113*, 834–841. [CrossRef]
27. Langer, H.F.; Stellos, K.; Steingen, C.; Froihofer, A.; Schonberger, T.; Kramer, B.; Bigalke, B.; May, A.E.; Seizer, P.; Muller, I.; et al. Platelet derived bFGF mediates vascular integrative mechanisms of mesenchymal stem cells in vitro. *J. Mol. Cell. Cardiol.* **2009**, *47*, 315–325. [CrossRef]
28. Kourtzelis, I.; Mitroulis, I.; von Renesse, J.; Hajishengallis, G.; Chavakis, T. From leukocyte recruitment to resolution of inflammation: The cardinal role of integrins. *J. Leukoc. Biol.* **2017**, *102*, 677–683. [CrossRef]
29. Yuan, W.; Ge, H.; He, B. Pro-inflammatory activities induced by CyPA-EMMPRIN interaction in monocytes. *Atherosclerosis* **2010**, *213*, 415–421. [CrossRef]
30. Yoshida, S.; Shibata, M.; Yamamoto, S.; Hagihara, M.; Asai, N.; Takahashi, M.; Mizutani, S.; Muramatsu, T.; Kadomatsu, K. Homo-oligomer formation by basigin, an immunoglobulin superfamily member, via its N-terminal immunoglobulin domain. *Eur. J. Biochem. FEBS* **2000**, *267*, 4372–4380. [CrossRef]
31. Seizer, P.; Gawaz, M.; May, A.E. Cyclophilin A and EMMPRIN (CD147) in cardiovascular diseases. *Cardiovasc. Res.* **2014**, *102*, 17–23. [CrossRef] [PubMed]
32. Xu, Q.; Leiva, M.C.; Fischkoff, S.A.; Handschumacher, R.E.; Lyttle, C.R. Leukocyte chemotactic activity of cyclophilin. *J. Biol. Chem.* **1992**, *267*, 11968–11971. [PubMed]
33. Kim, H.; Kim, W.J.; Jeon, S.T.; Koh, E.M.; Cha, H.S.; Ahn, K.S.; Lee, W.H. Cyclophilin A may contribute to the inflammatory processes in rheumatoid arthritis through induction of matrix degrading enzymes and inflammatory cytokines from macrophages. *Clin. Immunol.* **2005**, *116*, 217–224. [CrossRef] [PubMed]
34. Alexaki, V.I.; May, A.E.; Fujii, C.; V Ungern-Sternberg, S.N.; Mund, C.; Gawaz, M.; Chavakis, T.; Seizer, P. S100A9 induces monocyte/macrophage migration via EMMPRIN. *Thromb. Haemost.* **2017**, *117*, 636–639. [CrossRef]
35. Kourtzelis, I.; Kotlabova, K.; Lim, J.H.; Mitroulis, I.; Ferreira, A.; Chen, L.S.; Gercken, B.; Steffen, A.; Kemter, E.; Klotzsche-von Ameln, A.; et al. Developmental endothelial locus-1 modulates platelet-monocyte interactions and instant blood-mediated inflammatory reaction in islet transplantation. *Thromb. Haemost.* **2016**, *115*, 781–788.

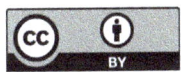

© 2020 by the authors. Licensee MDPI, Basel, Switzerland. This article is an open access article distributed under the terms and conditions of the Creative Commons Attribution (CC BY) license (http://creativecommons.org/licenses/by/4.0/).

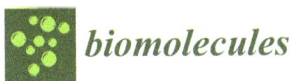

Article

Transient Expression of Reck Under Hepatic Ischemia/Reperfusion Conditions Is Associated with Mapk Signaling Pathways

Andrea Ferrigno [1], Laura G. Di Pasqua [1], Giuseppina Palladini [1,2], Clarissa Berardo [1], Roberta Verta [3], Plinio Richelmi [1], Stefano Perlini [1,4], Debora Collotta [3], Massimo Collino [3,†] and Mariapia Vairetti [1,†,*]

1. Department of Internal Medicine and Therapeutics, University of Pavia, 27100 Pavia, Italy; andrea.ferrigno@unipv.it (A.F.); lauragiuseppin.dipasqua01@universitadipavia.it (L.G.D.P.); giuseppina.palladini@unipv.it (G.P.); clarissa.berardo01@universitadipavia.it (C.B.); plinio.richelmi@unipv.it (P.R.); stefano.perlini@unipv.it (S.P.)
2. Fondazione IRCCS Policlinico San Matteo, 27100 Pavia, Italy
3. Department of Drug Science and Technology, University of Turin, 10125 Turin, Italy; roberta.verta@unito.it (R.V.); debora.collotta@unito.it (D.C.); massimo.collino@unito.it (M.C.)
4. Emergency Department, Fondazione IRCCS Policlinico San Matteo, 27100 Pavia, Italy
* Correspondence: mariapia.vairetti@unipv.it; Tel.: +39-0382-986398
† Both authors contributed equally.

Received: 8 January 2020; Accepted: 7 May 2020; Published: 11 May 2020

Abstract: In this study, we demonstrated the involvement of matrix metalloproteinases (MMPs) in hepatic ischemia/reperfusion (I/R) injury. Our aim is to evaluate the impact of reperfusion on I/R-related changes in RECK, an MMP modulator, and mitogen-activated protein kinase (MAPKs) pathways (ERK, p38, and JNK). Male Wistar rats were either subjected to 60 min partial-hepatic ischemia or sham-operated. After a 60 min or 120 min reperfusion, liver samples were collected for analysis of MMP-2 and MMP-9 by zymography and RECK, TIMP-1, and TIMP-2 content, MAPKs activation (ERK1/2, JNK1/2, and p38), as well as iNOS and eNOS by Western blot. Serum enzymes AST, ALT, and alkaline-phosphatase were quantified. A transitory decrease in hepatic RECK and TIMPs was associated with a transitory increase in both MMP-2 and MMP-9 activity and a robust activation of ERK1/2, JNK1/2, and p38 were detected at 60 min reperfusion. Hepatic expression of iNOS was maximally upregulated at 120 min reperfusion. An increase in eNOS was detected at 120 min reperfusion. I/R evoked significant hepatic injury in a time-dependent manner. These findings provide new insights into the underlying molecular mechanisms of reperfusion in inducing hepatic injury: a transitory decrease in RECK and TIMPs and increases in both MAPK and MMP activity suggest their role as triggering factors of the organ dysfunction.

Keywords: RECK; matrix metalloproteinase; MAPKs; ischemia/reperfusion; eNOS; iNOS

---

1. Introduction

Hepatic ischemia/reperfusion (I/R) injury may occur in a variety of clinical situations, including transplantation, liver resection, trauma, and vascular surgery. The reperfusion after ischemia may trigger I/R injury exacerbating cellular damage. The effects of reperfusion include excessive production of reactive oxygen species, oxidative stress, mitochondrial dysfunction, and systemic inflammatory response. Neutrophils play a critical role during the initial phase of I/R (0–6 h) triggering activation of pro-inflammatory intracellular cascades. One of the best characterized pathways within the context of organ I/R injury is the mitogen-activated protein kinase (MAPKs) family [1]. Among MAPKs, p38,

JNK1/2, and ERK 1/2, activated by a variety of cellular stressors including I/R, could potentially serve as potential targets in hepatic I/R injury [2,3].

Hepatic I/R injury is also connected with matrix metalloproteinases (MMPs) gene expression, activation, and release concomitant with alterations of tissue integrity [4]. The MMPs are a family of 24 proteases using zinc-dependent catalysis to breakdown extracellular matrix (ECM) components, allowing cell movement and tissue reorganization. Furthermore, MMP-2 and MMP-9 play a crucial role as they are the main components of Disse's space composed of loose extracellular matrix (ECM) [5]. We previously demonstrated that dysregulated expression and activation of MMPs are involved in hepatic injury and that changes in MMP activities already occur during the early phases of reperfusion [6]. Among different MMPs, MMP-9 is emerging as an important mediator of leukocyte traffic in hepatic I/R [7]. MMP-9 plays a crucial role in leukocyte recruitment and activation leading to liver I/R damage [8]. MMP-9(-/-) mice and mice treated with an anti MMP-9 antibody showed significantly reduced I/R damage, altered neutrophil migration, and depressed myeloperoxidase (MPO) activation [8]. Of note, the regulation of MMP activity appears as a multifaceted process; in particular, the relationship between the production of nitric oxide (NO) by inducible NO synthase (iNOS) and MMP-9 induction has obtained much attention over the last few years [9]. Selective iNOS inhibition down-regulates MMP-9 activity and disrupts leukocyte migration in hepatic I/R injury [10]. Most recent studies demonstrate that the activity of MMP-2 or MMP-9 is reduced by interaction with the reversion-inducing-cysteine-rich protein with kazal motifs (RECK) [11,12]. Recently, a study discovered RECK isoforms with opposing effects on cell migration: the short isoform appears to compete with MMP-9 for binding to the long RECK isoform [13]. RECK was identified as a transformation-suppressor gene which, regulating the expression of several MMPs, is involved in the inhibition of the tumor invasion and metastasis process [14]. RECK contains a glycosylphosphatidylinositol domain and a number of cysteine residues. It presents differences in the amino acid sequence when compared with the tissue inhibitors of metalloproteinases (TIMPs), which makes RECK an innovative membrane-targeted MMP regulator [14]. Besides, our understanding of the time course of activation of signaling cascades exerting a key role in liver injury following reperfusion remains incomplete and warrants further investigation.

Thus, the aim of the present study is to evaluate the impact of reperfusion on RECK and MAPK signaling pathways under hepatic I/R conditions. Their correlations with markers of organ dysfunction, such as MMP activity, iNOS, and eNOS were further investigated to better describe pathogenic mechanism(s) suitable for pharmacological modulation.

2. Materials and Methods

2.1. Materials

All reagents were of the highest grade of purity available and were obtained from Sigma-Aldrich (Milan, Italy).

2.2. Animals and Experimental Design

Male Wistar rats (Harlan-Nossan, Italy) were used in this study. The animals were allowed free access to water and food in all the experiments. The use and care of animals in this experimental study was approved by the Italian Ministry of Health and by the University of Pavia Commission for Animal Care (Document number 179/2017-PR). The effects of I/R were studied in vivo in a partial normothermic hepatic I/R model (n = 18). The rats were anesthetized with sodium pentobarbital (40 mg/kg i.p.), the abdomen was opened via a midline incision. Ischemia to the left and the median lobe was induced for 60 min with microvascular clips by clamping the branch of portal vein and the branch of the hepatic artery after the bifurcation to the right lobe, with the abdomen temporarily closed with a suture [6]. After 60 min of ischemia, the abdomen was reopened, the clips were removed, the abdomen was closed again, and the liver was allowed to reperfuse for 60 or 120 min. By using partial, rather than total, hepatic ischemia, portal vein congestion and subsequent bacterial translocation into the portal venous blood was avoided. Sham animals were subjected to the same procedure without clamping the vessels (n = 12). To prevent postsurgical dehydration and hypotension, 1 mL of saline was injected into the inferior vena cava. All the animals were maintained on a warm support to prevent heat loss with rectal temperature at 37 ± 0.1 °C. Animals were sacrificed under general anesthesia by exsanguination. Blood was drawn from the vena cava and allowed to clot at room temperature. After 15 min serum was centrifuged at 3000× g for 10 min at 4 °C. At the end of ischemia or after 60 min or 120 min reperfusion, hepatic biopsies were quickly removed from the median lobe and immediately frozen in liquid nitrogen, as were serum samples.

2.3. Biochemical Assays

Liver injury was assessed by serum levels of alanine transaminase (ALT), aspartate transaminase (AST), and alkaline phosphatase (ALP). Total and direct bilirubin were quantified using standard commercial kits (Merck, Italy).

2.4. Gelatin Zymography

Protein extraction from snap-frozen samples and gelatin zymography were performed as described previously [15]. To detect MMP lytic activity samples were homogenized in an ice-cold extraction buffer and protein content was normalized by a final concentration of 400 µg/mL in the sample loading buffer (0.25 M Tris-HCl, 4% sucrose w/v, 10% SDS w/v, and 0.1% bromphenol blue w/v, pH 6.8). After dilution, the samples were loaded onto electrophoretic gels (SDS-PAGE), containing gelatin, under nonreducing conditions. Following the electrophoretic run, the gels were washed twice and were incubated at 37 °C. To reveal zones of lysis, gels were stained with Coomassie Blue. The zymograms were analyzed by a densitometer (GS 900 Densitometer BIORAD, Hercules, CA, USA), and proteinases activity was expressed as optical density (OD), reported to 1 mg/mL protein content.

2.5. Western Blot Assay

Liver tissue samples were homogenized in an ice-cold Lysis Buffer supplemented with Protease Inhibitor Cocktail and centrifuged at 15,000 g for 10 min. The collected supernatant was stored at −80 °C. Samples of liver extracts containing the same amount of proteins were separated in SDS-PAGE on 7.5% acrylamide gels and transferred to PVDF membrane. Unspecific sites were blocked for 2 h with 5% Bovine Serum Albumin (BSA) in TBS Tween (20 mMTris/HCl, 500 mM NaCl, pH 7.5, 0.1% Tween 20) at 4 °C. The membranes were incubated with primary antibodies overnight at 4 °C, under gentle agitation. Primary antibodies against mouse monoclonal alpha tubulin (DM1A), mouse monoclonal anti-RECK, mouse monoclonal anti-eNOS, mouse monoclonal anti-Phospho-JNK (Thr183/Tyr185), mouse monoclonal anti-Phospho p38 (Thr180/Tyr182), rabbit monoclonal anti-Phospho-ERK1/2 (Thr202/Tyr204), rabbit monoclonal anti-ERK1/2, rabbit polyclonal antibody anti-iNOS, rabbit polyclonal anti-JNK, and rabbit polyclonal anti-p38 were used at 1:1000 dilution. Rabbit polyclonal anti TIMP-1 and TIMP-2 were used at 1:200. Membranes were washed in TBS Tween (Na2HPO4 8 mM, NaH2PO4-H2O 2 mM, NaCl 140 mM, pH 7.4, 0.1% Tween 20) and incubated with peroxidase-conjugated secondary anti-Rabbit or anti-Mouse antibodies at a 1:2000 dilution. The membranes were then stripped and incubated with tubulin monoclonal antibody (1:5000) and subsequently with anti-mouse (1:10,000) to assess uniformity of gel loading. Anti-iNOS was purchased from Cayman Chemical (Ann Arbor, Michigan, USA). RECK and eNOS were bought from Santa Cruz Biotechnology. Mouse monoclonal antibody against TIMP-1 and TIMP-2 were purchased from Thermo Fisher Scientific (USA For the detection of MAPKs, the antibodies were obtained from Cell Signaling Technology [LS1] (Leiden, the Netherlands). Immunostaining was revealed with BIO-RAD Chemidoc XRS+ visualized using the ECL Clarity BIO-RAD (Milan, Italy). Bands intensity quantification was performed by BIO-RAD Image Lab Software™ 6.0.1., and autoradiograms showing statistically significant differences in terms of gel-loading homogeneity were excluded from the following biomarkers analyses.

2.6. Liver Histology

Liver biopsies were rapidly removed, fixed in 2% p-formaldehyde in 0.1 M phosphate buffer at pH 7.4 for 24 h and processed routinely until they were embedded in Paraplast wax. Sections were cut at 7 µm and stained with Hematoxylin and Eosin (H&E) for histological examination [16]

2.7. Statistical Analysis

Results are expressed as means value ± standard error (SE) for all data. The value of $p < 0.05$ was considered the criterion for statistical significance. To assess normality of variance changes, the Kolmogorov–Shapiro normality test was used. Data were analyzed by ANOVA with Tukey's multiple comparison test as post-hoc test or Kruskall–Wallis and Dunn's test, as appropriate. Statistical Analysis was performed using MedCalc Statistical Software version 18.11.3 (MedCalc Software bvba, Ostend, Belgium; https://www.medcalc.org; 2019).

3. Results

3.1. Transient Expression of Reck, Mmps, and Timps in a Rat Model of Hepatic I/R Injury

To study the expression of RECK under hepatic I/R, we used a rat model of partial I/R injury. After 60 min reperfusion, a time-dependent increase in serum levels of AST, ALT, ALP, and total and direct bilirubin was observed (Table 1).

Table 1. Serum levels of AST, ALT, ALP (U/L), and total and direct bilirubin (mg/dL).

	Sham 60/60	I/R 60/60	Sham 60/120	I/R 60/120
AST	243 ± 57	3444 ± 1062	198 ± 43	10,387 ± 1158 *
ALT	66 ± 19	3830 ± 961	61 ± 28	9320 ± 1040 *
ALP	431 ± 50	605 ± 51	417 ± 55	769 ± 29 *
Total Bilirubin	0.13 ± 0.024	0.25 ± 0.070	0.12 ± 0.011	0.35 ± 0.043
Direct Bilirubin	0.045 ± 0.019	0.17 ± 0.032	0.04 ± 0.024	0.18 ± 0.013

Aspartate transaminase, AST; alanine transaminase, ALT; alkaline phosphatase, ALP; * $p < 0.05$.

This trend was supported by histological analysis (Figure 1). Livers from sham-operated animals showed well-preserved hepatic architecture while I/R caused marked injury to the parenchyma with sinusoid dilatation, extensive areas of cytoplasmic vacuolation, and wide areas of necrotic cells detached from the parenchyma, especially after 120 min reperfusion.

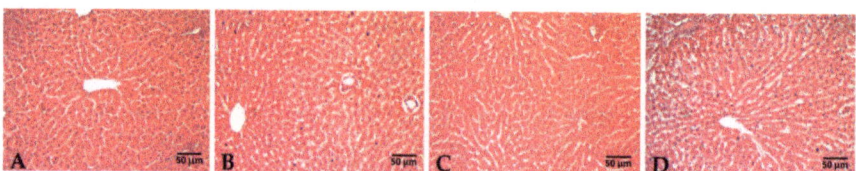

Figure 1. Liver histology at the end of reperfusion. Paraplast-embedded sections were cut at 7 µm and stained with H&E. Panel (**A**) and (**C**): 60/60 and 60/120 min sham-operated rats, respectively. Panel (**B**) and (**D**): rats submitted to ischemia followed by 60 or 120 min reperfusion, respectively.

The results of RECK protein analysis showed a significant decrease in RECK only at 60 min reperfusion when compared with 60 min ischemia or 120 min reperfusion or sham-operated groups; a complete recovery of RECK levels was found at 120 min reperfusion (Figure 2, Panel A). In addition, no changes in RECK content at the end of ischemia occurred when compared with sham-operated group. The opposite trend occurred for both MMP-2 and MMP-9 activities that increased after 60 min reperfusion when compared with sham-operated rats followed by a significant decrease in both hepatic

MMP activities detectable at 120 min reperfusion comparable with those found in sham-operated rats (Figure 2, Panel B). The analysis of TIMP-1 showed a decrease after 60 min reperfusion but was re-expressed at 120 min reperfusion relative to the 60 min time point. No differences in expression between TIMP-2 were detected between 60 min versus 120 min reperfusion (Figure 2, Panel C).

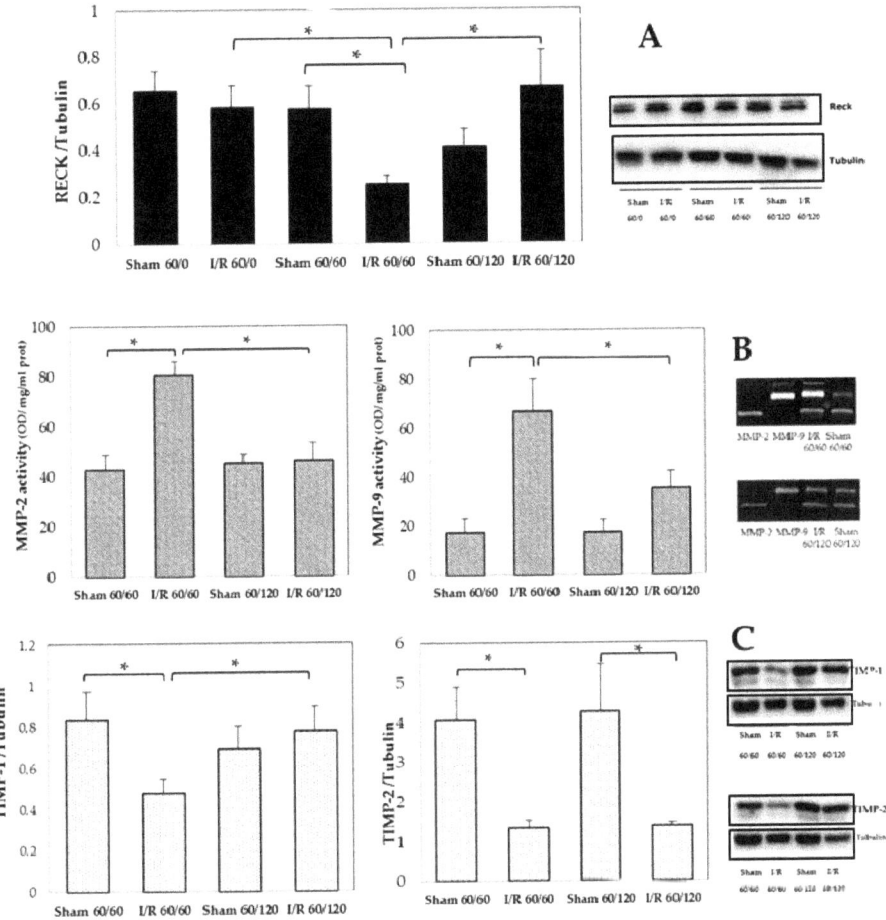

Figure 2. Hepatic MMP-2 and MMP-9 activity, RECK, TIMP-1, and TIMP-2 at the end of ischemia and after 60 min or 120 min of reperfusion. Panel (**A**): RECK, * $p = 0.02$; Panel (**B**): MMP-2, * $p = 0.006$; MMP-9: * $p = 0.007$; Panel (**C**): TIMP-1 * $p = 0.04$; TIMP-2, * $p = 0.03$. The results are reported as the mean ± SE of 6 different experiments. RECK, reversion-inducing cysteine-rich protein with Kazal motifs; TIMPs, tissue inhibitor of metalloproteinases.

3.2. Transient Expression of Mapks under Hepatic I/R

Animals that had undergone 60 min ischemia followed by 60 min reperfusion displayed higher phosphorylation of MAPKs (ERK1/2, JNK1/2 and p38) expression than ischemia or sham-operated animals (Figure 3 A–C), suggesting an early enhancement of the activation of these pathways by I/R injury. On the contrary, the longer I/R challenge resulted in lower expression levels of the MAPK phosphorylated forms, with values similar to those recorded in sham-operated animals, thus indicating a time-dependent quenching of I/R-injury. No significant changes in expression of total MAPK isoforms were recorded in ischemia group as well in sham-operated rats.

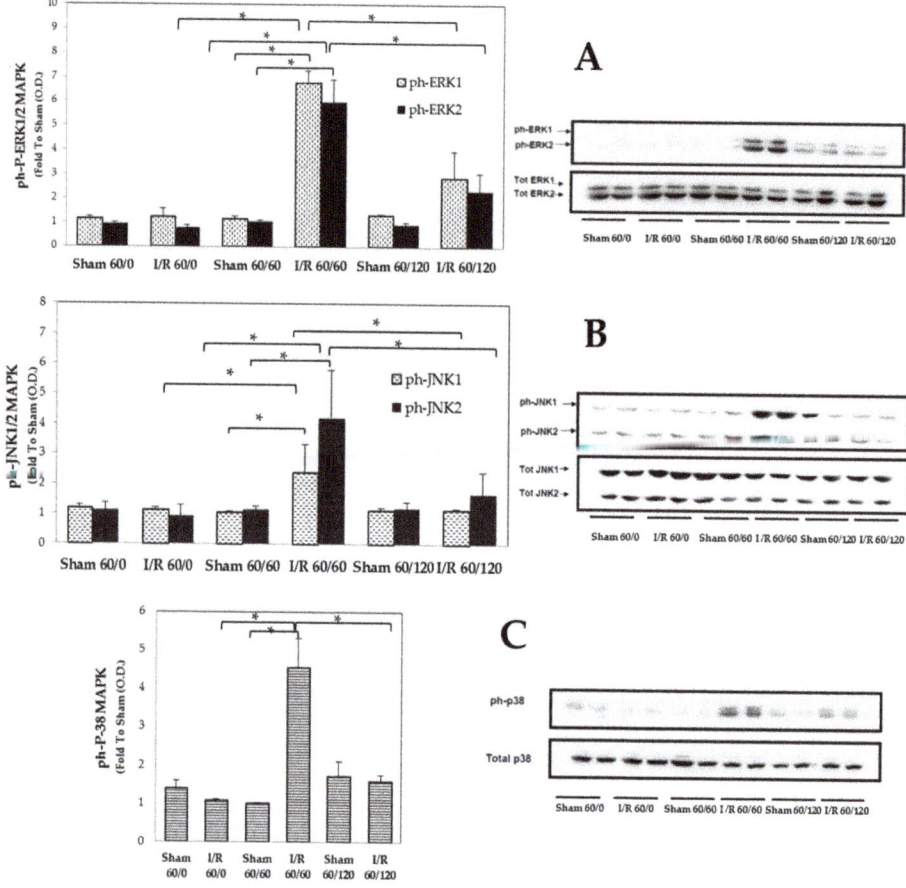

Figure 3. Hepatic MAPK pathways (ERK1/2, JNK1/2 and p38) at the end of ischemia and after 60 min or 120 min reperfusion. Panel (**A**): ERK1, * p = 0.025; ERK2, * p = 0.025; Panel (**B**): JNK1, * p = 0.028; JNK2, * p = 0.043; Panel (**C**): P-38, * p = 0.014. The results are reported as the mean ± SE of 6 different experiments.

3.3. Changes in Enos and Inos Expression Under Hepatic I/R

At 120 min reperfusion, a significant increase in eNOS expression was found and it was about 3-fold compared with sham-operated or 60 min reperfused animals (Figure 4, Panel A). Changes in iNOS expression emerged comparing sham and I/R treated groups both after 60 min or 120 min reperfusion: a time-dependent increase in iNOS content was found (Figure 4, Panel B).

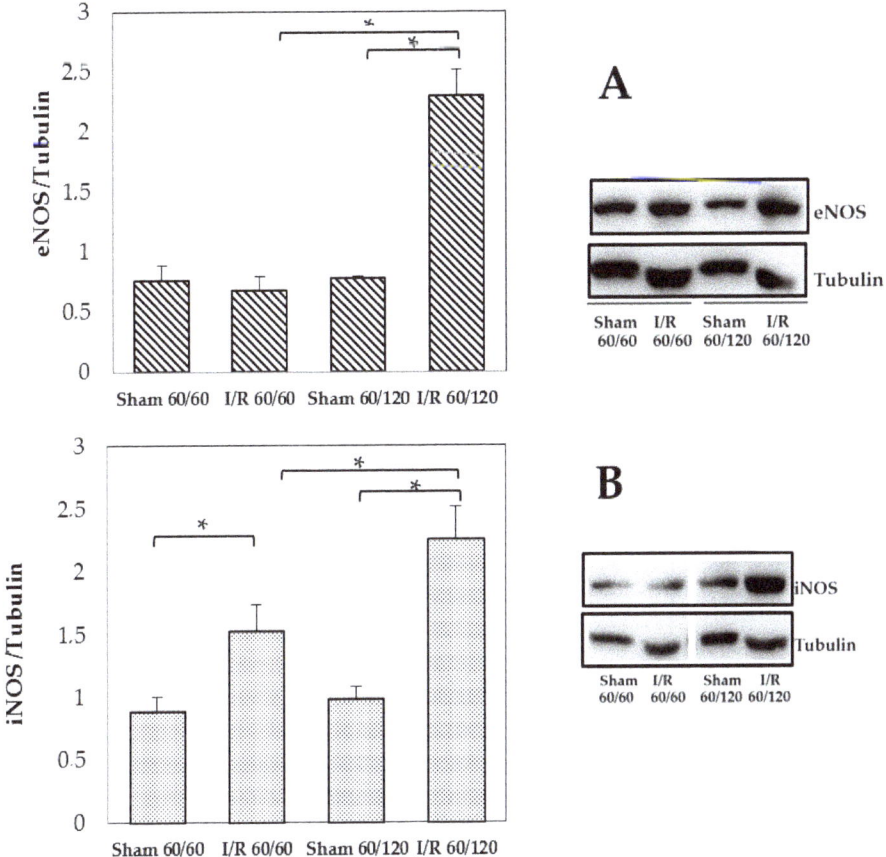

Figure 4. Hepatic eNOS and iNOS at the end of reperfusion. Panel (**A**): eNOS, * $p = 0.002$; Panel (**B**): iNOS, * $p = 0.004$. The results are reported as the mean ± SE of 6 different experiments.

4. Discussion

The present data provide new insights into the underlying molecular mechanisms that occur during reperfusion in hepatic I/R injury: a transitory decrease in RECK and TIMPs, concomitant with an increases in both MAPK and MMP activity, suggests their role as triggering factors of the organ dysfunction.

As previously documented, the kinetics of the reperfusion injury may also affect the entity of the expression and activation of MAPK signaling pathways involved in the I/R-induced damage [17]. A crucial intracellular step that can counteract the deleterious effects of I/R injury is the selective activation of MAPK. A time-course experiment of MAPK expression after liver I/R showed an increase in phosphorylation of each MAPK (ERK1/2, JNK1/2, and p38), detectable after 60 min reperfusion and the activation decreased after 3 h reperfusion, especially for JNK [18]. Here we confirmed the early and transient MAPK activation, coming back to values similar to those recorded in basal condition after 120 min reperfusion.

In keeping with the data on MAPK activation, when we measured MMP-2 and MMP-9 activity as well as the expression of their respective TIMP physiological inhibitors in the liver homogenates, we found a parallel between the early and transient activation of MMP-2 and MMP-9 and that observed for MAPKs, suggestive of simultaneous contribution to I/R-induced protein expression changes.

Here, for the first time, we demonstrated that both MMP-2 and MMP-9 over activation at 60 min was associated with RECK down-regulation, whereas the up-regulation of RECK expression was recorded at 120 min when no significant MMP activation was detectable. It has been reported that RECK overexpression decreases the amount of active MMP-2 and MMP-9 in conditioned medium and inhibits metastatic activity in vitro [19] and in vivo [12]. The evaluation of genotypes among hepatocellular carcinoma (HCC) patients suggested a possible involvement of RECK gene rs11788747 polymorphism in increasing the susceptibility of individuals to HCC [20]. In addition, RECK expression was found to be reduced in kidney epithelial cells subjected to hypoxia [21]. Here, for the first time, we demonstrated that modulation of RECK expression following liver I/R injury was paralleled by changes in MMP-2 and MMP-9 activation, thus suggesting a potential cross-talk mechanism linking these two signaling cascades. Our results were supported by findings reported in a recent study using a rat model of cerebral ischemia [22]. Besides, we did not measure activation of signaling cascades (neither at the very beginning of reperfusion, nor in non-ischemic liver lobes; thus, we cannot offer a comprehensive understanding here of all the kinetics factors potentially affecting their expression and activation. MMPs and TIMPs play also an important function in the preservation of liver homeostasis [23]. In particular, the major endogenous regulator of MMP-9, TIMP-1, exerts a protective role in the control of the survival of liver cells during I/R injury [24]. Curzio et al. reported that TIMP-1 was induced following liver I/R with an earlier induction so we can hypothesize that the failure to recover TIMP-2 at 120 min is due to slower induction times [25]. In addition, TIMP-1 has been reported to play the major protective role: the inability of TIMP-1$^{-/-}$ mice to express TIMP-1 resulted in enhanced liver damage and in lethal hepatic I/R injury [24]. Our data support these results: an opposite trend was found comparing MMP-9 activation versus TIMP-1 content.

RECK downregulation under hypoxic conditions has been demonstrated to be mediated by involvement of ERK1/2, JNK, and p38 MAPK signaling pathways [26]. The same authors demonstrated that inhibition of the MAPK signaling pathways restores RECK expression and its ability to affect MMP activity. In particular, activation of the p38 pathway and p38-associated inflammatory processes play a crucial role in post-ischemic damage [27]. Although several studies have demonstrated a detrimental role of JNK activation in I/R injury [28], the results about a protection by JNK inhibition are still controversial [27,29]. There are also studies indicating the potential involvement of ERK 1/2 in hepatic I/R injury [30]; to date, the potential role of ERK1/2 as a therapeutic target for liver I/R injury has not been clarified yet, because the molecules used are also able to modulate other pathways different from ERK1/2 [28]. However, liver protection against I/R injury was recently obtained via suppressing the MAPK signaling [1]. Although we demonstrated a time-dependent effect of reperfusion injury on the cross-talk mechanisms linking RECK expression to MAPK activity, we cannot rule out the potential impact of the kinetics of the ischemia injury on the activation/expression of the tested signaling cascades. In fact, as shown by Cursio and colleagues [18], a longer kinetics of ischemia (120 min of normothermic liver ischemia) resulted in sustained p38 MAPK activation until 3 h reperfusion, whereas, in keeping with our findings, ERK1/2 degree of activation already decreased after 1 h reperfusion.

We also showed no significant differences in RECK and MAPK content between ischemic livers without reperfusion and either the sham-operated and 120 min reperfusion groups, thus confirming that activation of the signaling cascades is mainly related to the reperfusion injury in our experimental conditions.

Once the MAPK pathway is activated, MAPKs phosphorylate downstream protein kinases and transcription factors, resulting in upregulation of both iNOS and eNOS. Under normal conditions, only eNOS is present in the liver, and low levels of NO regulate the hepatic perfusion [31]. Alternatively, the excess production of NO, generated primarily by iNOS, has been implicated as a mediator of cellular injury at sites of inflammation, including liver I/R injury [32]. Under these circumstances, NO reacts with molecular oxygen or superoxide and generates reactive nitrogen species, which may interfere with many biological functional and structural processes of liver injury evoked by hepatic I/R, including ECM degradation [10]. Here, we confirmed that the early MAPK activation resulted following overexpression of iNOS and eNOS, leading to excessive NO production, which contributes to the liver damage [33] and also remote organs [34]. Besides, specific iNOS inhibition has been demonstrated to down-regulate MMP-9 activity and disrupts leukocyte migration in hepatic I/R injury [10]. These findings further support the mechanistic loop linking MAPKs to MMPs here described. However, only the use of drugs that specifically inhibit these signaling cascades may allow to identify a causal relationship between these two pathways and their modulation by RECK. Unfortunately, the lack of knowledge of the in vivo pharmacological profile of highly selective pharmacological inhibitors limits further investigation.

5. Conclusions

In conclusion, we demonstrated that the kinetics of reperfusion selectively affect the activation of signaling pathways involved in hepatic I/R injury. Both MAPKs and MMPs showed an early and transient activation, which contribute to the development of organ dysfunction and injury. Our data show that reperfusion-induced modulation of RECK expression is paralleled by opposite changes in MAPK activation and MMP activity. These findings may contribute to better understanding intracellular pathways cross-regulation sensitive to liver I/R injury and, thus, to providing the rationale for much needed novel agents to fill the current therapeutic gaps. However, further studies are needed to better clarify the reciprocal interaction of these pathways for a wider understanding of the intricate network of cellular and functional interactions leading to I/R-related liver injury.

Author Contributions: Conceptualization, A.F., G.P. and M.V.; methodology, A.F., L.G.D.P., C.B., R.V. and D.C.; writing—original draft preparation, A.F.; writing—review and editing, G.P., M.C. and M.V.; visualization, P.R. and S.P.; supervision, M.C. and M.V. All authors have read and agreed to the published version of the manuscript.

Funding: Funds from the University of Pavia and the University of Turin (Ricerca Locale 2019) were used.

Acknowledgments: We thank Nicoletta Breda for editing assistance.

Conflicts of Interest: The authors declare no conflict of interest.

References

1. Xu, S.; Niu, P.; Chen, K.; Xia, Y.; Yu, Q.; Liu, N.; Li, J.; Li, S.; Wu, L.; Feng, J.; et al. The liver protection of propylene glycol alginate sodium sulfate preconditioning against ischemia reperfusion injury: Focusing MAPK pathway activity. *Sci. Rep.* **2017**, *7*, 15175. [CrossRef]
2. Kobayashi, M.; Takeyoshi, I.; Yoshinari, D.; Matsumoto, K.; Morishita, Y. P38 mitogen-activated protein kinase inhibition attenuates ischemia-reperfusion injury of the rat liver. *Surgery* **2002**, *131*, 344–349. [CrossRef]
3. Toledo-Pereyra, L.H.; Lopez-Neblina, F.; Toledo, A.H. Protein Kinases in Organ Ischemia and Reperfusion. *J. Investig. Surg.* **2008**, *21*, 215–226. [CrossRef]
4. Viappiani, S.; Sariahmetoglu, M.; Schulz, R. The role of matrix metalloproteinase inhibitors in ischemia-reperfusion injury in the liver. *Curr. Pharm. Des.* **2006**, *12*, 2923–2934. [CrossRef]
5. Khandoga, A.; Kessler, J.S.; Hanschen, M.; Burggraf, D.; Reichel, C.; Hamann, G.F.; Enders, G.; Krombach, F. Matrix metalloproteinase-9 promotes neutrophil and T cell recruitment and migration in the postischemic liver. *J. Leukoc. Boil.* **2006**, *79*, 1295–1305. [CrossRef]
6. Palladini, G.; Ferrigno, A.; Rizzo, V.; Boncompagni, E.; Richelmi, P.; Freitas, I.; Perlini, S.; Vairetti, M. Lobe-Specific Heterogeneity and Matrix Metalloproteinase Activation after Ischemia/Reperfusion Injury in Rat Livers. *Toxicol. Pathol.* **2012**, *40*, 722–730. [CrossRef]
7. Coito, A.J. Leukocyte transmigration across endothelial and extracellular matrix protein barriers in liver ischemia/reperfusion injury. *Curr. Opin. Organ Transplant.* **2011**, *16*, 34–40. [CrossRef]
8. Hamada, T.; Fondevila, C.; Busuttil, R.W.; Coito, A.J. Metalloproteinase-9 deficiency protects against hepatic ischemia/reperfusion injury. *Hepatology* **2007**, *47*, 186–198. [CrossRef]
9. O'Sullivan, S.; Medina, C.; Ledwidge, M.; Radomski, M.W.; Gilmer, J.F. Nitric oxide-matrix metaloproteinase-9 interactions: Biological and pharmacological significance. *Biochim. Biophys. Acta* **2014**, *1843*, 603–617. [CrossRef]

10. Hamada, T.; Duarte, S.; Tsuchihashi, S.; Busuttil, R.W.; Coito, A.J. Inducible Nitric Oxide Synthase Deficiency Impairs Matrix Metalloproteinase-9 Activity and Disrupts Leukocyte Migration in Hepatic Ischemia/Reperfusion Injury. *Am. J. Pathol.* **2009**, *174*, 2265–2277. [CrossRef]
11. Oh, J.; Takahashi, R.; Kondo, S.; Mizoguchi, A.; Adachi, E.; Sasahara, R.M.; Nishimura, S.; Imamura, Y.; Kitayama, H.; Alexander, D.B.; et al. The Membrane-Anchored MMP Inhibitor RECK is a Key Regulator of Extracellular Matrix Integrity and Angiogenesis. *Cell* **2001**, *107*, 789–800. [CrossRef]
12. Chang, C.-K.; Hung, W.-C.; Chang, H.-C. The Kazal motifs of RECK protein inhibit MMP-9 secretion and activity and reduce metastasis of lung cancer cells in vitro and in vivo. *J. Cell. Mol. Med.* **2008**, *12*, 2781–2789. [CrossRef]
13. Lee, H.N.; Mitra, M.; Bosompra, O.; Corney, D.C.; Johnson, E.L.; Rashed, N.; Ho, L.D.; Coller, H.A. RECK isoforms have opposing effects on cell migration. *Mol. Boil. Cell* **2018**, *29*, 1825–1838. [CrossRef]
14. Meng, N.; Li, Y.; Zhang, H.; Sun, X.-F. RECK, a novel matrix metalloproteinase regulator. *Histol. Histopathol.* **2008**, *23*, 1003–1010.
15. Ferrigno, A.; Palladini, G.; Bianchi, A.; Rizzo, V.; Di Pasqua, L.G.; Perlini, S.; Richelmi, P.; Vairetti, M. Lobe-Specific Heterogeneity in Asymmetric Dimethylarginine and Matrix Metalloproteinase Levels in a Rat Model of Obstructive Cholestasis. *BioMed Res. Int.* **2014**, *2014*, 1–8. [CrossRef]
16. Ferrigno, A.; Di Pasqua, L.G.; Berardo, C.; Siciliano, V.; Richelmi, P.; Vairetti, M. Oxygen tension-independent protection against hypoxic cell killing in rat liver by low sodium. *Eur. J. Histochem.* **2017**, *61*, 61. [CrossRef]
17. Mastrocola, R.; Penna, C.R.R.; Tullio, F.; Femminò, S.; Nigro, D.; Chiazza, F.; Serpe, L.; Collotta, D.; Alloatti, G.; Cocco, M.; et al. Pharmacological Inhibition of NLRP3 Inflammasome Attenuates Myocardial Ischemia/Reperfusion Injury by Activation of RISK and Mitochondrial Pathways. *Oxidative Med. Cell. Longev.* **2016**, *2016*, 1–11. [CrossRef]
18. Cursio, R.; Filippa, N.; Miele, C.; Van Obberghen, E.; Gugenheim, J. Involvement of protein kinase B and mitogen-activated protein kinases in experimental normothermic liver ischaemia–reperfusion injury. *BJS* **2006**, *93*, 752–761. [CrossRef]
19. Yan, K.H.; Lee, L.M.; Yan, S.H.; Huang, H.C.; Li, C.C.; Lin, H.T.; Chen, P.S. Tomadine inhibits invasion of human lung adenocarcinoma cell A549 by reducing matrix metalloproteinases expression. *Chem. Biol. Interact.* **2013**, *203*, 580–587. [CrossRef]
20. Bahgat, D.M.R.; Shahin, R.M.H.; Makar, N.N.; Aziz, A.O.A.; Hunter, S.S. Reversion-Inducing-Cysteine-Rich Protein With Kazal Motifs (RECK) Gene Single Nucleotide Polymorphism With Hepatocellular Carcinoma: A Case-Control Study. *J. Clin. Lab. Anal.* **2014**, *30*, 36–40. [CrossRef]
21. Lee, K.J.; Lee, K.Y.; Lee, Y.M. Downregulation of a tumor suppressor RECK by hypoxia through recruitment of HDAC1 and HIF-1α to reverse HRE site in the promoter. *Biochim. Biophys. Acta* **2010**, *1803*, 608–616. [CrossRef] [PubMed]
22. Tang, Y.; Zhang, Y.; Zheng, M.; Chen, J.; Chen, H.; Liu, N. Effects of treadmill exercise on cerebral angiogenesis and MT1-MMP expression after cerebral ischemia in rats. *Brain Behav.* **2018**, *8*, e01079. [CrossRef] [PubMed]
23. Duarte, S.; Baber, J.; Fujii, T.; Coito, A.J. Matrix metalloproteinases in liver injury, repair and fibrosis. *Matrix Boil.* **2015**, *44*, 147–156. [CrossRef] [PubMed]
24. Duarte, S.; Hamada, T.; Kuriyama, N.; Busuttil, R.W.; Coito, A.J. TIMP-1 deficiency leads to lethal partial hepatic ischemia and reperfusion injury. *Hepatol.* **2012**, *56*, 1074–1085. [CrossRef] [PubMed]
25. Cursio, R.; Mari, B.; Louis, K.; Rostagno, P.; Saint-Paul, M.-C.; Giudicelli, J.; Bottero, V.; Anglard, P.; Yiotakis, A.; Dive, V.; et al. Rat liver injury following normothermic ischemia is prevented by a phosphinic matrix metalloproteinase inhibitor. *FASEB J.* **2001**, *16*, 1–24. [CrossRef]
26. Jeon, H.W.; Lee, K.-J.; Lee, S.H.; Kim, W.-H.; Lee, Y.M. Attenuated expression and function of the RECK tumor suppressor under hypoxic conditions is mediated by the MAPK signaling pathways. *Arch. Pharmacal Res.* **2011**, *34*, 137–145. [CrossRef]
27. Deng, J.; Feng, J.; Liu, T.; Lu, X.; Wang, W.; Liu, N.; Lv, Y.; Liu, Q.; Guo, C.; Zhou, Y. Beraprost sodium preconditioning prevents inflammation, apoptosis, and autophagy during hepatic ischemia-reperfusion injury in mice via the P38 and JNK pathways. *Drug Des. Dev. Ther.* **2018**, *12*, 4067–4082. [CrossRef]
28. Jiménez-Castro, M.B.; Cornide-Petronio, M.E.; Gracia-Sancho, J.; Casillas-Ramírez, A.; Peralta, C. Mitogen Activated Protein Kinases in Steatotic and Non-Steatotic Livers Submitted to Ischemia-Reperfusion. *Int. J. Mol. Sci.* **2019**, *20*, 1785. [CrossRef]

29. Lee, K.-H.; Kim, S.-E.; Lee, Y.-S. SP600125, a selective JNK inhibitor, aggravates hepatic ischemia-reperfusion injury. *Exp. Mol. Med.* **2006**, *38*, 408–416. [CrossRef]
30. Yu, Q.; Wu, L.; Liu, T.; Li, S.; Feng, J.; Mao, Y.; Fan, X.; Guo, C.; Wu, J. Protective effects of levo-tetrahydropalmatine on hepatic ischemia/reperfusion injury are mediated by inhibition of the ERK/NF-κB pathway. *Int. Immunopharmacol.* **2019**, *70*, 435–445. [CrossRef]
31. Li, J.; Billiar, T.R., IV. Determinants of nitric oxide protection and toxicity in liver. *Am. J. Physiol. Liver Physiol.* **1999**, *276*, G1069–G1073. [CrossRef]
32. Isobe, M.; Katsuramaki, T.; Hirata, K.; Kimura, H.; Nagayama, M.; Matsuno, T. Beneficial Effects of Inducible Nitric Oxide Synthase Inhibitor on Reperfusion Injury in the Pig Liver. *Transplantation* **1999**, *68*, 803–813. [CrossRef] [PubMed]
33. Morisue, A.; Wakabayashi, G.; Shimazu, M.; Tanabe, M.; Mukai, M.; Matsumoto, K.; Kawachi, S.; Yoshida, M.; Yamamoto, S.; Kitajima, M. The role of nitric oxide after a short period of liver ischemia-reperfusion. *J. Surg. Res.* **2003**, *109*, 101–109. [CrossRef]
34. Cowled, P.A.; Khanna, A.; Laws, P.E.; Field, J.B.F.; Fitridge, R.A. Simvastatin Plus Nitric Oxide Synthase Inhibition Modulates Remote Organ Damage Following Skeletal Muscle Ischemia-Reperfusion Injury. *J. Investig. Surg.* **2008**, *21*, 119–126. [CrossRef] [PubMed]

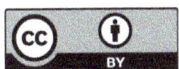

© 2020 by the authors. Licensee MDPI, Basel, Switzerland. This article is an open access article distributed under the terms and conditions of the Creative Commons Attribution (CC BY) license (http://creativecommons.org/licenses/by/4.0/).

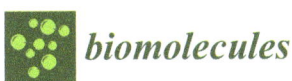

Article

Novel Barbiturate-Nitrate Compounds Inhibit the Upregulation of Matrix Metalloproteinase-9 Gene Expression in Intestinal Inflammation through a cGMP-Mediated Pathway

Shane O'Sullivan, Jun Wang, Marek W. Radomski, John F. Gilmer and Carlos Medina *

School of Pharmacy and Pharmaceutical Sciences, Trinity Biomedical Sciences Institute, Trinity College Dublin, 2 Dublin, Ireland; osullish@tcd.ie (S.O.); wangju@tcd.ie (J.W.); marek.radomski@usask.ca (M.W.R.); gilmerjf@tcd.ie (J.F.G.)
* Correspondence: carlos.medina@tcd.ie

Received: 29 April 2020; Accepted: 22 May 2020; Published: 25 May 2020

Abstract: Matrix metalloproteinase-9 is upregulated in inflammatory bowel disease. Barbiturate nitrate hybrid compounds have been designed to inhibit MMP secretion and enzyme activity. In this study, we investigated the mechanism of action of barbiturate-nitrate hybrid compounds and their component parts using models of intestinal inflammation in vitro. Cytokine-stimulated Caco-2 cells were used in all in vitro experiments. The NO donors SNAP and DETA-NONOate were used to study the effect of NO on MMP-9 mRNA. Mechanistic elucidation was carried out using the soluble guanylate cyclase (sGC) inhibitor, ODQ, and the cGMP analogue, 8-Bromo-cGMP. Further experiments were carried out to elucidate the role of NF-κB. NO donors exerted an inhibitory effect on MMP-9 mRNA in cytokine-stimulated cells. While the non-nitrate barbiturates had a limited effect on MMP-9 expression, the hybrid compounds inhibited MMP-9 expression through its NO-mimetic properties. No effect could be observed on mRNA for MMP-1 or MMP-2. The sGC inhibitior, ODQ, abolished the nitrate-barbiturate inhibition of MMP-9 gene expression, an effect which was reversed by 8-Br-cGMP. This study shows that the barbiturate scaffold is suitable for hybrid design as an MMP-9 inhibitor in cytokine-stimulated Caco-2 cells. The inhibition of MMP-9 levels was largely mediated through a reduction in its mRNA by a sGC/cGMP pathway mediated mechanism.

Keywords: inflammatory bowel disease; inflammation; NO; MMP-9; cGMP; Caco-2

1. Introduction

The matrix metalloproteinases are a group of endopeptidases capable of digesting the extracellular matrix (ECM), basement membrane as well as having an immunomodulatory role related to activation of other proteases and inflammatory mediators [1–3]. Inflammatory bowel disease (IBD), which encompasses ulcerative colitis (UC) and Crohn's disease (CD), is a chronic, relapsing condition involving inflammation of the gut leading to abdominal pain, diarrhoea, rectal bleeding and fever. MMP-9 is known to be up-regulated in IBD [4–7] and is associated with disruption of the epithelial barrier and activation of pro-inflammatory mediators [8–11]. Inhibition of this enzyme may therefore aid in reducing the severity of the disease. The development of clinically useful synthetic inhibitors has, to date, been disappointing, mainly due to dose-limiting side-effects but it is also true that the efficacy evident in animal models has not translated [12,13]. This has led to a revaluation of the precise role of specific MMPs in a given pathological setting and to investigate new strategies for modulating dysregulated MMP activity in disease tissue. Certain appropriately substituted barbiturates have been shown to possess MMP inhibitory characteristics [14,15] while being without sedative actions [16]. The barbiturates have, in general, better pharmacokinetic properties than other

MMP inhibitory compounds such as, for example, the hydroxamates. Our group reported a series of barbiturate-nitrate hybrid compounds that are potent inhibitors of MMP-2 and MMP-9 at the enzyme level [17]. Incorporation of a nitrate group as a nitric oxide (NO) donor or mimetic functionality was intended to confer on the compounds an ability to modulate the enzyme levels of inducible MMP in order to complement the purely enzyme inhibitory actions of the barbiturate zinc binding group. Interactions between NO and MMP-9, which have been recently reviewed, are complex and difficult to predict [18]. In our previous work we showed that the hybrid compounds were able to reduce MMP-9 activity in cell supernatants as measured by gelatin zymography, a property that was not shared by barbiturate inhibitors not bearing a nitrate group. Furthermore, the hybrid compounds were significantly more efficacious than the non-nitrate counterparts in a model of MMP-9 dependent cancer cell invasion [17]. Consistent with this, we subsequently found that one of the hybrid compounds was more effective in an animal model of IBD than the MMP inhibitor from which it was derived or its incorporated nitrate component [19]. The objective of the present study was to determine the mechanism by which the hybrid compounds influence MMP levels, to investigate the role of NO in this and to assess the selectivity for MMP-9 over other MMP enzymes. We found that the inhibition of MMP-9 mRNA was largely mediated through a reduction in its mRNA by a sGC/cGMP-mediated pathway.

2. Material and Methods

All chemicals and biological materials were supplied by Sigma Aldrich® (Dublin, Ireland) unless otherwise stated.

In this study, we used a group of barbiturate-nitrate hybrid compounds and their component parts that were previously synthesized in our lab [17].

2.1. Cell Culture

Caco-2 cells were supplied by the European Collection of Cell Cultures (ECACC, Salisbury, UK). Cells were cultured in minimum essential media (MEM) containing 20% fetal bovine serum (FBS), 1% sodium pyruvate, sodium bicarbonate 2.2 g/L, gentamicin 5 mg/L, streptomycin 10 mg/L, penicillin G 6 mg/L. Cells were maintained in a 37 °C, 5% CO_2 humidified incubator until approximately 75% confluent. All the following in vitro experiments were carried out in FBS-free media. Cells were incubated with 3 series of test compounds at 10 µM for 30 min. The dose of 10 µM was chosen in accordance with our previous study were toxicological studies were carried out [17]. Cytokines TNF-α and IL-1β 10 ng/mL were then added and the cells were incubated for 24 h. For NO-donor experiments, solutions of SNAP or DETA-NONOate were prepared daily when needed and incubated (in the concentration range 10 to 500 µM). For co-incubation experiments with ODQ, this was added with the nitrate-barbiturate hybrids to give a concentration in the serum-free media of 10 µM as with the compounds. In experiments where 8-Br-cGMP was used, this was added with the ODQ and compounds to give a final concentration of 10 µM in the serum-free media.

2.2. Gelatin Zymography

The conditioned media from cell experiments was removed, centrifuged at 13,000 rpm for 5 min to remove dead cells or floating debris and the resulting cell-free supernatants were stored at −80 °C until assayed for MMP-2 and MMP-9 using gelatin zymography. Briefly, samples were normalized with respect to protein content using a Bradford assay. The enzymatic activities of MMP-2 and MMP-9 were assayed by gelatin zymography in serum-free media. The samples were electrophoresed on an SDS–PAGE containing 2% gelatin. The gels were washed with 2.5% Triton X three times for 20 min cycles. The gels were then washed twice and finally incubated with zymography buffer (0.15 M NaCl, 5 mM $CaCl_2$, 0.05%NaN_3, and 50 mM Tris-HCl buffer, pH 7.5) at 37 °C for 48 h. After incubation, the gels were stained with 0.025% Coomassie Brilliant Blue G250 in 25% MeOH, 10% acetic acid, and H_2O and destained with acetic acid 8%, methanol 4%, and H_2O. The gelatinolytic activity was detected as a band of gelatin digestion and was quantified by densitometry using gel documentation system r (Bio-Rad, Dublin, Ireland, Universalhood II and Quantity One 4.6 software) and expressed as a percentage of the positive control.

2.3. Quantitative PCR

Quantitative PCR (qPCR) was used to study the effect of the different compounds on expression of MMP-1, MMP-2 and MMP 9 and NF-κB in cytokine-stimulated cells. Briefly, the RNA was isolated using RNAqueous-4PCR® kit from Ambion (Applied Biosystems, Waltham, MA, USA) according to the manufacturer's protocol. The concentration and purity of the RNA yielded was measured using the NanoDrop ND-1000. RNA samples were converted to single-stranded cDNA using a High Capacity cDNA Reverse Transcription kit (Applied Biosystems, Waltham, MA, USA). As target probes, TaqMan MGB human MMP-9 (Hs 00234579_m1), NOS (Hs 01075521_m1), NFKB1 (Hs 00949904_m1), RelA (Hs 01042014_m1) and IKBKG (Hs 01006763_m1) were used. Endogenous 18s rRNA was used as a control to normalize gene expression data, and an RQ value ($2^{-\Delta\Delta Ct}$, where Ct is the threshold cycle) was calculated for each sample. RQ values are presented as fold change in gene expression relative to the stimulated group, which was normalized to 1.

2.4. Nitrate and Nitrite Quantification–Modified Griess Assay

A spectrophotometric method was used to measure the nitrate and nitrite in conditioned media. Nitrate and nitrite standards were serially diluted to a range 1.6–200 μM in ddH$_2$O and 200 μL of each concentration was added to 12-well plates in duplicate. Nitrate was reduced to nitrite with the addition of 200 μL saturated vanadium (III) solution (400 mg VCl$_3$ in 50 mL 1M HCl) and then staining of the nitrite was carried out with rapid addition of 100 μL sulfanilamide (2% w/v in 5% v/v HCl) and 100 μL N-1-(naphthyl) ethylenediamine (NEDD) (0.1% w/v in ddH$_2$O). The plate was incubated with rocking for 45 min and absorbance was read at λ 540nm. Measurement of nitrite standards were carried out as above with ddH$_2$O added instead of VCL$_3$ solution and ddH$_2$O was used as a blank for both sets of standards. Conditioned media samples were normalised for protein concentration, and 200 μL loaded onto 12-well plates in duplicate for both methods described above used to measure the nitrite and nitrate levels. Addition of VCl$_3$ to the conditioned media samples will give a measure of total NO$_2^-$ and NO$_3^-$ given NO$_x^-$.

2.5. NF-κB (p65) Binding Activity

The binding activity of the p65 subunit was measured using an NF-κB (p65) Enzyme Linked Immunosorbent Assay (ELISA) kit (Cayman Chemicals, Dublin, Ireland). Nuclear extraction was first carried out from cultured and treated cells after 24 h using the nuclear extraction kit (Cayman Chemicals, Dublin, Ireland) according to the manufacturer's protocol. The biding of p65 in these nuclear extracts was then determined using the NF-κB (p65) transcription factor assay according to the manufacturer's instructions.

2.6. Statistical Analysis

Analysis of results was carried out using Graph Pad Prism® 5 for Windows (San Diego, CA, USA, Graph Pad software). All results shown represent $n \geq 3$ and were analyzed using a one way ANOVA and Dunnett's or Tukey post-test where appropriate. Graphs are presented as the mean ± the standard error of the mean (SEM) and statistical significance was judged as a p value of <0.05.

3. Results

3.1. Barbiturate-Nitrate Hybrids Reduce MMP-9 Expression in Cytokine-Stimulated Caco-2 Cells

We have previously demonstrated that the barbiturate-nitrate hybrids (series 1, Figure 1) can reduce supernatant MMP-9 activity as measured by gelatin zymography to a greater extent than the barbiturate-alcohols (series 2, Figure 1) [17]. Here we examine the effect of the hybrid compounds at the gene level and use the barbiturate-alcohols and nitrate side-chains (series 3, Figure 1) to measure the relative contributions of the component parts of the series of compounds.

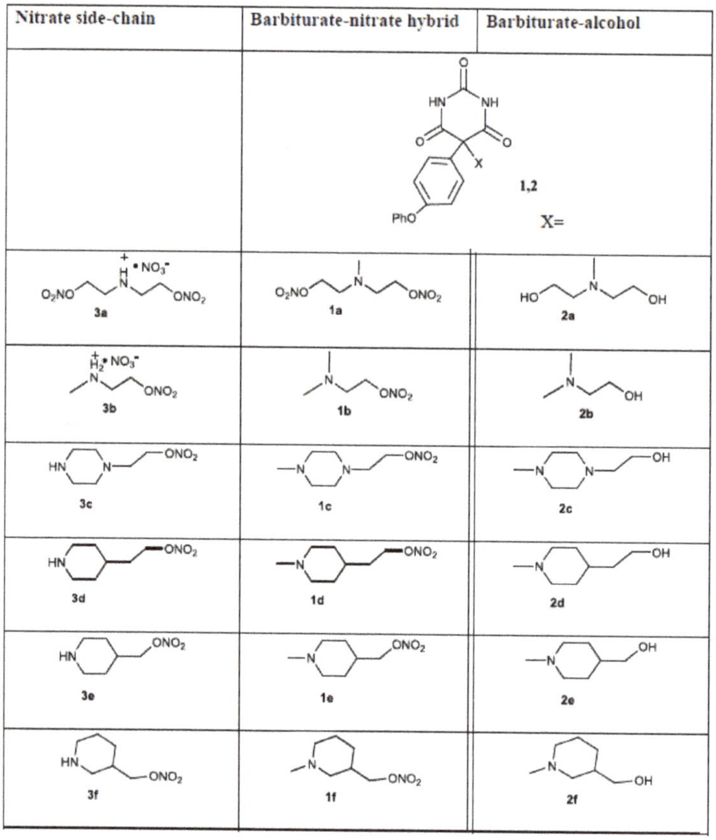

Nitrate side-chain	Barbiturate-nitrate hybrid	Barbiturate-alcohol
	1,2	X=
3a	1a	2a
3b	1b	2b
3c	1c	2c
3d	1d	2d
3e	1e	2e
3f	1f	2f

Figure 1. Structures of compounds used. Column one shows the nitrate side-chains. Columns two and three show the barbiturate scaffold and the nitrate and alcohol side-chains, respectively.

The nitrate-barbiturates (10 µM) caused a statistically significant reduction in MMP-9 mRNA in cytokine-stimulated Caco-2 cells after 24 h compared to the untreated, stimulated cells (Figure 2). Compounds **1c** and **1a** caused the greatest mean inhibition. The alcohol-barbiturates also inhibited the transcription of MMP-9 at 10 µM but to a lesser extent. The nitrate side-chains did reduce MMP-9 expression when tested at 10 µM (Figure 2), but this inhibition did not reach statistical significance except for compound **3f**. The compounds in parallel experiments did not affect mRNA levels of MMP-1 or MMP-2, showing selectivity for inhibition of MMP-9.

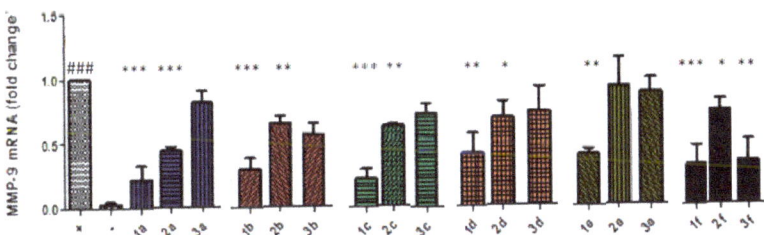

Figure 2. Barbiturate-nitrate hybrids (series 1) reduce MMP-9 mRNA to a greater extent than the barbiturate alcohols (series 2) or the nitrate side-chains (series 3). Caco-2 cells were incubated with series of the barbiturate-nitrate hybrids, barbiturate-alcohols or nitrate side-chains at 10 µM for 30 min prior to addition of TNF-α and IL-1β (10 ng/mL). ### $p < 0.001$ vs. unstimulated Caco-2 cells (negative control); * $p < 0.05$ vs. cytokine-stimulated Caco-2 cells (positive control); ** $p < 0.01$ vs. positive control; *** $p < 0.001$ vs. positive control.

3.2. Nitric Oxide Donors Reduce MMP-9 mRNA Levels in Cytokine-Stimulated Caco-2 Cells

In order to establish whether the effects that the nitrate-barbiturates had on MMP-9 mRNA in cytokine-stimulated Caco-2 cells were NO-mediated, we tested the effects of two NO-donors at a range of concentrations for 24 h. In this study we used the S-nitrosothiol, S-Nitroso-N-acetylpenicillamine (SNAP), which has been previously shown to have a half-life in aqueous media of approximately 4 h; the NO formation is high, where 100 µM yields about 1.4 µM NO/minute at 37 °C, and it is linear over a wide concentration range. In addition, we measured the effects of the diazeniumdiolate compound DETA-NONOate, which decomposes spontaneously and has been demonstrated to have a half-life of 20 h at pH 7.4 and 37 °C [20].

We found that DETA-NONOate reduced MMP-9 expression with the highest concentration tested (Figure 3A). Figure 3B shows the release of NO species. As expected from a NONOate NO-donor, there was a linear relationship between the concentration used and the NO released with correlation analysis results for NO_x^- ($p < 0.0001$, $R^2 = 0.9975$), NO_2^- ($p < 0.0001$, $R^2 = 0.9996$) and NO_3^- ($p < 0.0001$, $R^2 = 0.9828$) being statistically significant. There was little to no difference in NO yielded from the lower concentrations of DETA-NONOate used, which may reflect the limited sensitivity of the Griess assay. At a concentration of 500 µM, DETA-NONOate yielded statistically significantly more of all NO_x^- species than the positive control. The highest concentrations of nitrate and nitrite were produced from the highest concentration of DETA-NONOate, which also produced a significant inhibition of MMP-9 at the gene level.

We also found that the addition of SNAP caused a significant inhibition of MMP-9 at the gene level at all concentrations tested (Figure 4A). Figure 4B shows the release of NO species. Incubations with SNAP showed a linear correlation between the concentration used and the resultant nitrate and nitrite concentrations that were present in the conditioned media after 24 h. The results of correlation analysis of SNAP concentration and NO_x^- ($p < 0.0001$, $r^2 = 0.9964$), NO_2 ($p < 0.0001$, $r^2 = 0.9696$) and NO_3^- ($p = 0.0002$, $r^2 = 0.9525$) are unsurprising considering that SNAP is expected to spontaneously yield NO, which will be decomposed to nitrite and nitrate. At 500 µM SNAP, the difference in nitrite concentrations reached statistical significance for all groups. Similar results were observed for nitrate and NO_x^- concentrations, where 500 µM SNAP resulted in statistically significant differences with all other groups, and 200 µM was also statistically different from the controls and 10 µM SNAP. There is no obvious correlation between these results and the effect on MMP-9 gene expression.

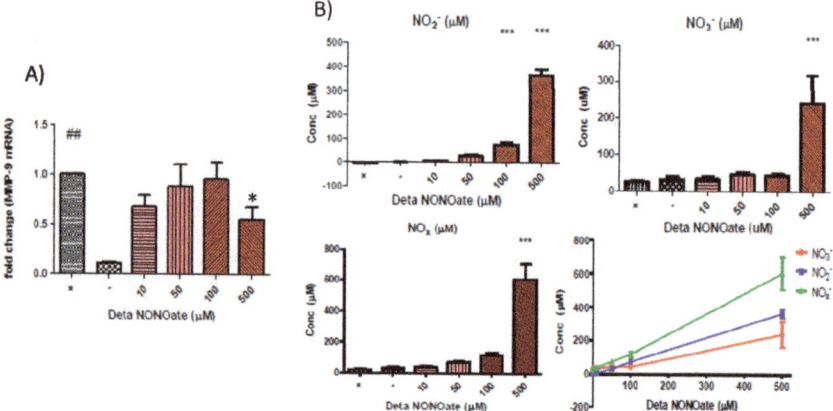

Figure 3. (**A**) DETA NONOate significantly reduced MMP-9 mRNA at high concentrations in cytokine-stimulated Caco-2 cells (## $p < 0.01$ vs. unstimulated Caco-2 cells (negative control); * $p < 0.05$ vs. cytokine-stimulated Caco-2 cells (positive control). (**B**) Measurements of nitrate and nitrite concentrations as breakdown products of NO by the Griess assay on the conditioned media of Caco-2 cells after 24 h of co-incubation with DETA-NONOate and pro-inflammatory cytokines TNF-α and IL-1β. Top left pane shows the nitrite concentration, top right panel shows the nitrate concentration, bottom left pane shows the combined reduced NO groups and bottom right shows the linear correlations of DETA-NONOate concentrations versus the concentration of measured NOx^- species (*** $p < 0.001$ vs. negative control).

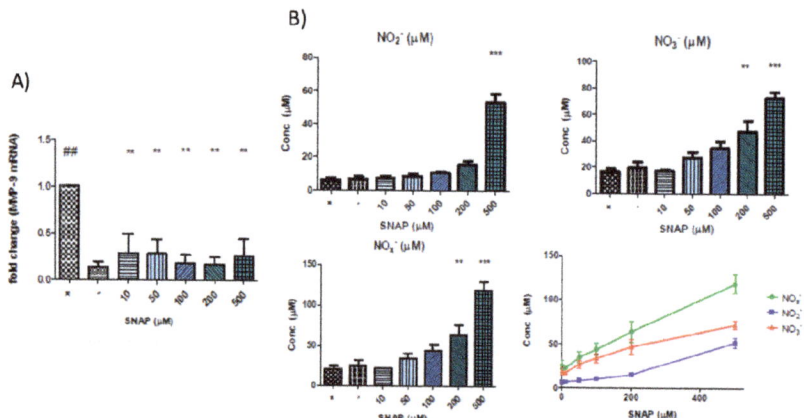

Figure 4. (**A**) SNAP significantly reduced MMP-9 mRNA at different concentrations tested in cytokine-stimulated Caco-2 cells: ## $p < 0.01$ vs. unstimulated Caco-2 cells (negative control); ** $p < 0.01$ vs. cytokine-stimulated Caco-2 cells (positive control). (**B**) Measurements of nitrate and nitrite concentrations as breakdown products of NO by the Griess assay on the conditioned media of Caco-2 cells after 24 h of co-incubation with SNAP and proinflammatory cytokines TNF-α and IL-1β. Top left pane shows the nitrite concentration, top right pane shows the nitrate concentration, bottom left pane shows the combined reduced NO groups and bottom right shows the linear correlations of SNAP concentrations versus the concentration of measured NOx^- species. (** $p < 0.01$ vs. negative control; *** $p < 0.001$ vs. negative control).

3.3. Barbiturate-Nitrate-Hybrids Inhibit MMP-9 Gene Expression in an NF-κB-Independent Manner

In this study, we examined the effect of the barbiturate-nitrate hybrids on gene expression of various components of the NF-κB pathway and the nuclear binding of the p65 subunit to test the hypothesis that the compounds could mimic the effect of NO on NF-κB.

A trend towards inhibition was observed for the nitrate-barbiturates that did not reach statistical significance (Figure 5A). Therefore, we decided to examine the effect of the compounds on the transcription of some of the elements of the NF-κB pathway.

The expression of RelA/p65, NF-κB1/p105 and IκBKG/NEMO, which forms part of the IKK complex, were assessed by qPCR (Figure 5B–D). However, the compounds showed a limited effect on RelA/p65, NF-κB1/p105 and IκBKG/NEMO with **1a**, **1b** and **1c** causing the greatest reduction in expression of these elements.

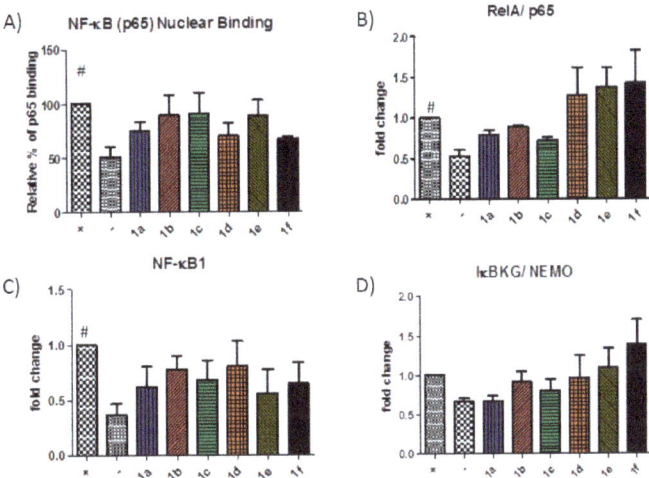

Figure 5. The barbiturate nitrate hybrids show little effect on the NF-κB pathway. The nuclear translocation and binding of the NF-κB subunit p65 was measured using ELISA (**A**) and the gene expression of RelA/p65, NF-κB1/p105 and a component of the IKK complex, IκBG/NEMO were measured using qPCR (**B–D**). # $p < 0.05$ vs. unstimulated Caco-2 cells (negative control).

3.4. Inhibition of MMP-9 by the Barbiturate-Nitrate Hybrids Is Partly Mediated Through a sGC/cGMP Pathway

Following the limited effect of the compounds in altering NF-κB nuclear binding or expression of components of the pathway, we focused on the role of the cGMP pathway in mediating the inhibition of MMP-9 by the nitrate-barbiturates. This was first achieved using the pharmacological inhibitor 1H-(1,2,4)oxadiazolo(4,3-a)quinoxalin-1-one (ODQ), which is a highly selective and irreversible heme site inhibitor of sGC and is competitive with NO [21,22]. As shown in Figure 6A, co-incubation of the nitrate-barbiturates with ODQ abolished any reduction in MMP-9 gene expression, an effect which was reversed by adding the cGMP analogue 8-Br-cGMP to the cells (Figure 6B). These effects correlated with MMP-9 protein activity as shown in Figure 6C,D.

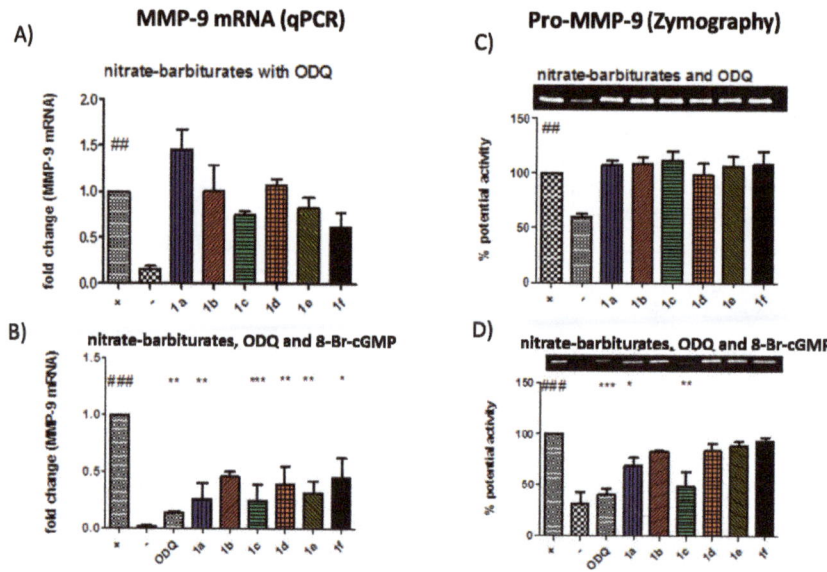

Figure 6. Barbiturate-nitrate hybrids inhibit MMP-9 via a soluble guanylate-cyclase-dependent pathway. (**A**) there was a significant up-regulation of the MMP-9 gene when inducing Caco-2 cells with the pro-inflammatory cytokines. When cells were activated in the presence of ODQ (0.05 µM), this resulted in a reversion of MMP-9 mRNA levels in barbiturate-nitrate hybrid-treated cells. (**B**) Exogenously added 8-bromo-cGMP restored the effect of ODQ (0.5 µM). These results correlated with the pro-MMP-9 protein activity as shown by zymography (**C,D**) ## $p < 0.01$ vs. unstimulated Caco-2 cells (negative control); ### $p < 0.001$ vs. negative control; * $p < 0.05$ vs. cytokine-stimulated Caco-2 cells (positive control); ** $p < 0.01$ vs. positive control; *** $p < 0.001$ vs. positive control.

4. Discussion

Understanding that MMP-9 remains an attractive target for inhibition in a variety of inflammatory conditions, our group designed a series of barbiturate-based hybrids that are intrinsically active as MMP inhibitors at the enzyme level but have additional effects on MMP activity through a nitrate moiety [17]. The present findings indicate that the hybrid compounds, which inhibit at the enzyme level, also reduce MMP-9 at the gene level in response to inflammatory stimuli. These effects are mediated by NO mimicry in cGMP activation and they are selective for MMP-9 inhibition over MMP-1 and MMP-2.

MMPIs have failed in clinical trials due to disappointing clinical efficacy results compared to animal trials and dose-limiting side-effects of MSS; but we can now reflect on how little was known of the complex protease network or the net effect of inhibition of certain enzymes in a given setting. The trials added MMPIs as co-therapies for patients with invasive or metastatic cancer, which may not have been appropriate considering that metastasis was already established and also, the genetic diversity of the disease [13]. It is now known that the MMPs may play a protective role in tumour progression [23,24] including MMP-8 and indeed much broader roles in inflammation than previously appreciated, many of which are protective [25,26]. Setting will be crucial to the success of MMPIs, and so as we understand more about the interactions of the MMP network and the roles of individual MMPs in a given disease setting, we may be better able to appropriately target them for inhibition. While broad spectrum inhibition may be appropriate in certain acute inflammatory settings, selectivity may be important in reducing side-effects in chronic inflammatory conditions. With the difficulties in finding selective and clinically useful active-site inhibitors, alternative strategies such as blocking upstream pathways of activation [27,28] or indeed targeting the transcriptional upregulation of the enzyme is of utmost importance. Xanthine-derivatives, NSAIDs and 3-hydroxy-3-methylglutaryl coenzyme A (HMG-CoA) reductase inhibitors have all been studied as inhibitors of MMP-9 expression [9]. Doxycycline, the only clinically approved drug acting through MMP inhibition [29], is a weak enzyme level inhibitor [30] which exerts its effects mainly at the transcriptional level [31–33].

In previous studies, we established that the hybrid compounds affect MMP-9 secretion [17], but it was unclear if this was at the storage, secretory or transcriptional level. In this study, we found a profound reduction of MMP-9 mRNA with the hybrid compounds on cytokine-stimulated cells. These effects were not observed on MMP-1 and MMP-2 mRNA. We also found a smaller but significant reduction in MMP-9 transcription with the alcohol-barbiturates. The inhibitory effect of the non-nitrates on MMP transcription is probably due to a general anti-inflammatory effect associated with MMP-9 inhibition at enzyme level. The MMPs catalyse the activation of a broad range of substrates [2,34], which can promote the transcriptional up-regulation of pro-inflammatory mediators, including MMPs themselves. MMPs have become common read-outs for inflammation in cell and animal models of IBD. For example, in a rat model of UC, the broad spectrum hydroxamate MMP inhibitor, ilomastat, was shown to inhibit MMP-1 expression in the colon [35]. The nitrate side-chains tested alone also reduced MMP-9 levels with a similar order of magnitude to the alcohol-barbiturates. The striking effect of the hybrid compounds on MMP-9 expression may be attributed to an indirect inhibitory action at the enzyme level and an additional NO-mediated effect at the mRNA level.

Next, we tested the effects of NO-donors on MMP-9 in our model of intestinal epithelial inflammation in order to ascribe some of the MMP-9 inhibitory action of the compounds to the nitrate moiety. In our experiments, SNAP and DETA-NONOate were chosen as NO-donors to represent varying NO release profiles. There was a linear relationship between the concentration of the compound used and the concentration of nitrate and nitrite, breakdown products of NO, that were in the media after 24 h. Cytokine-stimulated cells that were incubated with SNAP showed a large inhibition of MMP-9 gene expression. DETA-NONOate was used in the same range of concentrations as SNAP but did not result in the same effect on MMP-9. It is interesting to note that while there was a direct correlation between the concentration of donor used and the NO_x^- species measured, this did not correlate with the effect on MMP-9 despite both NO-donors having some inhibitory effect. The half-life of NO in a biological setting is in the range of seconds and so the measurement of its breakdown products after 24 h may not necessarily be relevant. SNAP is expected to breakdown spontaneously and has a shorter half-life than DETA-NONOate and will likely produce a higher concentration of NO that may be sustained for a shorter period of time and it may be this property that resulted in the inhibition of MMP-9 mRNA.

Knowing that the nitrate-barbiturates can inhibit MMP-9 transcription, that NF-κB is involved in the upregulation of MMP-9 and that NF-κB is sensitive to NO, we decided to assess the effect of the compounds on the NF-κB pathway. NF-κB exists in the cytoplasm as an inactive dimer bound to its inhibitor IκB. Activation of the IKK complex liberates the dimer to migrate to the nucleus and interact with κB binding sites in the promoter regions of certain genes. The MMP-9 gene contains at least two of these binding sites in its promoter region [36] and NF-κB has been shown to be essential for MMP-9 upregulation [37–39]. NF-κB can induce the expression of iNOS when activated and NO is a known regulator of NF-κB, likely functioning in a concentration-dependent negative feedback loop [40,41]. We have previously reviewed the evidence for the NO's modulation of NF-κB in the context of MMP-9 [18]. Therefore, we decided to assess the effect of the compounds on the NF-κB pathway. An ELISA of the p65 subunit was used to measure the nuclear binding of the NF-κB complex. There was a trend of inhibition for all the compounds with a maximum mean reduction of 32%, but the observed reductions were not statistically significant. To further investigate the effect on p65 nuclear binding, we measured the effect of the compounds on the expression of some of the components of the NF-κB pathway. RelA and NF-κB1 are common components of the NF-κB complex, a protein dimer that will bind to its response element on certain genes. Although the primary mechanism of regulation is its liberation from IκB, it is still under transcriptional control and these two components are both upregulated by pro-inflammatory cytokines in Caco-2 cells. IκBKG is part of the IKK complex, which can phosphorylate IκB, leaving the NF-κB complex free to migrate to the nucleus. The difference between the sham and stimulated controls was small, which reflects the fact that transcriptional control is not the primary mechanism of regulation of IκBKG. The compounds exerted a limited effect on RelA/p65, NF-κB1/p105 and IκBKG/NEMO.

We next turned our attention to cGMP as a candidate for the NO-mediated effect. The cGMP pathway is one of the most well-defined ways that NO exerts many of its effects such as vasodilation and inhibition of platelet aggregation. NO can react with the heme centre of sGC, increasing the rate of catalytic conversion of GTP to cGMP [42]. sGC can mediate the transcriptional upregulation of COX-2, TNF, plasminogen activator inhibitor-1 (PAI-1), vascular endothelial growth factor receptor-1 (VEGFR1), mitogen-activated protein kinase phosphatase-1 (MKP-1) and MMP-9. The exact mechanism by which cGMP exerts its transcription regulatory functions has not been fully explained but it can alter the function of cGMP-regulated ion channels, cGMP-regulated phosphodiesterases and cGMP-dependent protein kinases (PKG) [43]. Several lines of evidence suggest PKG as the mediator of sGC action on MMP-9 gene transcription [44–47]. Co-incubation of the hybrid compounds with the sGC inhibitor ODQ, abolished their MMP-9 inhibitory effects and no differences were observed between the compound treated cells and the positive control at the level of gene transcription or enzyme activity. We could therefore deduce that the nitrate-barbiturates inhibited MMP-9 transcription in a sGC-dependent manner. To confirm this result and further elucidate the pathway, the cGMP analogue, 8-Br-cGMP, was added with the compounds along with ODQ, and it was found that the inhibitory properties of the compounds were restored to what they were with the compounds alone. We can therefore conclude that nitrate-barbiturates exert their inhibitory action on MMP-9 transcription through a sGC-cGMP pathway.

In summary, both control NO donors were able to exert some inhibitory effect on MMP-9 transcription in cytokine-stimulated Caco-2 cells, but this effect was independent of the NO_x^- concentration after 24 h. The barbiturate-nitrate hybrids, which are established enzyme level inhibitors, also inhibit MMP-9 at the gene level, an effect that is partly mediated by the nitrate group through a sGC-cGMP pathway. This discovery highlights the potential of these drugs in treating colonic inflammation and also represents a novel mechanism for correcting MMP dysregulation in inflammatory diseases. New studies are guaranteed to test these new compounds in other inflammatory conditions where MMP-9 upregulation plays an important role.

Author Contributions: S.O., J.W., M.W.R., J.F.G. and C.M. have contributed to the design of the work; acquisition, analysis and interpretation of data; drafting the work; final approval of the version; and agreement to be accountable for all aspects of the work. All authors have read and agreed to the published version of the manuscript.

Funding: This work was supported by Science Foundation Ireland (SFI-RFP/BMT2781) awarded to C.M. and J.F.G.

Conflicts of Interest: The authors declare no conflict of interest.

References

1. Vandooren, J.; Steen, P.E.V.D.; Opdenakker, G. Biochemistry and molecular biology of gelatinase B or matrix metalloproteinase-9 (MMP-9): The next decade. *Crit. Rev. Biochem. Mol. Biol.* **2013**, *48*, 222–272. [CrossRef] [PubMed]
2. Rodríguez, D.; Morrison, C.J.; Overall, C.M. Matrix metalloproteinases: What do they not do? New substrates and biological roles identified by murine models and proteomics. *Biochim. Biophys. Acta* **2010**, *1803*, 39–54. [CrossRef] [PubMed]
3. Mehana, E.-S.E.; Khafaga, A.F.; El-Blehi, S.S.; El-Sayed, M.E.; Khafaga, A.F.; Samar, E.-B.S. The role of matrix metalloproteinases in osteoarthritis pathogenesis: An updated review. *Life Sci.* **2019**, *234*, 116786. [CrossRef] [PubMed]

4. Medina, C.; Videla, S.; Radomski, A.; Radomski, M.W.; Antolín, M.; Guarner, F.; Vilaseca, J.; Salas, A.; Malagelada, J.-R. Increased activity and expression of matrix metalloproteinase-9 in a rat model of distal colitis. *Am. J. Physiol. Liver Physiol.* **2003**, *284*, G116–C122. [CrossRef]
5. Medina, C.; Santana, A.; Paz, M.C.; Díaz-González, F.; Farre, E.; Salas, A.; Radomski, M.W.; Quintero, E Matrix metalloproteinase-9 modulates intestinal injury in rats with transmural colitis. *J. Leukoc. Biol.* **2006**, *79*, 954–962. [CrossRef]
6. Castaneda, F.E.; Walia, B.; Vijay–Kumar, M.; Patel, N.R.; Roser, S.; Kolachala, V.L.; Rojas, M.; Wang, L.; Oprea, G.; Garg, P.; et al. Targeted Deletion of Metalloproteinase 9 Attenuates Experimental Colitis in Mice: Central Role of Epithelial-Derived MMP. *Gastroenterology* **2005**, *129*, 1991–2008. [CrossRef]
7. Al-Sadi, R.; Youssef, M.; Rawat, M.; Guo, S.; Dokladny, K.; Haque, M.; Watterson, M.D.; Ma, T.Y.; Watterson, D.M. MMP-9-induced increase in intestinal epithelial tight permeability is mediated by p38 kinase signaling pathway activation of MLCK gene. *Am. J. Physiol. Liver Physiol.* **2019**, *316*, G278–G290. [CrossRef]
8. Opdenakker, G.; Steen, P.E.V.D.; Van Damme, J. Gelatinase B: A tuner and amplifier of immune functions. *Trends Immunol.* **2001**, *22*, 571–579. [CrossRef]
9. Atkinson, J.J.; Senior, R.M. Matrix Metalloproteinase-9 in Lung Remodeling. *Am. J. Respir. Cell Mol. Biol.* **2003**, *28*, 12–24. [CrossRef]
10. Mohan, R.; Chintala, S.K.; Jung, J.-C.; Villar, W.V.L.; McCabe, F.; Russo, L.A.; Lee, Y.; McCarthy, B.E.; Wollenberg, K.R.; Jester, J.V.; et al. Matrix Metalloproteinase Gelatinase B (MMP-9) Coordinates and Effects Epithelial Regeneration. *J. Biol. Chem.* **2001**, *277*, 2065–2072. [CrossRef]
11. Fini, M.E.; Parks, W.C.; Rinehart, W.B.; Girard, M.T.; Matsubara, M.; Cook, J.R.; West-Mays, J.A.; Sadow, P.M.; Burgeson, R.E.; Jeffrey, J.J.; et al. Role of matrix metalloproteinases in failure to re-epithelialize after corneal injury. *Am. J. Pathol.* **1996**, *149*, 1287–1302. [PubMed]
12. Hu, J.; Steen, P.E.V.D.; Sang, Q.-X.A.; Opdenakker, G. Matrix metalloproteinase inhibitors as therapy for inflammatory and vascular diseases. *Nat. Rev. Drug Discov.* **2007**, *6*, 480–498. [CrossRef] [PubMed]
13. Winer, A.; Adams, S.; Mignatti, P. Matrix Metalloproteinase Inhibitors in Cancer Therapy: Turning Past Failures Into Future Successes. *Mol. Cancer Ther.* **2018**, *17*, 1147–1155. [CrossRef] [PubMed]
14. Grams, F.; Brandstetter, H.; Dalò, S.; Geppert, D.; Krell, H.-W.; Leinert, H.; Livi, V.; Menta, E.; Oliva, A.; Zimmermann, G. Pyrimidine-2,4,6-Triones: A New Effective and Selective Class of Matrix Metalloproteinase Inhibitors. *Biol. Chem.* **2001**, *382*, 1277–1285. [CrossRef] [PubMed]
15. Breyholz, H.-J.; Schäfers, M.; Wagner, S.; Höltke, C.; Faust, A.; Rabeneck, H.; Levkau, B.; Schober, O.; Kopka, K. C-5-Disubstituted Barbiturates as Potential Molecular Probes for Noninvasive Matrix Metalloproteinase Imaging. *J. Med. Chem.* **2005**, *48*, 3400–3409. [CrossRef] [PubMed]
16. Foley, L.H.; Palermo, R.; Dunten, P.; Wang, P. Novel 5,5-disubstitutedpyrimidine-2,4,6-triones as selective MMP inhibitors. *Bioorganic Med. Chem. Lett.* **2001**, *11*, 969–972. [CrossRef]
17. Wang, J.; O'Sullivan, S.; Harmon, S.; Keaveny, R.; Radomski, M.W.; Medina, C.; Gilmer, J.F. Design of Barbiturate–Nitrate Hybrids that Inhibit MMP-9 Activity and Secretion. *J. Med. Chem.* **2012**, *55*, 2154–2162. [CrossRef]
18. O'Sullivan, S.; Medina, C.; Ledwidge, M.; Radomski, M.W.; Gilmer, J.F. Nitric oxide-matrix metalloproteinase-9 interactions: Biological and pharmacological significance. *Biochim. Biophys. Acta* **2014**, *1843*, 603–617. [CrossRef]
19. O'Sullivan, S.; Wang, J.; Pigott, M.T.; Docherty, N.; Boyle, N.; Lis, S.K.; Gilmer, J.F.; Medina, C. Inhibition of matrix metalloproteinase-9 by a barbiturate-nitrate hybrid ameliorates dextran sulphate sodium-induced colitis: Effect on inflammation-related genes. *Br. J. Pharmacol.* **2017**, *174*, 512–524. [CrossRef]
20. Webb, D.J.; Megson, I. Nitric oxide donor drugs: Current status and future trends. *Expert Opin. Investig. Drugs* **2002**, *11*, 587–601. [CrossRef]
21. Schrammel, A.; Behrends, S.; Schmidt, K.; Koesling, D.; Mayer, B. Characterization of 1H-(1,2,4)oxadiazolo(4,3-a)quinoxalin-1-one as a heme-site inhibitor of nitric oxide-sensitive guanylyl cyclase. *Mol. Pharmacol.* **1996**, *50*, 1–5. [PubMed]
22. Garthwaite, J.; Southam, E.; Boulton, C.L.; Nielsen, E.B.; Schmidt, K.; Mayer, B. Potent and selective inhibition of nitric oxide-sensitive guanylyl cyclase by 1H-(1,2,4)oxadiazolo(4,3-a)quinoxalin-1-one. *Mol. Pharmacol.* **1995**, *48*, 184–188. [PubMed]
23. Martin, M.D.; Matrisian, L.M. The other side of MMPs: Protective roles in tumor progression. *Cancer Metastasis Rev.* **2007**, *26*, 717–724. [CrossRef] [PubMed]

24. Juurikka, K.; Butler, G.S.; Salo, T.; Nyberg, P.; Åström, P. The Role of MMP8 in Cancer: A Systematic Review. *Int. J. Mol. Sci.* **2019**, *20*, 4506. [CrossRef] [PubMed]
25. Dufour, A.; Overall, C.M. Missing the target: Matrix metalloproteinase antitargets in inflammation and cancer. *Trends Pharmacol. Sci.* **2013**, *34*, 233–242. [CrossRef] [PubMed]
26. Takahashi, Y.; Kobayashi, T.; D'Alessandro-Gabazza, C.N.; Toda, M.; Fujiwara, K.; Okano, T.; Fujimoto, H.; Asayama, K.; Takeshita, A.; Yasuma, T.; et al. Protective Role of Matrix Metalloproteinase-2 in Allergic Bronchial Asthma. *Front. Immunol.* **2019**, *10*, 1795. [CrossRef]
27. Gong, Y.; Hart, E.; Shchurin, A.; Hoover-Plow, J. Inflammatory macrophage migration requires MMP-9 activation by plasminogen in mice. *J. Clin. Investig.* **2008**, *118*, 3012–3024. [CrossRef]
28. Fayard, B.; Bianchi, F.; Dey, J.; Moreno, E.; Djaffer, S.; E Hynes, N.; Monard, D. The Serine Protease Inhibitor Protease Nexin-1 Controls Mammary Cancer Metastasis through LRP-1-Mediated MMP-9 Expression. *Cancer Res.* **2009**, *69*, 5690–5698. [CrossRef]
29. Dormán, G.; Kocsis-Szommer, K.; Spadoni, C.; Ferdinandy, P. MMP Inhibitors in Cardiac Diseases: An Update. *Recent Patents Cardiovasc. Drug Discov.* **2007**, *2*, 186–194. [CrossRef]
30. Garcia, R.A.; Pantazatos, D.P.; Gessner, C.R.; Go, K.V.; Woods, V.L.; Villarreal, F.J. Molecular Interactions between Matrilysin and the Matrix Metalloproteinase Inhibitor Doxycycline Investigated by Deuterium Exchange Mass Spectrometry. *Mol. Pharmacol.* **2005**, *67*, 1128–1136. [CrossRef]
31. Egeblad, M.; Werb, Z. New functions for the matrix metalloproteinases in cancer progression. *Nat. Rev. Cancer* **2002**, *2*, 161–174. [CrossRef] [PubMed]
32. Ramamurthy, N.S.; Rifkin, B.R.; Greenwald, R.A.; Xu, J.-W.; Liu, Y.; Turner, G.; Golub, L.M.; Vernillo, A. Inhibition of Matrix Metalloproteinase-Mediated Periodontal Bone Loss in Rats: A Comparison of 6 Chemically Modified Tetracyclines. *J. Periodontol.* **2002**, *73*, 726–734. [CrossRef] [PubMed]
33. Paemen, L.; Martens, E.; Norga, K.; Masure, S.; Roets, E.; Hoogmartens, J.; Opdenakker, G. The gelatinase inhibitory activity of tetracyclines and chemically modified tetracycline analogues as measured by a novel microtiter assay for inhibitors. *Biochem. Pharmacol.* **1996**, *52*, 105–111. [CrossRef]
34. Sternlicht, M.D.; Werb, Z. How Matrix Metalloproteinases Regulate Cell Behavior. *Annu. Rev. Cell Dev. Biol.* **2001**, *17*, 463–516. [CrossRef] [PubMed]
35. Wang, Y.-D.; Wang, W. Protective effect of ilomastat on trinitrobenzenesulfonic acid-induced ulcerative colitis in rats. *World J. Gastroenterol.* **2008**, *14*, 5683–5688. [CrossRef] [PubMed]
36. St-Pierre, Y.; Couillard, J.; Van Themsche, C. Regulation of MMP-9 gene expression for the development of novel molecular targets against cancer and inflammatory diseases. *Expert Opin. Ther. Targets* **2004**, *8*, 473–489. [CrossRef]
37. Eberhardt, W.; Huwiler, A.; Beck, K.F.; Walpen, S.; Pfeilschifter, J. Amplification of IL-1 beta-induced matrix metalloproteinase-9 expression by superoxide in rat glomerular mesangial cells is mediated by increased activities of NF-kappa B and activating protein-1 and involves activation of the mitogen-activated protein kinase pathways. *J. Immunol.* **2000**, *165*, 5788–5797.
38. Bond, M.; Fabunmi, R.P.; Baker, A.H.; Newby, A. Synergistic upregulation of metalloproteinase-9 by growth factors and inflammatory cytokines: An absolute requirement for transcription factor NF-kappa B. *FEBS Lett.* **1998**, *435*, 435. [CrossRef]
39. Bond, M.; Chase, A.J.; Baker, A.H.; Newby, A. Inhibition of transcription factor NF-kappaB reduces matrix metalloproteinase-1, -3 and -9 production by vascular smooth muscle cells. *Cardiovasc. Res.* **2001**, *50*, 556–565. [CrossRef]
40. Chen, X.; Chang, L.; Li, X.; Huang, J.; Yang, L.; Lai, X.; Huang, Z.; Wang, Z.; Wu, X.; Zhao, J.; et al. Tc17/IL-17A Up-Regulated the Expression of MMP-9 via NF-κB Pathway in Nasal Epithelial Cells of Patients with Chronic Rhinosinusitis. *Front. Immunol.* **2018**, *9*, 2121. [CrossRef]
41. Janssen-Heininger, Y.M.W.; E Poynter, M.; A Baeuerle, P. Recent advances towards understanding redox mechanisms in the activation of nuclear factor kappaB. *Free. Radic. Biol. Med.* **2000**, *28*, 1317–1327. [CrossRef]
42. Dijkstra, G.; Moshage, H.; Jansen, P.L.M. Blockade of NF-κ B Activation and Donation of Nitric Oxide: New Treatment Options in Inflammatory Bowel Disease? *Scand. J. Gastroenterol.* **2002**, *37*, 37–41. [CrossRef] [PubMed]
43. Pfeilschifter, J.; Eberhardt, W.; Beck, K.-F. Regulation of gene expression by nitric oxide. *Pflüger* **2001**, *442*, 479–486. [CrossRef] [PubMed]

44. Ahern, G. cGMP and S-nitrosylation: Two routes for modulation of neuronal excitability by NO. *Trends Neurosci.* **2002**, *25*, 510–517. [CrossRef]
45. Gudi, T.; Hong, G.K.-P.; Vaandrager, A.B.; Lohmann, S.M.; Pilz, R.B. Nitric oxide and cGMP regulate gene expression in neuronal and glial cells by activating type II cGMP-dependent protein kinase. *FASEB J.* **1999**, *13*, 2143–2152. [CrossRef] [PubMed]
46. Huvar, I. Regulation of Gene Expression by cGMP-dependent Protein Kinase. *J. Biol. Chem.* **1996**, *271*, 4597–4600. [CrossRef]
47. Gudi, T.; Lohmann, S.M.; Pilz, R.B. Regulation of gene expression by cyclic GMP-dependent protein kinase requires nuclear translocation of the kinase: Identification of a nuclear localization signal. *Mol. Cell. Biol.* **1997**, *17*, 5244–5254. [CrossRef]

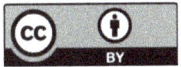

© 2020 by the authors. Licensee MDPI, Basel, Switzerland. This article is an open access article distributed under the terms and conditions of the Creative Commons Attribution (CC BY) license (http://creativecommons.org/licenses/by/4.0/).

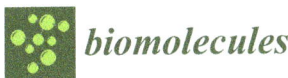

Review

The Association of Matrix Metalloproteinases with Chronic Kidney Disease and Peripheral Vascular Disease: A Light at the End of the Tunnel?

Michele Provenzano [1], Michele Andreucci [1], Carlo Garofalo [2], Teresa Faga [1], Ashour Michael [1], Nicola Ielapi [3,4,5], Raffaele Grande [6], Paolo Sapienza [6], Stefano de Franciscis [3,7], Pasquale Mastroroberto [8] and Raffaele Serra [3,7,*]

1. Department of Health Sciences, Renal Unit, "Magna Graecia" University, 88100 Catanzaro, Italy; michiprov@hotmail.it (M.P.); andreucci@unicz.it (M.A.); teresa_faga@yahoo.it (T.F.); ashourmichael@yahoo.com (A.M.)
2. Division of Nephrology, University of Campania "Luigi Vanvitelli", 80100 Naples, Italy; carlo.garofalo@hotmail.it
3. Interuniversity Center of Phlebolymphology (CIFL), "Magna Graecia" University, 88100 Catanzaro, Italy; infermierenicola@hotmail.it (N.I.); defranci@unicz.it (S.d.F.)
4. Department of Public Health and Infectious Disease, "Sapienza" University of Rome, 00185 Rome, Italy
5. Department of Radiology, Vibo Valentia Hospital, 89900 Vibo Valentia, Italy
6. Department of Surgery "P. Valdoni", "Sapienza" University of Rome, 00161 Rome, Italy; raffaele.grandeprospero@gmail.com (R.G.); paolo.sapienza@uniroma1.it (P.S.)
7. Department of Medical and Surgical Sciences, "Magna Graecia" University, 88100 Catanzaro, Italy
8. Department of Experimental and Clinical Medicine, "Magna Graecia" University, 88100 Catanzaro, Italy; mastroroberto@unicz.it
* Correspondence: rserra@unicz.it

Received: 16 December 2019; Accepted: 14 January 2020; Published: 17 January 2020

Abstract: Chronic Kidney Disease (CKD) represents a risk factor for fatal and nonfatal cardiovascular (CV) events, including peripheral vascular disease (PVD). This occurs because CKD encompasses several factors that lead to poor prognoses, mainly due to a reduction of the estimated glomerular filtration rate (eGFR), the presence of proteinuria, and the uremic inflammatory milieu. The matrix metalloproteinases (MMPs) are a group of zinc-containing endopeptidases implicated in extracellular matrix (ECM) remodeling, a systemic process in tissue homeostasis. MMPs play an important role in cell differentiation, angiogenesis, inflammation, and vascular damage. Our aim was to review the published evidence regarding the association between MMPs, PVD, and CKD to find possible common pathophysiological mechanisms. MMPs favor ECM deposition through the glomeruli, and start the shedding of cellular junctions and epithelial-mesenchymal transition in the renal tubules. MMP-2 and -9 have also been associated with the presence of systemic vascular damage, since they exert a pro-inflammatory and proatherosclerotic actions. An imbalance of MMPs was found in the context of PVD, where MMPs are predictors of poor prognoses in patients who underwent lower extremity revascularization. MMP circulating levels are increased in both conditions, i.e., that of CKD and PVD. A possible pathogenic link between these conditions is represented by the enhanced production of transforming growth factor-β that worsens vascular calcifications and atherosclerosis and the development of proteinuria in patients with increased levels of MMPs. Proteinuria has been recognized as a marker of systemic vascular damage, and this may explain in part the increase in CV risk that is manifest in patients with CKD and PVD. In conclusion, MMPs can be considered a useful tool by which to stratify CV risk in patients with CKD and PVD. Further studies are needed to investigate the causal-relationships between MMPs, CKD, and PVD, and to optimize their prognostic and predictive (in response to treatments) roles.

Keywords: metalloproteinases; MMPs; TIMPs; CKD; peripheral vascular disease; biomarkers; proteinuria; eGFR; PAD

1. Introduction

Chronic Kidney Disease (CKD) is defined as the presence of abnormalities in kidney function or structure for at least 3 months [1]. The Kidney Disease: Improving Global Outcomes (KDIGO) guidelines classify CKD according to the level of estimated glomerular filtration rate (eGFR), a marker of kidney function, and the amount of urine protein (proteinuria or albuminuria), which represents the principal marker of kidney damage and the primary cause of CKD [2]. The onset of CKD exerts a deleterious impact on individual health. Indeed, it has been demonstrated that either an eGFR reduction < 60 mL/min/1.73 m^2 or a small increase in proteinuria are associated with a poor prognosis, as shown by the increased rate of cardiovascular (CV) fatal and nonfatal events, all-cause mortality, and the progression of kidney disease resulting in the need for renal replacement therapies (kidney transplantation or dialysis) [3,4].

CV risk is severely increased in patients with CKD, and the impact of CV events in this population is crucial if one considers that the rate of CV events (such as myocardial infarction, stroke, arrhythmias, peripheral vascular disease, and chronic heart failure) over time is higher than the risk for kidney disease progression [5]. This strong association has been attributed to the coexistence of traditional and nontraditional CV risk factors in CKD patients, with the former being represented by hypertension, smoking, hypercholesterolemia, and metabolic abnormalities, and the latter by the two main prognostic measures of CKD, i.e., proteinuria and eGFR [6,7].

Among the wide spectrum of CV events, a relevant role is portrayed by peripheral vascular disease (PVD). It has been demonstrated that the presence of mild-to-moderate CKD increases the risk of peripheral artery disease, leg revascularization, leg amputation, and hospitalizations [8]. Either an eGFR reduction below 60 mL/min/1.73 m^2 or slight increases of albuminuria (>30 mg/g) have been associated with a 1.5 to 4 times higher risk of peripheral artery disease (PAD). This evidence is strong, being derived from patients without PAD at basal visit, and reproducible, being confirmed in the general population, as well as in high-risk populations, regardless of the geographic area. Notably, the rate of PVD among patients with End-Stage Kidney Disease (ESKD) is higher than the incidence of acute myocardial infarction, stroke, and arrhythmias [9]. Hence, CKD patients warrant clinical surveillance and prompt the need for strategies to prevent the onset of PVD.

The magnitude of the association is so important that research has recently focused on discovering new biomarkers that are potentially useful in the clinical management of CKD patients at increased risk for PVD. Matrix Metalloproteinases (MMPs) are zinc-containing endopeptidases that are involved in regulating tissue development and homeostasis [10]. Although all MMPs are better acknowledged for their role in remodeling the extracellular matrix (ECM), they actually interact with both ECM and non-ECM substrates. Cell adhesion molecules and growth factors or their receptors represent these latter group of substrates. The wide range of interactions in which MMPs play an active role also explains why these endopeptidases participate in a number of functions such as cell differentiation, migration, apoptosis, and angiogenesis. On the other hand, MMPs have also been attributed to a profibrotic and pro-inflammatory role. MMP-2 and MMP-7 were increased in plasma and urine samples of CKD patients, and may affect direct damage to the kidney with the onset of albuminuria [11]. Moreover, imbalances in the expression and the levels of MMPs or their inhibitors have been linked to the structural changes that occur in the development of PAD, atherosclerotic plaque maturation, and arterial remodeling [12].

The purpose of this review is to examine the role of MMPs in increasing the risk of peripheral vascular disease by the specific aggravating condition of Chronic Kidney Disease.

2. Materials and Methods

The PubMed and ISI Web of science databases were searched for articles by using the following terms: 'chronic kidney disease", "chronic renal insufficiency", "metalloproteinases", "MMP" "atherosclerosis" "peripheral vascular disease". Titles and abstracts were screened by three authors (Michele Provenzano, Michele Andreucci, and Raffaele Serra) to identify potentially relevant studies. All potentially eligible studies were subsequently evaluated in detail by one reviewer and three authors (Michele Provenzano, Michele Andreucci, Carlo Garofalo, and Raffaele Serra) through consideration of the full text. Reference lists of retrieved articles were also searched for relevant publications. Clinical trial, meta-analyses, narrative review, and systematic reviews published in the last 10 years were included. Bibliographies of relevant articles and reviews were manually screened to identify additional studies. Studies were excluded if they were not in the English language, if they did not fit the research question, or if they had insufficient data.

3. Results

3.1. Study Selection

Initial database searches yielded 180 studies from PubMed and 445 from ISI Web of Science in the last 10 years. After the evaluation of the bibliographies of the relevant articles, we evaluated 67 eligible full text articles. The current evidence on MMP expression and kidney disease, the link between MMPs and CV risk specifically in CKD patients, and the association between MMPs and peripheral vascular disease are described below.

3.2. Metalloproteinases and the Kidney

MMPs are classified, according to their structure (or function) and the substrate selectivity, into six groups: Collagenases (MMP-1, MMP-8 and MMP-13), which cleave native collagen and with possible antifibrotic function; Gelatinases (MMP-2 and MMP-9), whose function is to cleave denatured collagens, type IV collagens in basement membranes and some chemokines; Stromelysins (MMP-3, MMP-10, MMP-11 and MMP-19), which degrade a number of substances such as fibronectin, laminin but are unable to cleave native collagen; Matrilysins (MMP-7 and MMP-26) act by degrading ECM components (laminin and entactin); Membrane-type MMPs (MMP-14, -15, -16, -17, -24, and -25), so called because they are anchored to the exterior of the cell membrane; and other MMPs that are tissue or cell-type specific [10,13]. The MMP activity is modulated by a series of four known enzymes called tissue inhibitors of metalloproteinases (TIMPs). TIMPs participate either in the activation or inhibition of MMP activity and, like MMPs, regulate several cellular functions such as cell proliferation, apoptosis, and angiogenesis [14]. It has been demonstrated that MMPs exert a role in the development of proteinuric kidney diseases in humans. Indeed, a number of studies depicted increased serum and urine levels of MMP-2, -8, and -9 in diabetic patients, with MMP-9 in particular being positively correlated with the degree of proteinuria in these patients [15–18]. It is remarkable that, in addition to MMP-9, urinary levels of neutrophil gelatinase-associated lipocalin (NGAL) have been found to increase in patients with diabetic nephropathy [19]. NGAL and MMP-9 are coexpressed, and their interaction prevents the degradation of MMP-9. It has, thus, been postulated that the increase in NGAL may prolong the action of MMP-9 as a trigger of kidney damage [20]. MMP-7, which is normally expressed in the proximal and distal convoluted tubules, as well as in the collecting duct, is found to be overexpressed in diabetic patients where it is also inversely correlated with the degree of kidney function [21]. Other than in diabetic patients, MMP expression is altered in many other glomerular diseases. Typical patterns of MMP-2 and MMP-9 are differentially expressed in patients with focal segmental glomerulosclerosis, minimal change disease, membranous nephropathy, and ANCA-associated vasculitis [22–26]. Regardless of the specific kidney disease involved, several mechanisms of damage have been put forward to explain the pathophysiologic effects of MMPs (Figure 1).

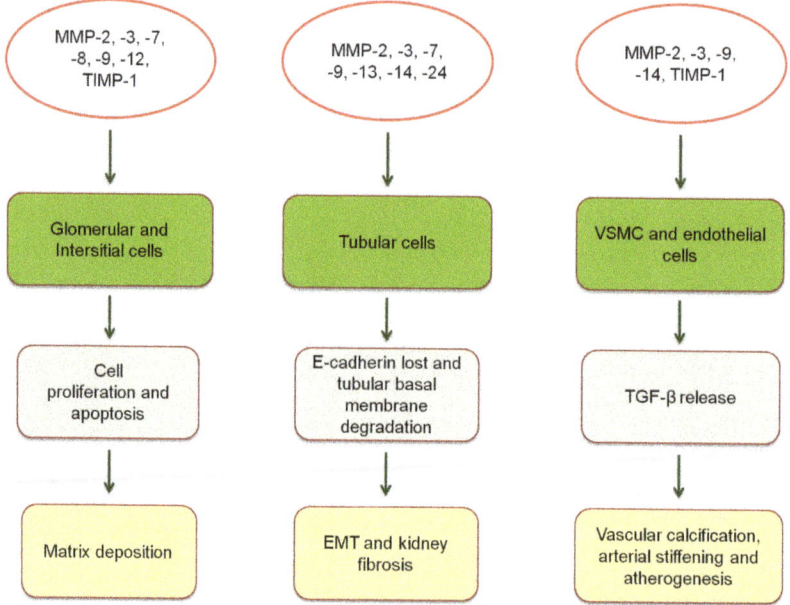

Figure 1. Expression of MMPs and TIMPs, and pathophysiological mechanisms of vascular and kidney damage [10,11,27–31]. EMT, epithelial-mesenchymal transition; VSMC, vascular smooth muscle cells; TGF-β, transforming growth factor-β.

MMPs intervene in all phases of renal fibrosis, from infiltration of mononuclear cells to cells proliferation and scarring. All these processes lead to a progressive decline of renal function in CKD patients. Henger and Colleagues performed a hierarchical clustering analysis to assess the differential gene expression in human kidney fibrosis. Interestingly, they observed that several MMP (MMP-3, -13, -14) genes were upregulated in different degrees of fibrosis [32]. With respect to inflammation, different MMPs play different, often opposing, actions. MMP-7 and MMP-9 expand inflammatory processes, particularly by their chemotactic effect on human dendritic cells [33,34]. Conversely, MMP-13 and MMP-14 have been hypothesized to act as anti-inflammatory mediators [35]. MMP-3 may also promote epithelial-to-mesenchymal transition, the conversion of tissue phenotype, from the epithelial to fibroblastic, thereby accelerating fibrosis [36]. Abnormalities in the accumulation/degradation of ECM due to imbalanced levels of MMPs and TIMPs have also been described in rat and humans [37–39]. Indeed, downregulation of MMP-1 and the overexpression of TIMP-1, MMP-2, MMP-7, and MMP-9 are associated with a profibrotic effect, as well as with a destructive effect on renal parenchyma [38,39]. Moreover, increased TIMP-1 plasma levels were predictors of incident CKD, regardless of other systemic and inflammatory biomarkers (C-Reactive Protein or Brain Natriuretic Peptide) and many clinical parameters (liver function, concomitant lipid-lowering, or antihypertensive medications) [40].

3.3. Vascular Effects of Metalloproteinases in CKD Patients

The structural remodeling of ECM, together with the profibrotic effect of MMPs, are detrimental for other organs apart from the kidney. Elevated blood concentrations of TIMP-1 have been associated with an increased risk of developing chronic heart failure (CHF) and, in patients already diagnosed with CHF, they were predictors of poor prognoses [41,42]. Moreover, the increase in MMP-9 and TIMP-1 conferred risk of all-cause mortality and incident CV disease in community studies [43,44]. Possible explanations for the relationship between MMPs and CV risk are varied. Whereas all MMPs are likely risk factors for atherosclerosis and cardiac dysfunction, a more specific mechanism of damage has been postulated for MMP-9 and TIMP-1. Indeed, MMP-9 is involved in the intracellular cleavage of myosin filaments, a mechanism that leads to ventricular hypertrophy [45]. TIMP-1 has shown a direct relation with the left ventricular mass in the Framingham Heart Study participants [41]. The CKD condition is associated with an increased prevalence of CV morbidity and mortality. The United States Renal Data System (USRDS) showed that the frequency of each CVD, including myocardial infarction, coronary artery disease, and peripheral vascular disease was higher among patients with CKD compared with those without (Figure 2) [9].

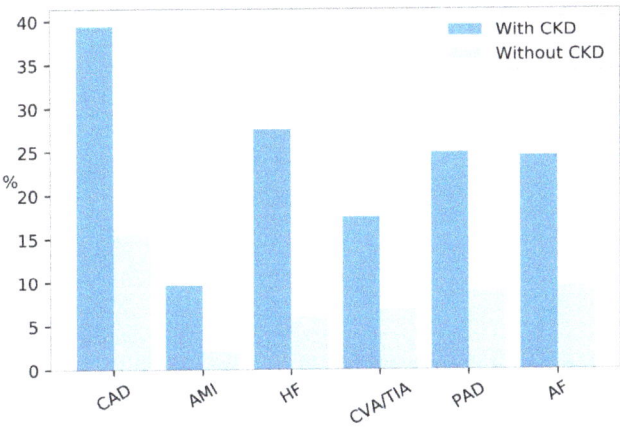

Figure 2. Prevalence of cardiovascular diseases according to the presence (dark blue bars) or absence (turquoise bars) of Chronic Kidney Disease (CKD) in the United States, in the year 2015. AF, atrial fibrillation; AMI, acute myocardial infarction; CAD, coronary artery disease; CVA/TIA, cerebrovascular accident/transient ischemic attack; HF, heart failure; PAD, peripheral arterial disease.

The CV burden in these patients is significant if one considers that the rate of CV events is similar to that of reaching ESKD [46,47]. As a result of this epidemiological and public health evidence, great effort has been placed in finding early atherosclerosis biomarkers that predict CV events in CKD patients and serve as a possible target for new therapeutic agents [48]. MMPs were included in the set of investigated substances. Indeed, MMP-2 was positively associated with carotid Intima-Media Thickness (cIMT) and abdominal aortic calcification, suggesting that an association between this MMP and subclinical atherosclerosis is plausible [49–51]. Moreover, MMP-2 was also found to be higher in patients with a positive history of CV disease vs no history of CV disease [52,53]. MMP-9 was also strongly associated with cIMT, the development of carotid plaques, and systemic atherosclerosis [49,50]. MMP deregulation is intensified in patients with advanced CKD stages that are also associated with a reduction of their clearance. All these mechanisms enhance the inflammatory process that is chronically activated in CKD patients, due to oxidative stress, the uremic milieu, and the metabolic acidosis [54]. The combination of uremic status and imbalance in pro-inflammatory substances (such as MMPs) accelerates the atherosclerotic process, arterial stiffness, and vascular calcification, and impairs the vascular repair process as well [55]. Circulating MMP-2, -9, and -10 have been found to increase in CKD patients, and have been implicated in the vascular damage process. Moreover, MMP-2 and -9 are able to reduce the plaque stability in advanced CKD stages, thus rendering the plaque itself more prone to rupture [56,57].

3.4. Metalloproteinases and Peripheral Vascular Disease

MMPs play a role in the pathogenesis and prognosis of arterial and venous disease. With respect to the damage occurring in the arterial tissue, multiple studies have shown that MMPs are involved in one or more steps of atherogenesis and aneurysm development [58]. Evidence that confirms this hypothesis comes from both basic and clinical studies. During the progression of atherosclerotic plaques, a number of MMPs are produced, including TIMP-1, MMP-1, -2, -3, -9, and -14 [59]. An in vivo study on Fischer male rats showed that TIMP-1 directly regulates the smooth muscle cell migration [27]. A similar function has been recognized in human studies on MMP-14 and TIMP-1, with being both involved in the process of cellular migration to the plaque fibrous cap and plaque inflammation [28,29]. MMP-9 also contributes to the destruction of the fibrous cap itself in patients with increased CV risk [30]. Interestingly, increased concentrations of MMP-2, -3, and -9 have been found within the aneurysm human tissue, being mainly produced by the macrophages localized in the aneurysm wall [31]. These different enzymes are differentially expressed according to the aneurysm dimensions and severity [60,61]. MMP-2 is increased in small aneurysms (<5.5 cm), whereas MMP-9 is dominant in large aneurysms (5.5–7 cm). Moreover, it has also been shown that different localizations of MMP activity within the aneurysm wall modify the risk of rupture [60]. In clinical studies, abnormal circulating levels of MMP-1, -2, -8, -9, and TIMP-1 were found in patients with Peripheral Arterial Disease; their increase was attributed to the presence of ischemic tissue [12,62,63]. Circulating levels of MMP-1 and -8 were also found as predictors of poor prognosis, in terms of major amputation or death, in patients who underwent lower extremity bypass [64]. These multiple findings enhanced the importance of MMPs as biomarkers of arterial disease severity that also provide important prognostic information in clinical practice.

Regarding venous diseases, it has been observed that alterations in ECM remodeling are common in the case of varicose veins and chronic venous insufficiency (CVI). With regards to varicose veins, the expression of MMP-1, -2, -3, -7, and -9 is increased, particularly in the smooth muscular cell of the vein wall, both in human and mice models [65,66]. Moreover, an analysis of human saphenous vein showed that this expression is even higher in varicose veins with inflammation, as compared to those without inflammation [65]. Mechanisms underlying the association between MMPs and varicose vein physiopathology might involve the effect of MMPs on ECM degradation and the relaxation of the venous wall [66]. An upregulation of MMP-1, -2, -9, and -13, together with a downregulation of TIMP-1 and TIMP-2, have been described in patients with CVI [67,68]. The distribution of MMP varies based upon the stage (from CVI to active wound) and cells, suggesting that MMP-1 and TIMP-1 are needed in the re-epithelialization phase, while MMP-9 and -13 primarily participate in the remodeling of the collagenous matrix [69]. A summary of the principal pieces of evidence provided from this paper is depicted in Table 1.

Table 1. Summary of main paper results.

	Key-Messages
MMPs and CKD	• The metalloproteinases (MMPs) are associated with kidney damage. Increased levels of MMP-2 and MMP-9 mediate the deposition of extracellular matrix (ECM) in the glomerular cells while inducing the loss of cellular junctions, and start epithelial-mesenchymal transition (EMT) in the tubular cells. These processes result in tubular atrophy and fibrosis [52,70]. • In the pathogenesis of renal damage, a crucial role is played by the downregulation of MMP-1 and the overexpression of TIMP-1, MMP-2, MMP-7, MMP-9, and neutrophil gelatinase-associated lipocalin (NGAL). These molecules are involved in the inflammatory process and in all phases of renal fibrosis, which, taken together, lead to a progressive decline in renal function. Furthermore, MMP-3 could also promote EMT [32,37–39]. • The cardiovascular risk among patients with Chronic Kidney Disease (CKD) is not trivial. These patients experience a higher rate of cardiovascular events over time than kidney disease progression [5–7]. • In CKD patients, the combination of uremic milieu, oxidative stress, and imbalance in pro-inflammatory substances, such as MMPs and metalloproteinase tissue inhibitors (TIMPs), amplifies the atherosclerotic process, arterial stiffness and vascular calcification. MMP-2 and MMP-9 have been implicated in carotid Intima-Media Thickness (cIMT) and plaque instability. Moreover, increased levels of TIMP-1 have been associated with a higher risk of CHF [49–52].

Table 1. *Cont.*

	Key-Messages
MMPs and PVD	• MMPs play a role in the pathogenesis of peripheral vascular disease. It has been demonstrated that TIMP-1, MMP-1, -2, -3, -9, and -14 favor the progression of atherosclerotic plaques. Increased levels of MMP-2, -3, and -9 are involved in the weakening of the aneurysm wall. In relation to varicose veins, the expression of MMP-1, -2, -3, -7, and -9 is increased. Therefore, the amount of these MMPs is related to a major risk of amputation or death in patients who underwent lower extremity bypass, making that parameter a good predictor of poor prognosis [27–31,59]. • Circulating levels of MMP-2 and MMP-9 were found in patients with acute and chronic lower limb ischemia. These MMPs induce the release of transforming growth factor beta (TGF-β). TGF-β affects the balance between endothelial cells and smooth muscle cells [71].

3.5. Synthetic Metalloproteinases Inhibitors in Experimental and Clinical Research

MMP activity is regulated at different levels, including either intracellular (mRNA expression and post-translational modification of MMP structure) or extracellular (stimulation or inhibition of their enzymatic activity from endogenous or exogenous substrates) process. The net activity of MMPs is a crucial step, since its up- or down- regulation could affect MMP activity, and ultimately lead to metabolic diseases, cancer, cardiovascular, and renal disorders [72]. For these reasons, new pharmacological agents that interfere with MMP activity have been developed and utilized as potential tools that could benefit a wide spectrum of patients. Synthetic MMPs inhibitors (MMPs-I) include broad-spectrum and specific MMPs-I. The vast majority of these compounds contain Zn^{2+} in their structure, and have structured as Zn^{2+} binding globulin (ZBG). Indeed, ZBGs inactivate MMPs by displacing the Zn^{2+}- bound water in the MMPs, and favor the anchorage of the drug to the MMPs substrate binding-pocket [73]. ZBGs encompass hydroxamic acids Batimastat (BB-94), Marimastat (BB-2516), and Ilomastat (GM6001), that displays a broad-spectrum inhibition of MMPs. More selective ZBGs molecules have also been developed, and include hydrazides and sulfonylhydrazides that specifically inhibit MMP-1, -2, and -9. Hydroxamic ZBGs are effective, but they have poor oral bioavailability and, by inhibiting multiple MMPs, cause several musculoskeletal side effects [74]. Hence, heterocyclic bidentate chelators have been developed that have shown more biostability and lower toxicity in cells assays. Tetracyclines are antibiotic molecules that, by chelating Zn^{2+} ion, are able to inhibit MMPs. Doxycycline inhibits MMP-2 and-9 [75]. Chemically-modified tetracyclines reach higher plasma levels for prolonged periods of time, require less frequent administration, are associated with lower rate of side effects when administered orally, and are thus preferred over conventional tetracyclines [76]. Apart from zinc-based compounds, several MMPs-I act by a noncompetitive, nonzinc-binding, mechanism of inhibition. They show high selectivity that minimizes the side effects, and thus, are considered very promising molecules [77]. MMPs-Is have already been used in pilot studies in mice and in human models of kidney damage [11]. MMPs-I BB-1101 has shown to reduce proteinuria in rats with anti-Thy1.1 nephritis, an experimental model of glomerular damage induced by antibody against Thy 1 gene [78]. A similar effect on proteinuria was found with the MMPs-I BB-94 in an experimental model of kidney allograft rejection in mice and the tetracycline antibiotic doxycycline in human patients with diabetic nephropathy already under renin-angiotensin-aldosterone inhibition [79,80]. Interestingly, doxycycline also reduced the aneurysm expansion in small randomized clinical trials enrolling patients with abdominal aortic aneurysm [81,82].

4. Discussion

The evidence for how the circulating levels or the expression of MMPs increase cardiovascular risk is well documented in both basic and clinical studies. However, to our knowledge, this represents the first review to encapsulate and describe the dual association between MMPs and CKD and MMPs and PVD.

Two large meta-analyses have separately summarized the strength of the relationship between MMP-2, TIMP-1, and subclinical atherosclerosis in CKD patients or between MMPs and vascular risk, regardless of the level of kidney function [58,83]. They concluded that imbalances in MMPs/TIMPS were implicated in the pathogenesis, clinical manifestations, and prognosis of arterial and venous diseases.

According to our results, we can also affirm that the CKD condition contributes to reinforcing the risk-pathways oriented from MMPs toward PVD. Numerous pieces of evidence support this: (1) Numerous MMP molecules are likely responsible for both CV (including PVD) and kidney damage and related clinical manifestations. Hence, such biomarkers warrant further investigation. The Gelatinases MMP-2 and MMP-9 are produced by both intrinsic glomerular and tubular cells [52,70]. It has been shown that the increased activity of MMP-2 and MMP-9 across the kidney tubules may lead to structural alterations in the tubular basement membrane, which starts epithelial-mesenchymal transition (EMT). EMT consists of the process in which a component of adherent junctions, the E-cadherin, and cell adhesion are mislaid, whereas epithelial cells acquire a mesenchymal phenotype by expressing and producing α-smooth muscle actin (αSMA) and matrix protein. All these mechanisms subsequently trigger tubular atrophy and fibrosis [71,84]. Moreover, Pulskerova and coworkers have demonstrated that levels of MMP-2 were significantly higher in CKD patients Stage III–V as compared to those with Stage I–II, and correlated with fibroblast growth factor 23 (FGF-23) and levels of serum phosphate, two important surrogates of oxidative stress and CV risk in these patients [52,71]. Similarly, gelatinases have also been implicated in the onset of structural changes associated with PAD. Circulating levels of MMP-2 and MMP-9 have been found to increase in patients with acute and chronic lower limb ischemia (i.e., intermittent claudication and critical ischemia), as well as in patients with hyperlipidemia when compared with healthy subjects [12,85,86]. The connecting link between CKD, gelatinases, and PAD is mainly represented by the increased atherosclerotic risk and arterial remodeling due to the imbalance of ECM enzymes. Indeed, MMP-2 and MMP-9 are capable of releasing latent transforming growth factor beta (TGF-β), which acts as a mediator in the cross-talk between endothelial cells and vascular smooth muscle cells [71]. Imbalances in MMPs and alterations in endothelial cells are a direct causative factor of abnormal extracellular matrices, vascular calcification with arterial stiffness, atherogenesis, and high pulse pressure [71,87]. TIMP-1 has been shown to exert a similar role. In CKD patients, TIMP-1 serum concentrations were significantly increased from Stage I–III to IV–V [88]. Moreover, TIMP-1 has been found to be a predictor of the new onset of CKD and heart failure, regardless of age, gender, and biomarkers of systemic inflammation (c-reactive protein and brain natriuretic peptide) [40]. TIMP-1 is also increased in patients with PAD, with ischemic muscle being a possible source for this enzyme [12]. Interestingly, an association between TIMP-1 levels and TGF-β was described in young patients with CKD, suggesting that this factor may be involved in the pathogenesis of inflammation and CV damage even at an early stage of the disease [89].

A further crucial role in the link between metalloproteinases, CKD, and PVD is indicated by NGAL. It has been shown that NGAL levels are increased in atherosclerosis and chronic inflammatory processes, and in particular, are overexpressed in atherosclerotic plaques which are vulnerable to rupture [90]. Moreover, NGAL circulating levels have been found to increase in patients with CKD, being directly related to diabetic status and inversely to the eGFR levels [91]. From a prognostic perspective, in both CKD and general populations, plasma NGAL was a significant predictor of CV fatal and nonfatal events, including PVD [92,93]. These findings were globally reinforced by the evidence that plasma and tissue NGAL expression contribute to the pathogenesis and severity of central and peripheral aneurismal disease [94]. In this context, it has been proposed that NGAL reflects the leukocyte-mediated inflammatory response, with higher values being associated with weakness of the vascular wall and impaired vascular damage [95]. (2) CKD is characterized by a persistent low-grade inflammation with the production of pro-inflammatory cytokines, and MMP activity has been implicated in these pathways. The uremic milieu may also induce oxidative stress and recurrences in thrombotic events and infections, as well as impairment in arterial stiffening and calcification of both the intima and media of the arterial wall [55]. In the pathogenesis of all these processes, a crucial step is represented by ECM remodeling. MMPs are directly involved in ECM processes in almost all tissues. (3) In patients with already diagnosed CKD, serum levels of MMPs have been found to be significantly associated with the degree of proteinuria. This means that MMPs may be directly implicated in the development of glomerular or tubular damage typical of a wide spectrum of kidney diseases. The presence of proteinuria is a strong predictor of CV events (and PVD as well), and is recognized as a marker of endothelial systemic damage. Moreover, its prognostic role is even stronger than that attributed to the traditional CV risk factors in CKD patients (i.e., Framingham risk factors) [7,8,48]. Indeed, MMPs are detected and elevated in human kidneys with nephritic syndrome, which is a high-risk condition with severe proteinuria [51,96]. (4) It should not be excluded that MMPs play a predictive other than a prognostic role in patients with CKD or PVD. This means that the reduction of MMPs following a selective treatment could be associated with a better prognosis in these patients. Recently, several therapeutic agents that modulate the function of MMPs have been developed. The tetracycline antibiotic doxycycline and the nonselective inhibitors of MMPs, Batimastat and Marimastat, have been shown to cut vascular tissue remodeling by reducing MMP activity [97,98]. However, larger clinical studies are needed to generalize and translate these effects to clinical application. Moreover, the reduction in proteinuria that followed the use of doxycycline was associated with a reduction in the glomerular expression of MMP [58]. Also, the Renin-Angiotensin-Aldosterone system inhibitors (RAAS-I), that are currently considered the most effective renoprotective drugs against the risk of ESKD and CV events in CKD patients, have been shown to decrease the MMPs levels [99–101]. However, all these important pieces of evidence have led to the hypothesis that MMPs could be one of the causal links between CKD and CV risk, including PVD. (5) In the era of precision medicine, the need to ameliorate prognoses in patients with chronic diseases is currently increasing [102]. To this end, a number of clinical trials evaluating the beneficial effect of new drugs on cardiovascular (including peripheral vascular disease) and renal outcomes have been started [103]. Interventions varied between studies, with the effect of blood pressure lowering drugs, albuminuria lowering agents, diuretics, and endothelin receptor antagonist being tested. Results from these first studies increased the interest in a relatively new drug class, Sodium–glucose cotransporter 2 (SGLT-2) inhibitors. SGLT2-Is reduce the reabsorption of glucose from the proximal tubules of the kidney. The SGLT2-Is canagliflozin and empagliflozin reduced the risk of developing fatal and nonfatal CV events in previous trials, with this effect being associated with a reduction of albuminuria in the first 3 to 6 months of treatment [104,105]. However, an interesting recent analysis of human proximal tubular epithelial cells showed that empagliflozin is also able to reverse the renal suppression of Reversion Inducing Cysteine Rich Protein with Kazal Motifs (RECK), a membrane anchored endogenous MMP inhibitor whose expression is induced by hyperglycemia in animal and human models of diabetic kidney disease [106]. Interestingly, empagliflozin reduced the epithelial-to-mesenchymal transition, a mechanism that is strictly linked to MMPs activity and that anticipates kidney fibrosis, by directly reducing migration of tubular cells and expression of pro-inflammatory mediators (TRAF3IP2, NF-κB, p38MAPK, miR-21, and IL-1β, IL-6, TNF-α, and MCP-1). This means that SGLT2-Is may exert a protective effect on renal tubules that is independent from the albuminuria reduction. Thus, new large intervention studies evaluating the effect of drugs that interfere with MMPs activity are expected in the future to evaluate their impact on prognoses of albuminuric and nonalbuminuric CKD patients. This would be particularly important considering that nonalbuminuric CKD patients are growing in prevalence as referred patients in nephrology clinics [47,107]. In the context of intervention studies, MMPs may play a role as "predictive" biomarkers, since their assessment could identify a population of patients which is more likely to benefit from a specific drug. This point is crucial, since the development and optimization of new treatments that reduce CV risk in CKD patients may help to overcome the variability in response to the old standard treatments [108].

In addition to clinical trials perspective, further efforts are needed in the context of observational studies and risk stratification. Indeed, risk stratification of CKD patients may improve prevention strategies, acting to slow down CKD progression and reduce the high residual risk in CKD patients. In observational research, it may be useful to evaluate the potential role of MMPs as "prognostic" biomarkers used to identify the likelihood of a patient to develop a clinical outcome, regardless of treatment (i.e., under the standard of care). Such a measure may improve physicians' abilities to identify patients with poor prognoses [109]. One approach involves the discovery of novel biomarkers that may add proper prognostic information on top of already known risk factors [46,107,110–113]. Investigators from the Steno Diabetes Center, a prospective cohort that contributed to the comprehension of prognosis of diabetic patients with or without CKD, showed that MMP-1 and MMP-2 are associated with an increased risk of CV events and CV mortality, regardless of age, gender, eGFR, and albuminuria [114]. A similar effort in improving risk stratification is ongoing in the case of PAD management. It has indeed been demonstrated that patients suffering from PAD are exposed to a higher risk of CV events than those with coronary heart disease [115,116]. Hence, ameliorating prognoses of these patients is mandatory and urgent. A previous recent analysis showed that variations in the serum levels of MMPs before and after lower limb surgical revascularization in patients with critical limb ischemia are significantly associated with the subsequent outcome (major amputations or death). From our research, we can also assert that measuring the serum levels of MMPs could be even more useful in patients with CKD, PVD, or both conditions, as they potentiate the risk of progression for these conditions.

Author Contributions: Conceptualization, M.P., M.A., C.G., and R.S.; methodology, R.S.; validation, M.P., M.A., C.G., and R.S.; formal analysis, T.F., A.M., N.I., R.G., P.S. and S.d.F.; investigation, M.P., M.A., C.G., P.M. and R.S.; data curation, P.M., and P.S.; writing—original draft preparation, M.P., M.A., C.G., T.F., A.M., N.I., R.G., P.S., P.M., S.d.F., and R.S.; writing—review and editing, M.P., M.A., C.G., and R.S.; supervision, M.A., and R.S. All authors have read and agreed to the published version of the manuscript.

Funding: The work was not founded.

Conflicts of Interest: The authors declare no conflict of interest.

References

1. Levey, A.S.; Coresh, J. Chronic kidney disease. *Lancet* **2012**, *379*, 165–180. [CrossRef]
2. Kidney Disease: Improving Global Outcomes (KDIGO) CKD Work Group. KDIGO 2012 Clinical Practice Guideline for the Evaluation and Management of Chronic Kidney Disease. *Kidney Int.* **2013**, *3* (Suppl. 2013), 1–150.
3. Matsushita, K.; van der Velde, M.; Astor, B.C.; Woodward, M.; Levey, A.S.; de Jong, P.E.; Coresh, J.; Gansevoort, R.T. Association of estimated glomerular filtration rate and albuminuria with all-cause and cardiovascular mortality in general population cohorts: A collaborative meta-analysis. *Lancet* **2010**, *375*, 2073–2081. [CrossRef] [PubMed]
4. Gansevoort, R.T.; Matsushita, K.; van der Velde, M.; Astor, B.C.; Woodward, M.; Levey, A.S.; de Jong, P.E.; Coresh, J. Lower estimated GFR and higher albuminuria are associated with adverse kidney outcomes. A collaborative meta-analysis of general and high-risk population cohorts. *Kidney Int.* **2011**, *80*, 93–104. [CrossRef]
5. Go, A.S.; Chertow, G.M.; Fan, D.; McCulloch, C.E.; Hsu, C.Y. Chronic kidney disease and the risks of death, cardiovascular events, and hospitalization. *N. Engl. J. Med.* **2008**, *351*, 1296–1305, Erratum in *N. Engl. J. Med.* **2008**, *18*, 4. [CrossRef]
6. De Nicola, L.; Minutolo, R.; Chiodini, P.; Zoccali, C.; Castellino, P.; Donadio, C.; Strippoli, M.; Casino, F.; Giannattasio, M.; Petrarulo, F.; et al. Global approach to cardiovascular risk in chronic kidney disease: Reality and opportunities for intervention. *Kidney Int.* **2006**, *69*, 538–545. [CrossRef]
7. Matsushita, K.; Coresh, J.; Sang, Y.; Chalmers, J.; Fox, C.; Guallar, E.; Jafar, T.; Jassal, S.K.; Landman, G.W.; Muntner, P.; et al. Estimated glomerular filtration rate and albuminuria for prediction of cardiovascular outcomes: A collaborative meta-analysis of individual participant data. *Lancet Diabetes Endocrinol.* **2015**, *3*, 514–525. [CrossRef]

8. Matsushita, K.; Ballew, S.H.; Coresh, J.; Arima, H.; Ärnlöv, J.; Cirillo, M.; Ebert, N.; Hiramoto, J.S.; Kimm, H.; Shlipak, M.G.; et al. Measures of chronic kidney disease and risk of incident peripheral artery disease: A collaborative meta-analysis of individual participant data. *Lancet Diabetes Endocrinol.* **2017**, *5*, 718–728. [CrossRef]
9. United States Renal Data System. 2017. Available online: https://www.usrds.org/2017/view/Default.aspx (accessed on 6 November 2019).
10. Tan, R.J.; Liu, Y. Matrix metalloproteinases in kidney homeostasis and diseases. *Am. J. Physiol. Renal Physiol.* **2012**, *302*, F1351–F1361. [CrossRef]
11. Parrish, A.R. Matrix Metalloproteinases in Kidney Disease: Role in Pathogenesis and Potential as a Therapeutic Target. *Prog. Mol. Biol. Transl. Sci.* **2017**, *148*, 31–65. [CrossRef]
12. Tayebjee, M.H.; Tan, K.T.; Mac Fadyen, R.J.; Lip, G.Y. Abnormal circulating levels of metalloprotease 9 and its tissue inhibitor 1 in angiographically proven peripheral arterial disease: Relationship to disease severity. *J. Intern. Med.* **2005**, *257*, 110–116. [CrossRef] [PubMed]
13. Catania, J.M.; Chen, G.; Parrish, A.R. Role of matrix metalloproteinases in renal pathophysiologies. *Am. J. Physiol. Renal Physiol.* **2007**, *292*, F905–F911. [CrossRef] [PubMed]
14. Nagase, H.; Visse, R.; Murphy, G. Structure and function of matrix metalloproteinases and TIMPs. *Cardiovasc. Res.* **2006**, *69*, 562–573. [CrossRef] [PubMed]
15. Gharagozlian, S.; Svennevig, K.; Bangstad, H.J.; Winberg, J.O.; Kolset, S.O. Matrix metalloproteinases in subjects with type 1 diabetes. *BMC Clin. Pathol.* **2009**, *9*, 7:1–7:5. [CrossRef] [PubMed]
16. Lauhio, A.; Sorsa, T.; Srinivas, R.; Stenman, M.; Tervahartiala, T.; Stenman, U.H.; Gronhagen-Riska, C.; Honkanen, E. Urinary matrix metallo-proteinase-8, -9, -14 and their regulators (TRY-1, TRY-2, TATI) in patients with diabetic nephropathy. *Ann. Med.* **2008**, *40*, 312–320. [CrossRef] [PubMed]
17. Li, Y.; Kang, Y.S.; Dai, C.; Kiss, L.P.; Wen, X.; Liu, Y. Epithelial-to-mesenchymal transition is a potential pathway leading to podocyte dysfunction and proteinuria. *Am. J. Pathol.* **2008**, *172*, 299–308. [CrossRef]
18. Tashiro, K.; Koyanagi, I.; Ohara, I.; Ito, T.; Saitoh, A.; Horikoshi, S.; Tomino, Y. Levels of urinary matrix metalloproteinase-9 (MMP-9) and renal injuries in patients with type 2 diabetic nephropathy. *J. Clin. Lab. Anal.* **2004**, *18*, 206–210. [CrossRef]
19. Thrailkill, K.M.; Moreau, C.S.; Cockrell, G.E.; Jo, C.H.; Bunn, R.C.; Morales-Pozzo, A.E.; Lumpkin, C.K.; Fowlkes, J.L. Disease and gender-specific dysregulation of NGAL and MMP-9 in type 1 diabetes mellitus. *Endocrine* **2010**, *37*, 336–343. [CrossRef]
20. Tschesche, H.; Zolzer, V.; Triebel, S.; Bartsch, S. The human neutrophil lipocalin supports the allosteric activation of matrix metalloproteinases. *Eur. J. Biochem.* **2001**, *268*, 1918–1928. [CrossRef]
21. Ban, C.R.; Twigg, S.M.; Franjic, B.; Brooks, B.A.; Celermajer, D.; Yue, D.K.; McLennan, S.V. Serum MMP-7 is increased in diabetic renal disease and diabetic diastolic dysfunction. *Diabetes Res. Clin. Pract.* **2010**, *87*, 335–341. [CrossRef]
22. Huja, T.S.; Gopalani, A.; Davies, P.; Ahuja, H. Matrix metalloproteinase-9 expression in renal biopsies of patients with HIV-associated nephropathy. *Nephron. Clin. Pract.* **2003**, *95*, c100–c104.
23. Bauvois, B.; Mothu, N.; Nguyen, J.; Nguyen-Khoa, T.; Noel, L.H.; Jungers, P. Specific changes in plasma concentrations of matrix metalloproteinase-2 and -9, TIMP-1 and TGF-beta1 in patients with distinct types of primary glomerulonephritis. *Nephrol. Dial. Transplant.* **2007**, *22*, 1115–1122. [CrossRef] [PubMed]
24. Czech, K.A.; Bennett, M.; Devarajan, P. Distinct metalloproteinase excretion patterns in focal segmental glomerulosclerosis. *Pediatr. Nephrol.* **2011**, *26*, 2179–2184. [CrossRef]
25. Sanders, J.S.; Huitema, M.G.; Hanemaaijer, R.; van Goor, H.; Kallenberg, C.G.; Stegeman, C.A. Urinary matrix metalloproteinases reflect renal damage in anti-neutrophil cytoplasm autoantibody-associated vasculitis. *Am. J. Physiol. Renal Physiol.* **2007**, *293*, F1927–F1934. [CrossRef] [PubMed]
26. Sanders, J.S.; van Goor, H.; Hanemaaijer, R.; Kallenberg, C.G.; Stegeman, C.A. Renal expression of matrix metalloproteinases in human ANCA- associated glomerulonephritis. *Nephrol. Dial. Transplant.* **2004**, *19*, 1412–1419. [CrossRef]
27. Forough, R.; Koyama, N.; Hasenstab, D.; Lea, H.; Clowes, M.; Nikkari, S.T.; Clowes, A.W. Overexpression of tissue inhibitor of matrix metalloproteinase-1 inhibits vascular smooth muscle cell functions in vitro and in vivo. *Circ. Res.* **1996**, *79*, 812–820. [CrossRef]

28. Sritharan, K.; Essex, D.; Sandison, A.; Ellis, M.; Monaco, C.; Davies, A.H. Membrane Type-1 matrix metalloproteinase: A key player in carotid plaque instability and symptomatic carotid atherosclerotic disease. *Br. J. Surg.* **2008**, *95*, 2.
29. Sritharan, K.; Navin, T.; Ellis, M.; Monaco, C.; Davies, A.H. Membrane type-1 matrix metalloproteinase is upregulated in symptomatic carotid atherosclerotic disease and along with other members of the quarternary complex regulated by pro-inflammatory cytokines. *Br. J. Surg.* **2008**, *95*, 934.
30. Blankenberg, S.; Rupprecht, H.J.; Poirier, O.; Bickel, C.; Smieja, M.; Hafner, G.; Meyer, J.; Cambien, F.; Tiret, L. Plasma concentrations and genetic variation of matrix metalloproteinase 9 and prognosis of patients with cardiovascular disease. *Circulation* **2003**, *107*, 1579–1585. [CrossRef]
31. Newman, K.M.; Jean-Claude, J.; Li, H.; Scholes, J.V.; Ogata, Y.; Nagase, H.; Tilson, M.D. Cellular localization of matrix metalloproteinases in the abdominal aortic aneurysm wall. *J. Vasc. Surg.* **1994**, *20*, 814–820. [CrossRef]
32. Henger, A.; Kretzler, M.; Doran, P.; Bonrouhi, M.; Schmid, H.; Kiss, E.; Cohen, C.D.; Madden, S.; Porubsky, S.; Gröne, E.F.; et al. Gene expression fingerprints in human tubulointerstitial inflammation and fibrosis as prognostic markers of disease progression. *Kidney Int.* **2004**, *65*, 904–917. [CrossRef] [PubMed]
33. Hu, Y.; Ivashkiv, L.B. Costimulation of chemokine receptor signaling by matrix metalloproteinase-9 mediates enhanced migration of IFN-alpha dendritic cells. *J. Immunol.* **2006**, *176*, 6022–6033. [CrossRef] [PubMed]
34. Li, Q.; Park, P.W.; Wilson, C.L.; Parks, W.C. Matrilysin shedding of syndecan-1 regulates chemokine mobilization and transepithelial efflux of neutrophils in acute lung injury. *Cell* **2002**, *111*, 635–646. [CrossRef]
35. Essick, E.; Sithu, S.; Dean, W.; D'Souza, S. Pervanadate-induced shedding of the intercellular adhesion molecule (ICAM)-1 ectodomain is mediated by membrane type-1 matrix metalloproteinase (MT1-MMP). *Mol. Cell Biochem.* **2008**, *314*, 151–159. [CrossRef] [PubMed]
36. Yamashita, C.M.; Dolgonos, L.; Zemans, R.L.; Young, S.K.; Robertson, J.; Briones, N.; Suzuki, T.; Campbell, M.N.; Gauldie, J.; Radisky, D.C.; et al. Matrix metalloproteinase 3 is a mediator of pulmonary fibrosis. *Am. J. Pathol.* **2011**, *179*, 1733–1745. [CrossRef]
37. Gagliano, N.; Arosio, B.; Santambrogio, D.; Balestrieri, M.R.; Padoani, G.; Tagliabue, J.; Masson, S.; Vergani, C.; Annoni, G. Age-dependent expression of fibrosis-related genes and collagen deposition in rat kidney cortex. *J. Gerontol. A Biol. Sci. Med. Sci.* **2000**, *55*, B365–B372. [CrossRef]
38. Kim, H.; Oda, T.; Lopez-Guisa, J.; Wing, D.; Edwards, D.R.; Soloway, P.D.; Eddy, A.A. TIMP-1 deficiency does not attenuate interstitial fibrosis in obstructive nephropathy. *J. Am. Soc. Nephrol.* **2001**, *12*, 736–748.
39. Lu, Y.; Liu, S.; Zhang, S.; Cai, G.; Jiang, H.; Su, H.; Li, X.; Hong, Q.; Zhang, X.; Chen, X. Tissue inhibitor of metalloproteinase-1 promotes NIH3T3 fibroblast proliferation by activating p-Akt and cell cycle progression. *Mol. Cells* **2011**, *31*, 225–230. [CrossRef]
40. Lieb, W.; Song, R.J.; Xanthakis, V.; Vasan, R.S. Association of Circulating Tissue Inhibitor of Metalloproteinases-1 and Procollagen Type III Aminoterminal Peptide Levels With Incident Heart Failure and Chronic Kidney Disease. *J. Am. Heart Assoc.* **2019**, *8*, e011426. [CrossRef]
41. Sundstrom, J.; Evans, J.C.; Benjamin, E.J.; Levy, D.; Larson, M.G.; Sawyer, D.B.; Siwik, D.A.; Colucci, W.S.; Wilson, P.W.; Vasan, R.S. Relations of plasma total TIMP-1 levels to cardiovascular risk factors and echocardiographic measures: The Framingham Heart Study. *Eur. Heart J.* **2004**, *25*, 1509–1516. [CrossRef]
42. Morishita, T.; Uzui, H.; Mitsuke, Y.; Amaya, N.; Kaseno, K.; Ishida, K.; Fukuoka, Y.; Ikeda, H.; Tama, N.; Yamazaki, T.; et al. Association between matrix metalloproteinase-9 and worsening heart failure events in patients with chronic heart failure. *ESC Heart Fail.* **2017**, *4*, 321–330. [CrossRef] [PubMed]
43. Hansson, J.; Vasan, R.S.; Arnlov, J.; Ingelsson, E.; Lind, L.; Larsson, A.; Michaelsson, K.; Sundstrom, J. Biomarkers of extracellular matrix metabolism (MMP-9 and TIMP-1) and risk of stroke, myocardial infarction, and cause-specific mortality: Cohort study. *PLoS ONE* **2011**, *6*, e16185. [CrossRef] [PubMed]
44. Agarwal, I.; Glazer, N.L.; Barasch, E.; Biggs, M.L.; Djousse, L.; Fitzpatrick, A.L.; Gottdiener, J.S.; Ix, J.H.; Kizer, J.R.; Rimm, E.B.; et al. Fibrosis-related biomarkers and risk of total and cause-specific mortality: The Cardiovascular Health Study. *Am. J. Epidemiol.* **2014**, *179*, 1331–1339. [CrossRef] [PubMed]
45. Rouet-Benzineb, P.; Buhler, J.M.; Dreyfus, P.; Delcourt, A.; Dorent, R.; Perennec, J.; Crozatier, B.; Harf, A.; Lafuma, C. Altered balance between matrix gelatinases (MMP-2 and MMP-9) and their tissue inhibitors in human dilated cardiomyopathy: Potential role of MMP-9 in myosin-heavy chain degradation. *Eur. J. Heart Fail.* **1999**, *1*, 337–352. [CrossRef]

46. Provenzano, M.; Mancuso, C.; Garofalo, C.; De Nicola, L.; Andreucci, M. Temporal variation of Chronic Kidney Disease's epidemiology. *G. Ital. Nefrol.* **2019**, *36*, 2019-vol2.
47. Minutolo, R.; Gabbai, F.B.; Provenzano, M.; Chiodini, P.; Borrelli, S.; Garofalo, C.; Sasso, F.C.; Santoro, D.; Bellizzi, V.; Conte, G.; et al. Cardiorenal prognosis by residual proteinuria level in diabetic chronic kidney disease: Pooled analysis of four cohort studies. *Nephrol. Dial. Transplant.* **2018**, *33*, 1942–1949. [CrossRef]
48. Matsushita, K.; Sang, Y.; Ballew, S.H.; Shlipak, M.; Katz, R.; Rosas, S.E.; Peralta, C.A.; Woodward, M.; Kramer, H.J.; Jacobs, D.R.; et al. Subclinical atherosclerosis measures for cardiovascular prediction in CKD. *J. Am. Soc. Nephrol.* **2015**, *26*, 439–447. [CrossRef]
49. Pawlak, K.; Pawlak, D.; Mysliwiec, M. Extrinsic coagulation pathway activation and metalloproteinase-2/TIMPs system are related to oxidative stress and atherosclerosis in hemodialysis patients. *Thromb. Haemost.* **2004**, *92*, 646–653. [CrossRef]
50. Pawlak, K.; Pawlak, D.; Mysliwiec, M. Urokinase-type plasminogen activator and metalloproteinase-2 are independently related to the carotid atherosclerosis in haemodialysis patients. *Thromb. Res.* **2008**, *121*, 543–548. [CrossRef]
51. Nagano, M.; Fukami, K.; Yamagishi, S.; Ueda, S.; Kaida, Y.; Matsumoto, T.; Yoshimura, J.; Hazama, T.; Takamiya, Y.; Kusumoto, T.; et al. Circulating matrix metalloproteinase-2 is an independent correlate of proteinuria in patients with chronic kidney disease. *Am. J. Nephrol.* **2009**, *29*, 109–115. [CrossRef]
52. Peiskerová, M.; Kalousová, M.; Kratochvílová, M.; Dusilová-Sulková, S.; Uhrová, J.; Bandúr, S.; Malbohan, I.M.; Zima, T.; Tesař, V. Fibroblast growth factor 23 and matrix-metalloproteinases in patients with chronic kidney disease: Are they associated with cardiovascular disease? *Kidney Blood Press. Res.* **2009**, *32*, 276–283. [CrossRef] [PubMed]
53. Pawlak, K.; Tankiewicz, J.; Mysliwiec, M.; Pawlak, D. Systemic levels of MMP2/TIMP2 and cardiovascular risk in CAPD patients. *Nephron. Clin. Pract.* **2010**, *115*, c251–c258. [CrossRef] [PubMed]
54. Akchurin, O.M.; Kaskel, F. Update on inflammation in chronic kidney disease. *Blood Purif.* **2015**, *39*, 384–392. [CrossRef] [PubMed]
55. Brunet, P.; Gondouin, B.; Duval-Sabatier, A.; Dou, L.; Cerini, C.; Dignat-George, F.; Jourde-Chiche, N.; Argiles, A.; Burtey, S. Does uremia cause vascular dysfunction? *Kidney Blood Press. Res.* **2011**, *34*, 284–290. [CrossRef]
56. Newby, A.C. Dual role of matrix metalloproteinases (matrix-ins) in intimal thickening and atherosclerotic plaque rupture. *Physiol. Rev.* **2005**, *85*, 1–31. [CrossRef]
57. Libby, P. Collagenases and cracks in the plaque. *J. Clin. Investig.* **2013**, *123*, 3201–3203. [CrossRef]
58. Lim, C.S.; Shalhoub, J.; Gohel, M.S.; Shepherd, A.C.; Davies, A.H. Matrix metalloproteinases in vascular disease—A potential therapeutic target? *Curr. Vasc. Pharmacol.* **2010**, *8*, 75–85. [CrossRef]
59. Monaco, C.; Andreakos, E.; Kiriakidis, S.; Mauri, C.; Bicknell, C.; Foxwell, B.; Chesire, N.; Paleolog, E.; Feldmann, M. Canonical pathway of nuclear factor kappa B activation selectively regulates proinflammatory and prothrombotic responses in human atherosclerosis. *Proc. Natl. Acad. Sci. USA* **2004**, *101*, 5634–5639. [CrossRef]
60. McMillan, W.D.; Tamarina, N.A.; Cipollone, M.; Johnson, D.A.; Parker, M.A.; Pearce, W.H. Size matters: The relationship between MMP 9 expression and aortic diameter. *Circulation* **1997**, *96*, 2228–2232. [CrossRef]
61. Freestone, T.; Turner, R.J.; Coady, A.; Higman, D.J.; Greenhalgh, R.M.; Powell, J.T. Inflammation and matrix metalloproteinases in the enlarging abdominal aortic aneurysm. *Arterioscler. Thromb. Vasc. Biol.* **1995**, *15*, 1145–1151. [CrossRef]
62. Martinez-Aguilar, E.; Gomez-Rodriguez, V.; Orbe, J.; Rodriguez, J.A.; Fernández-Alonso, L.; Roncal, C.; Páramo, J.A. Matrix metalloproteinase 10 is associated with disease severity and mortality in patients with peripheral arterial disease. *J. Vasc. Surg.* **2015**, *61*, 428–435. [CrossRef] [PubMed]
63. Morishita, T.; Uzui, H.; Nakano, A.; Mitsuke, Y.; Geshi, T.; Ueda, T.; Lee, J.D. Number of endothelial progenitor cells in peripheral artery disease as a marker of severity and association with pentraxin-3, malondialdehyde-modified low-density lipoprotein and membrane type-1 matrix metalloproteinase. *J. Atheroscler. Thromb.* **2012**, *19*, 149–158. [CrossRef] [PubMed]
64. De Caridi, G.; Massara, M.; Spinelli, F.; David, A.; Gangemi, S.; Fugetto, F.; Grande, R.; Butrico, L.; Stefanelli, R.; Colosimo, M.; et al. Matrix metalloproteinases and risk stratification in patients undergoing surgical revascularisation for critical limb ischaemia. *Int. Wound J.* **2016**, *13*, 493–499. [CrossRef] [PubMed]

65. Woodside, K.J.; Hu, M.; Burke, A.; Murakami, M.; Pounds, L.L.; Killewich, L.A.; Daller, J.A.; Hunter, G.C. Morphologic characteristics of varicose veins: Possible role of metalloproteinases. *J. Vasc. Surg.* **2003**, *38*, 162–169. [CrossRef]
66. Raffetto, J.D.; Qiao, X.; Koledova, V.V.; Khalil, R.A. Prolonged increases in vein wall tension increase matrix metalloproteinases and decrease constriction in rat vena cava: Potential implications in varicose veins. *J. Vasc. Surg.* **2008**, *48*, 447–456. [CrossRef]
67. Herouy, Y.; Mellios, P.; Bandemir, E.; Dichmann, S.; Nockowski, P.; Schöpf, E.; Norgauer, J. Inflammation in stasis dermatitis upregulates MMP-1, MMP-2 and MMP-13 expression. *J. Dermatol. Sci.* **2001**, *25*, 198–205. [CrossRef]
68. Herouy, Y.; May, A.E.; Pornschlegel, G.; Stetter, C.; Grenz, H.; Preissner, K.T.; Schöpf, E.; Norgauer, J.; Vanscheidt, W. Lipodermatosclerosis is characterized by elevated expression and activation of matrix metalloproteinases: Implications for venous ulcer formation. *J. Investig. Dermatol.* **1998**, *111*, 822–827. [CrossRef]
69. Vaalamo, M.; Leivo, T.; Saarialho-Kere, U. Differential expression of tissue inhibitors of metalloproteinases (TIMP-1, -2, -3, and -4) in normal and aberrant wound healing. *Hum. Pathol.* **1999**, *30*, 795–802. [CrossRef]
70. Chung, A.W.; Booth, A.D.; Rose, C.; Thompson, C.R.; Levin, A.; van Breemen, C. Increased matrix metalloproteinase 2 activity in the human internal mammary artery is associated with ageing, hypertension, diabetes and kidney dysfunction. *J. Vasc. Res.* **2008**, *45*, 357–362. [CrossRef]
71. Ravarotto, V.; Simioni, F.; Pagnin, E.; Davis, P.A.; Calò, L.A. Oxidative stress—chronic kidney disease—cardiovascular disease: A vicious circle. *Life Sci.* **2018**, *210*, 125–131. [CrossRef]
72. Raffetto, J.D.; Khalil, R.A. Matrix metalloproteinases and their inhibitors in vascular remodeling and vascular disease. *Biochem. Pharmacol.* **2008**, *75*, 346–359. [CrossRef] [PubMed]
73. Rao, B.G. Recent developments in the design of specific Matrix Metalloproteinase inhibitors aided by structural and computational studies. *Curr. Pharm. Des.* **2005**, *11*, 295–322. [CrossRef] [PubMed]
74. Vihinen, P.; Ala-aho, R.; Kahari, V.M. Matrix metalloproteinases as therapeutic targets in cancer. *Curr. Cancer Drug Targets* **2005**, *5*, 203–220. [CrossRef] [PubMed]
75. Acharya, M.R.; Venitz, J.; Figg, W.D.; Sparreboom, A. Chemically modified tetracyclines as inhibitors of matrix metalloproteinases. *Drug Resist. Updates* **2004**, *7*, 195–208. [CrossRef] [PubMed]
76. Zakeri, B.; Wright, G.D. Chemical biology of tetracycline antibiotics. *Biochem. Cell Biol.* **2008**, *86*, 124–136. [CrossRef]
77. Morales, R.; Perrier, S.; Florent, J.M.; Beltra, J.; Dufour, S.; De Mendez, I.; Manceau, P.; Tertre, A.; Moreau, F.; Compere, D.; et al. Crystal structures of novel non-peptidic, non-zinc chelating inhibitors bound to MMP-12. *J. Mol. Biol.* **2004**, *341*, 1063–1076. [CrossRef]
78. Steinmann-Niggli, K.; Ziswiler, R.; Kung, M.; Marti, H.P. Inhibition of matrix metalloproteinase attenuates anti-Thy1.1 nephritis. *J. Am. Soc. Nephrol.* **1998**, *9*, 397–407.
79. Ermolli, M.; Schumacher, M.; Lods, N.; Hammoud, M.; Marti, H.P. Differential expression of MMP-2/MMP-9 and potential benefit of an MMP inhibitor in experimental acute kidney allograft rejection. *Transpl. Immunol.* **2003**, *11*, 137–145. [CrossRef]
80. Aggarwal, H.K.; Jain, D.; Talapatra, P.; Yadav, R.J.; Gupta, T.; Kathuria, K.L. Evaluation of role of doxycycline (a matrix metalloproteinase inhibitor) on renal functions in patients of diabetic nephropathy. *Ren. Fail.* **2010**, *32*, 941–946. [CrossRef]
81. Mosorin, M.; Juvonen, J.; Biancari, F.; Satta, J.; Surcel, H.M.; Leinonen, M.; Saikku, P.; Juvonen, T. Use of doxycycline to decrease the growth rate of abdominal aortic aneurysms: A randomized, double-blind, placebo-controlled pilot study. *J. Vasc. Surg.* **2001**, *34*, 606–610. [CrossRef]
82. Lindeman, J.H.; Abdul-Hussien, H.; van Bockel, J.H.; Wolterbeek, R.; Kleemann, R. Clinical trial of doxycycline for matrix metalloproteinase-9 inhibition in patients with an abdominal aneurysm: Doxycycline selectively depletes aortic wall neutrophils and cytotoxic T cells. *Circulation* **2009**, *119*, 2209–2216. [CrossRef] [PubMed]
83. Kousios, A.; Kouis, P.; Panayiotou, A.G. Matrix Metalloproteinases and Subclinical Atherosclerosis in Chronic Kidney Disease: A Systematic Review. *Int. J. Nephrol.* **2016**, *2016*, 9498013. [CrossRef] [PubMed]
84. Cheng, S.; Pollock, A.S.; Mahimkar, R.; Olson, J.L.; Lovett, D.H. Matrix metalloproteinase 2 and basement membrane integrity: A unifying mechanism for progressive renal injury. *FASEB J.* **2006**, *20*, 1898–1900. [CrossRef] [PubMed]

85. Beaudeux, J.; Giral, P.; Bruckert, E.; Bernard, M.; Foglietti, M.; Chapman, M. Serum matrix metalloproteinase-3 and tissue inhibitor of metalloproteinases-1 as potential markers of carotid atherosclerosis in infraclinical hyperlipidemia. *Atherosclerosis* **2003**, *169*, 139–146. [CrossRef]
86. Muhs, B.; Plits, G.; Delgado, Y.; Ianus, I.; Shaw, J.P.; Adelman, M.A.; Lamparello, P.; Shamamian, P.; Gagne, P. Temporal expression and activation of matrix metalloproteinases-2, -9, and membrane type 1—Matrix metalloproteinase following acute hind limb ischemia. *J. Surg. Res.* **2003**, *111*, 8–15. [CrossRef]
87. Zakiyanov, O.; Kalousová, M.; Zima, T.; Tesař, V. Matrix Metalloproteinases in Renal Diseases: A Critical Appraisal. *Kidney Blood Press. Res.* **2019**, *44*, 298–330. [CrossRef]
88. Coll, B.; Rodríguez, J.A.; Craver, L.; Orbe, J.; Martínez-Alonso, M.; Ortiz, A.; Díez, J.; Beloqui, O.; Borras, M.; Valdivielso, J.M.; et al. Serum levels of matrix metalloproteinase-10 are associated with the severity of atherosclerosis in patients with chronic kidney disease. *Kidney Int.* **2010**, *78*, 1275–1280. [CrossRef]
89. Musiał, K.; Zwolińska, D. Novel indicators of fibrosis-related complications in children with chronic kidney disease. *Clin. Chim. Acta* **2014**, *430*, 15–19. [CrossRef]
90. Van der Wal, A.C.; Becker, A.E.; Van der Loos, C.M.; Das, P.K. Site of intimal rupture or erosion of thrombosed coronary atherosclerotic plaques is characterized by an inflammatory process irrespective of the dominant plaque morphology. *Circulation* **1994**, *89*, 36–44. [CrossRef]
91. Bolignano, D.; Donato, V.; Coppolino, G.; Campo, S.; Buemi, A.; Lacquaniti, A.; Buemi, M. Neutrophil gelatinase-associated lipocalin (NGAL) as a marker of kidney damage. *Am. J. Kidney Dis.* **2008**, *52*, 595–605. [CrossRef]
92. Helmersson-Karlqvist, J.; Larsson, A.; Carlsson, A.C.; Venge, P.; Sundström, J.; Ingelsson, E.; Lind, L.; Arnlöv, J. Urinary neutrophil gelatinase-associated lipocalin (NGAL) is associated with mortality in a community-based cohort of older Swedish men. *Atherosclerosis* **2013**, *227*, 408–413. [CrossRef]
93. Solak, Y.; Yilmaz, M.I.; Siripol, D.; Saglam, M.; Unal, H.U.; Yaman, H.; Gok, M.; Cetinkaya, H.; Gaipov, A.; Eyileten, T.; et al. Serum neutrophil gelatinase-associated lipocalin is associated with cardiovascular events in patients with chronic kidney disease. *Int. Urol. Nephrol.* **2015**, *47*, 1993–2001. [CrossRef]
94. Serra, R.; Grande, R.; Montemurro, R.; Butrico, L.; Caliò, F.G.; Mastrangelo, D.; Scarcello, E.; Gallelli, L.; Buffone, G.; de Franciscis, S. The role of matrix metalloproteinases and neutrophil gelatinase-associated lipocalin in central and peripheral arterial aneurysms. *Surgery.* **2015**, *157*, 155–162. [CrossRef]
95. Ramos-Mozo, P.; Madrigal-Matute, J.; Vega de Ceniga, M.; Blanco-Colio, L.M.; Meilhac, O.; Feldman, L.; Michel, J.B.; Clancy, P.; Golledge, J.; Norman, P.E.; et al. Increased plasma levels of NGAL, a marker of neutrophil activation, in patients with abdominal aortic aneurysm. *Atherosclerosis* **2012**, *220*, 552–556. [CrossRef]
96. Urushihara, M.; Kagami, S.; Kuhara, T.; Tamaki, T.; Kuroda, Y. Glomerular distribution and gelatinolytic activity of matrix metalloproteinases in human glomerulonephritis. *Nephrol. Dial. Transplant.* **2002**, *17*, 1189–1196. [CrossRef]
97. Kenagy, R.D.; Vergel, S.; Mattsson, E.; Bendeck, M.; Reidy, M.A.; Clowes, A.W. The role of plasminogen, plasminogen activators, and matrix metalloproteinases in primate arterial smooth muscle cell migration. *Arterioscler. Thromb. Vasc. Biol.* **1996**, *16*, 1373–1382. [CrossRef]
98. Sansilvestri-Morel, P.; Rupin, A.; Jullien, N.D.; Lembrez, N.; Mestries-Dubois, P.; Fabiani, J.N.; Verbeuren, T.J. Decreased production of collagen type III in cultured smooth muscle cells from varicose vein patients is due to a degradation by MMPs: Possible implication of MMP-3. *J. Vasc. Res.* **2005**, *42*, 388–398. [CrossRef]
99. Kang, S.Y.; Li, Y.; Dai, C.; Kiss, L.P.; Wu, C.; Liu, Y. Inhibition of integrin-linked kinase blocks podocyte epithelial-mesenchymal transition and ameliorates proteinuria. *Kidney Int.* **2010**, *78*, 363–373. [CrossRef]
100. Sorbi, D.; Fadly, M.; Hicks, R.; Alexander, S.; Arbeit, L. Captopril inhibits the 72 kDa and 92 kDa matrix metalloproteinases. *Kidney Int.* **1993**, *44*, 1266–1272. [CrossRef]
101. Lods, N.; Ferrari, P.; Frey, F.J.; Kappeler, A.; Berthier, C.; Vogt, B.; Marti, H.P. Angiotensin converting enzyme inhibition but not angiotensin II receptor blockade regulates matrix metalloproteinase activity in patients with glomerulonephritis. *J. Am. Soc. Nephrol.* **2003**, *14*, 2861–2872. [CrossRef]
102. Provenzano, M.; Chiodini, P.; Minutolo, R.; Zoccali, C.; Bellizzi, V.; Conte, G.; Locatelli, F.; Tripepi, G.; Del Vecchio, L.; Mallamaci, F.; et al. Reclassification of chronic kidney disease patients for end-stage renal disease risk by proteinuria indexed to estimated glomerular filtration rate: Multicenter prospective study in nephrology clinics. *Nephrol. Dial. Transplant.* **2018**. [CrossRef] [PubMed]

103. Provenzano, M.; Coppolino, G.; De Nicola, L.; Serra, R.; Garofalo, C.; Andreucci, M.; Bolignano, D. Unraveling Cardiovascular Risk in Renal Patients: A New Take on Old Tale. *Front. Cell Dev. Biol.* **2019**, *7*, 314:1–314:14. [CrossRef] [PubMed]
104. Neal, B.; Perkovic, V.; Mahaffey, K.W.; de Zeeuw, D.; Fulcher, G.; Erondu, N.; Shaw, W.; Law, G.; Desai, M.; Matthews, D.R. Canagliflozin and Cardiovascular and Renal Events in Type 2 Diabetes. *N. Engl. J. Med.* **2017**, *377*, 644–657. [CrossRef] [PubMed]
105. Zinman, B.; Wanner, C.; Lachin, J.M.; Fitchett, D.; Bluhmki, E.; Hantel, S.; Mattheus, M.; Devins, T.; Johansen, O.E.; Woerle, H.J.; et al. Empagliflozin, Cardiovascular Outcomes, and Mortality in Type 2 Diabetes. *N. Engl. J. Med.* **2015**, *373*, 2117–2128. [CrossRef]
106. Das, N.A.; Carpenter, A.J.; Belenchia, A.; Aroor, A.R.; Noda, M.; Siebenlist, U.; Chandrasekar, B.; DeMarco, V.G. Empagliflozin reduces high glucose-induced oxidative stress and miR-21-dependent TRAF3IP2 induction and RECK suppression, and inhibits human renal proximal tubular epithelial cell migration and epithelial-to-mesenchymal transition. *Cell. Signal.* **2019**, *68*, 109506. [CrossRef]
107. De Nicola, L.; Provenzano, M.; Chiodini, P.; Borrelli, S.; Russo, L.; Bellasi, A.; Santoro, D.; Conte, G.; Minutolo, R. Epidemiology of low-proteinuric chronic kidney disease in renal clinics. *PLoS ONE* **2017**, *12*, e0172241. [CrossRef]
108. Petrykiv, S.I.; de Zeeuw, D.; Persson, F.; Rossing, P.; Gansevoort, R.T.; Laverman, G.D.; Heerspink, H.J.L. Variability in response to albuminuria-lowering drugs: True or random? *Br. J. Clin. Pharmacol.* **2017**, *83*, 1197–1204. [CrossRef]
109. Simon, R.M.; Subramanian, J.; Li, M.C.; Menezes, S. Using cross-validation to evaluate predictive accuracy of survival risk classifiers based on high-dimensional data. *Brief. Bioinform.* **2011**, *12*, 203–214. [CrossRef]
110. Tangri, N.; Grams, M.E.; Levey, A.S.; Coresh, J.; Appel, L.J.; Astor, B.C.; Chodick, G.; Collins, A.J.; Djurdjev, O.; Elley, C.R.; et al. Multinational assessment of accuracy of equations for predicting risk of kidney failure: A meta-analysis. *JAMA* **2016**, *315*, 164–174. [CrossRef]
111. De Nicola, L.; Provenzano, M.; Chiodini, P.; D'Arrigo, G.; Tripepi, G.; Del Vecchio, L.; Conte, G.; Locatelli, F.; Zoccali, C.; Minutolo, R.; et al. Prognostic role of LDL cholesterol in non-dialysis chronic kidney disease: Multicenter prospective study in Italy. *Nutr. Metab. Cardiovasc. Dis.* **2015**, *25*, 756–762. [CrossRef]
112. Russo, D.; Morrone, L.F.; Errichiello, C.; De Gregorio, M.G.; Imbriaco, M.; Battaglia, Y.; Russo, L.; Andreucci, M.; Di Iorio, B.R. Impact of BMI on cardiovascular events, renal function, and coronary artery calcification. *Blood Purif.* **2014**, *38*, 1–6. [CrossRef]
113. Russo, D.; Corrao, S.; Battaglia, Y.; Andreucci, M.; Caiazza, A.; Carlomagno, A.; Lamberti, M.; Pezone, N.; Pota, A.; Russo, L.; et al. Progression of coronary artery calcification and cardiac events in patients with chronic renal disease not receiving dialysis. *Kidney Int.* **2011**, *80*, 112–118. [CrossRef]
114. Peeters, S.A.; Engelen, L.; Buijs, J.; Jorsal, A.; Parving, H.H.; Tarnow, L.; Rossing, P.; Schalkwijk, C.G.; Stehouwer, C.D.A. Plasma matrix metalloproteinases are associated with incident cardiovascular disease and all-cause mortality in patients with type 1 diabetes: A 12-year follow-up study. *Cardiovasc. Diabetol.* **2017**, *16*, 55:1–55:12. [CrossRef]
115. Criqui, M.H.; Langer, R.D.; Fronek, A.; Feigelson, H.S.; Klauber, M.R.; McCann, T.J.; Browner, D. Mortality over a period of 10 years in patients with peripheral arterial disease. *N. Engl. J. Med.* **1992**, *326*, 381–386. [CrossRef]
116. Caro, J.; Migliaccio-Walle, K.; Ishak, K.J.; Proskorovsky, I. The morbidity and mortality following a diagnosis of peripheral arterial disease: Long-term follow-up of a large database. *BMC Cardiovasc. Disord.* **2005**, *5*, 14:1–14:8. [CrossRef]

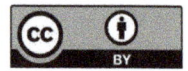

© 2020 by the authors. Licensee MDPI, Basel, Switzerland. This article is an open access article distributed under the terms and conditions of the Creative Commons Attribution (CC BY) license (http://creativecommons.org/licenses/by/4.0/).

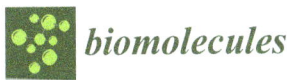

Review

Challenges in Matrix Metalloproteinases Inhibition

Helena Laronha [1,2], Inês Carpinteiro [1], Jaime Portugal [3], Ana Azul [1], Mário Polido [1], Krasimira T. Petrova [2], Madalena Salema-Oom [1,2] and Jorge Caldeira [1,2,*]

1. Centro de Investigação Interdisciplinar Egas Moniz, Instituto Universitário Egas Moniz, 2829-511 Caparica, Portugal; h.laronha@campus.fct.unl.pt (H.L.); icarpinteiro@egasmoniz.edu.pt (I.C.); aazul@egasmoniz.edu.pt (A.A.); mpolido@egasmoniz.edu.pt (M.P.); moom@egasmoniz.edu.pt (M.S.-O.)
2. UCIBIO and LAQV, Requimte, Faculdade de Ciências e Tecnologia, Universidade Nova de Lisboa, 2829-516 Caparica, Portugal; k.petrova@fct.unl.pt
3. Faculdade de Medicina Dentária Universidade de Lisboa, 1649-003 Lisboa, Portugal; jaime.portugal@fmd.ulisboa.pt
* Correspondence: jcaldeira@egasmoniz.edu.pt; Tel.: +351-919553592

Received: 9 April 2020; Accepted: 30 April 2020; Published: 5 May 2020

Abstract: Matrix metalloproteinases are enzymes that degrade the extracellular matrix. They have different substrates but similar structural organization. Matrix metalloproteinases are involved in many physiological and pathological processes and there is a need to develop inhibitors for these enzymes in order to modulate the degradation of the extracellular matrix (ECM). There exist two classes of inhibitors: endogenous and synthetics. The development of synthetic inhibitors remains a great challenge due to the low selectivity and specificity, side effects in clinical trials, and instability. An extensive review of currently reported synthetic inhibitors and description of their properties is presented.

Keywords: matrix metalloproteinases; TIMP; synthetic inhibitors

---

1. Introduction

Matrix metalloproteinases (MMPs) are a protein family within the metzincin superfamily, comprising zinc-dependent endopeptidases with similar structural characteristics but with different substrate preferences. MMPs are produced and secreted from cells as inactive proenzymes depending, herein, on a structural alteration for activation [1–6]. In human tissues, there are 23 different types of MMPs expressed and they can be subdivided according to their substrate specificity, sequential similarity, and domain organization [1,2,4,7–17] (Table 1).

The most common structural features shared by MMPs are [1,2,4,5,7,8,10–14,16,18] (Figure 1) a pro-domain, a catalytic domain, a hemopexin-like domain, and a transmembrane domain for membrane type MMPs (MT-MMPs) although some MMPS do not have all the structural features represented in the figure. The pro-domain keeps MMP inactive by a cysteine switch, which interacts with the catalytic zinc making it impossible to connect the substrate. The catalytic domain has two zinc ions, three calcium ions, and three histidine residues, which are highly conserved [1–9,11–20]. In the terminal zone of the catalytic domain there is a region that forms the outer wall of the S_1' pocket [1,14,17]. This pocket is the most variable region in MMPs and it is a determining factor for substrate specificity [1,2,6,7,11,17,18]. However, there are six pockets (P_1, P_2, P_3, P_1', P_2', and P_3') and the fragments of the substrates or inhibitors are named depending on the interaction with these pockets (R_1, R_2, R_3, R_1' or R_a, R_2', and R_3'). The linker is proline-rich, of variable length, allowing inter-domain flexibility and enzyme stability [4,8,12,13]. The hemopexin-like domain is necessary for collagen triple helix degradation and is important for substrate specificity [3,4,7,9,19].

Table 1. Matrix metalloproteinases (MMPs) classes.

Class	MMP	
Collagenases	MMP-1, Collagenase-1, Interstitial or Fibroblast collagenases MMP-8, Collagenase-2, or Neutrophil collagenases MMP-13 or Collagenase 3	
Gelatinases	MMP-2 or Gelatinase A MMP-9 or Gelatinase B	
Stromelysin	MMP-3 or Stromelysin-1 MMP-10 or Stromelysin-2 MMP-11	
Matrilysin	MMP-7 MMP-26, Matrilysin-2, or Endometase	
Membrane-type	Type I transmembrane protein	MMP-14 or MT1-MMP MMP-15 or MT2-MMP MMP-16 or MT3-MMP MMP-24 or MT5-MMP
	Glycosylphosphatidylinositol (GPI)-anchored	MMP17 or MT4-MMP MMP-25 or MT6-MMP
Other MMPs	MMP-12 MMP-19 MMP-20 MMP-21 MMP-23 MMP-27 MMP-28	

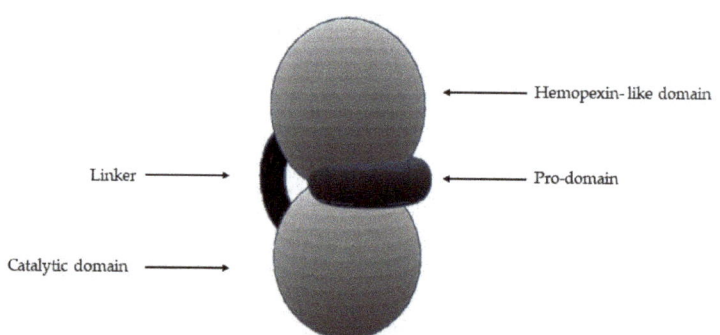

Figure 1. Schematic representation of the general structure of MMP.

The MMPs can process ECM proteins and glycoproteins, membrane receptors, cytokines, hormones, chemokines, adhesion molecules, and growth factors [1,3,4,6,7,9–11,13,14,20–26]. However, the presence and the activity of MMPs have been demonstrated to be intracellular [25,26]. For example, some studies show intracellular localization of MMP-2 in cardiac myocytes and colocalization of MMP-2 with troponin I in cardiac myofilaments [23]. The MMP-2 activity has also been detected in nuclear extracts from human heart and rat liver [23]. The MMPs are involved in many biologic processes, such as tissue repair and remodulation, cellular differentiation, embryogenesis, angiogenesis, cell mobility, morphogenesis, wound healing, inflammatory response, apoptosis, ovulation, and endometrial proliferation [1,2,4,6,8,10,11,13,16–18,20,27]. The deregulation of MMPs activity leads to the progression of various pathologies depending on which enzyme is involved [1,6,10,13–17,20,27]: cancer and metastasis, inflammatory processes, arthritis, ulcers, periodontal diseases, brain degenerative diseases, liver cirrhosis, fibrotic lung diseases, otosclerosis, atherosclerosis, multiple sclerosis, dilated cardiomyopathy, aortic aneurysm, or varicose veins.

Although therapeutic strategies for specific inhibition of MMPs have been long researched, they are difficult to develop because these enzymes are involved in a myriad of pathways [2,5]. However, this inhibition can be done at the biomolecular expression and active enzyme terms [2,5,18]. The MMPs inhibitors can be divided into endogenous inhibitors, which can be specific or non-specific, and synthetic inhibitors [1,2,4,7,10,12–14,16,20,28,29] (Table 2).

Table 2. MMPs inhibitors classification.

	Specific Inhibitor	Tissue Inhibitor of Metalloproteinases (TIMP)
Endogenous inhibitor	Non-specifics inhibitors	α2-macroglobulin Tissue factor pathway inhibitor (TFPI) Membrane-bound β-amyloid precursor protein C-terminal proteinases enhancer protein Reversion-inducing cystein-rich protein with Kasal domain motifs (RECK) GPI-anchored glycoprotein
Synthetic inhibitor		Hydroxamate-based inhibitors Non-hydroxamate-based inhibitors Catalytic domain (non-zinc binding) inhibitors Allosteric and exosite inhibitors Antibody-based inhibitors

2. Specific Endogenous Inhibitor-Tissue Inhibitors of Metalloproteinases (TIMPs)

Tissue inhibitors of metalloproteinases (TIMPs) are endogenous proteins responsible for the regulation of MMPs activity, but also of families such as the disintegrin metalloproteinases (ADAM and with thrombospondin motifs ADAMTS) and therefore for maintaining the physiological balance between ECM degradation and MMPs activity [1,2,8,9,18,30]. There are four TIMPs (TIMP-1, -2, -3, and -4) (Table 3), with 22–29 KDa and 41%–52% sequential similarity [2,4,12,13,16,20,31].

Table 3. Tissue inhibitors of metalloproteinases (TIMPs) classification.

TIMP	Expression	Inhibition	Inhibition Mode
1	Several tissues with transcription inducible by cytokines and hormones	Strong interaction with MMP-1, -2, -3, and -9 Weak interaction with MT1-MMP, MT3-MMP, MT5-MMP, and MMP-19	TIMP-1 forms a complex with pro-MMP-9 by binding to the hemopexin domain
2	Constitutive expression	Strong interaction with MMP-2	TIMP-2 has four residues in the N-terminal domain and an adjacent CD-loop region, which allows interaction between TIMP and the active center of MMP-2
3	In response to mitogenic stimulation and during cell cycle progression	MMP-1, -2, -3, -9, and -13	The inhibition mode is different from the other TIMPs for its unusual localization, as it is largely sequestered into the extracellular matrix or at the cell surface via heparan sulphate proteoglycans
4	Especially abundant in the heart, but is also expressed in injured tissue	MMP-2 and -14	-

TIMPs consist of a N- and C-terminal domain with 125 and 65 amino acids, respectively, each containing six conserved cysteine residues, which form three conserved disulphide bonds [2,4,7–9,12,31,32] (Figure 2a). The N-terminal domain is an independent unit, which can be inhibited by MMPs, in a 1:1 ratio [2,4,8–10,12,13,16,20]. This domain has two groups of four residues: Cys-Thr-Cys-Val and Glu-Ser-Val-Cys (Figure 2b), which are connected by disulphide bounds which are important for TIMP activity [7,12]. This is the main domain responsible for MMP inhibition through its binding to the catalytic site in a substrate-like manner [31]. The several domains allow the TIMP and pro-gelatinases interactions [4].

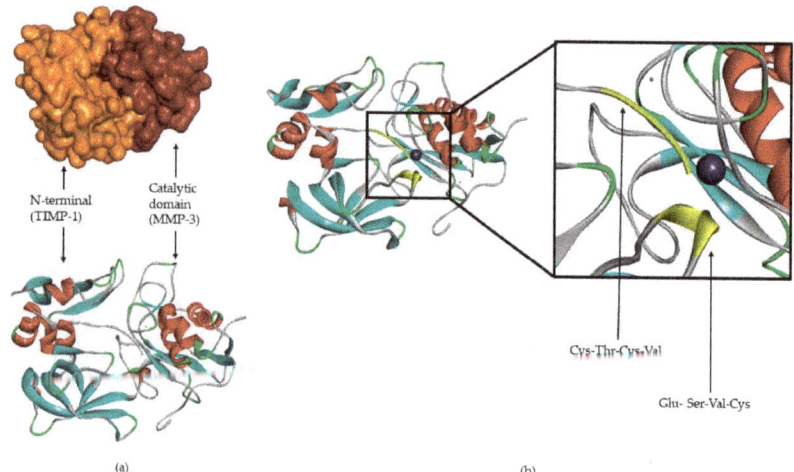

Figure 2. (a) TIMP-1-catalytic domain of the MMP-3 complex. (b) TIMP-1-catalytic domain of the MMP-3 complex, where two conserved groups, Cys-Thr-Cys-Val and Glu-Ser-Val-Cys, are represented in yellow.

3. Non-Specific Endogenous Inhibitors

Non-specific endogenous inhibitors have been reported to inhibit MMPs (Table 4), however, the inhibition mechanism details have only been partially discovered [7,12].

Table 4. Non-specific endogenous inhibitors [4,7,12,13,33,34].

Non-Specific Inhibitor	Inhibition
α2-macroglobulin	MMP-2 and -9
Tissue factor pathway inhibitor	MMP-1 and -2
Membrane-bound β-amyloid precursor protein	MMP-2
C-terminal proteinase enhancer protein	MMP-2
Reversion-inducing-cysteine-rich protein with Kasal motifs (RECK)	MMP-2, -9, and -14
GPI-anchored glycoprotein	-

Human α2-macroglobulin is a glycoprotein with four identical subunits that act by entrapping MMP and the complex is cleared by endocytosis [2]. The α2-macroglobulin has been found in blood and tissue fluid [2,31]. The tissue factor pathway inhibitor (TFPI) is a serine proteinase inhibitor, which targets MMP-1 and -2, but this inhibition mode is still unknown [7,12]. The C-terminal proteinase enhancer protein and tissue factor pathway inhibitor have sequences with certain similarities to the N-terminal domain of TIMPs [31].

4. Synthetic Inhibitors

MMPs are molecular targets for the development of therapeutic and diagnostic agents [14]. The development of synthetic MMP inhibitors was initially based on the peptide sequence, recognized by proteases, with different chemical functionalities, capable of interacting potently with zinc ion [11–13,19]. The requirements for an effective inhibitor are [2,11,13,17,19,35]:

- A functional group able to chelate the zinc ion (II)-zinc binding group (ZBG). The first generation inhibitors used hydroxamate (CONHO⁻) but the second generation use carboxylate (COO⁻), thiolates (S⁻), phosphonyls (PO₂⁻), for example (Figure 3);
- At least one functional group that promotes hydrogen bonding with the protein backbone;
- One or more side chains undergoing Van der Waals interactions with enzyme subsites.

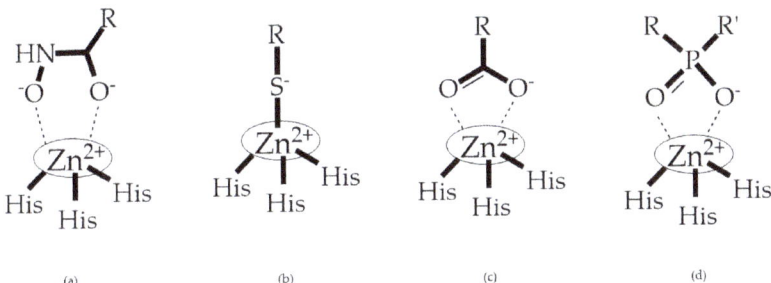

Figure 3. Examples of zinc binding groups (ZBGs). (**a**) Hydroxamate-based inhibitor; (**b**) thiolate-based inhibitor; (**c**) carboxylate-based inhibitor; (**d**) phosphorous-based inhibitor. The R group is the scaffold of inhibitor.

ZBGs have negative charges that prevent their penetration in the cell, restricting their activity to the extracellular space which reduces their cell toxicity [2]. Changes in the ZBG structure or in the point of attachment of the ZBG to the backbone of the MMP inhibitor can change its potency and selectivity [2]. When comparing what selectivity or potency of different ZBGs leaving the structure constant, Castelhano et al. arrived at the following list [36]: hydroxamic acid >> formylhydroxylamine > sulfhydryl > aminocarboxylates > carboxylate.

The selectivity of inhibitor is a primordial goal of MMPs' inhibitors (MMPis) design to increase efficacy and prevent side effects [2]. This selectivity is based on two molecular characteristics [11]: a chelating capacity for catalytic zinc and the presence of hydrophobic bridges of the active center for the S₁' pocket. Numerous strategies have been suggested for creating selective MMP inhibitors [27] (Figure 4): endogenous-like inhibitors, exosite targeting inhibitors, a combination of exosite binding and metal chelating inhibitors, and function-blocking antibodies.

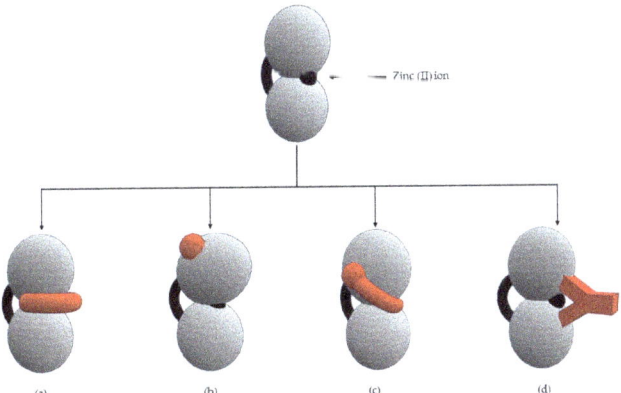

Figure 4. Types of MMPs' inhibitors: (**a**) endogenous-like inhibitors that chelate the catalytic zinc (II) ion; (**b**) exosite targeting inhibitors that alter the conformation of the enzyme; (**c**) a combination of exosite binding and metal chelating inhibitors; (**d**) antibodies inhibitors.

The synthetic inhibitors have had a great challenge in their development since first it is necessary to identify the enzymes that are involved in disease progression. Moreover, this goal has an additional difficulty as there are more than 50 human metalloproteinases (23 MMPs, 13 ADAM, and 19 ADAMTS) [2].

4.1. Hydroxamate-Based Inhibitors

The first generation of MMPis (1995–1999 [16]) were designed based on the knowledge of the triple helix collagen amino acid sequence (cleavage site) and the information derived from specific substrates [6,15,19,31,35,37]. These compounds contain a hydroxamic acid group as ZBG [5,6,15,18,27,28,31,37]. Hydroxamic acids (HA) were first described in 1986 [38,39]. They are easy to synthesize, are monoanionic compounds, bidentate chelating agents, and due the excellent zinc-chelating capability they are the more popular ZBG for MMPs [2,6,17,18,27–29]. The hydroxamic group established interactions with zinc ions, through two oxygens and two hydrogen bonds (NH and OH groups of HA with Ala and Glu, respectively), forming a distorted triangular bipyramid [2,5,18,19,28,29] (Figure 5a). Reich et al., in 1988 [40], used a hydroxamic acid compound, SC-44463 (Figure 5b), to block collagenase and prevent metastasis in a mouse model, which initiated the era of MMP inhibition therapeutics [40].

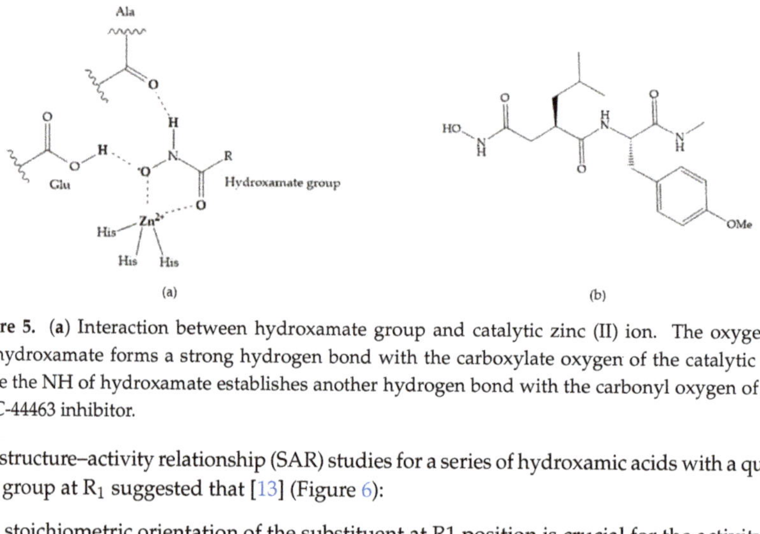

Figure 5. (a) Interaction between hydroxamate group and catalytic zinc (II) ion. The oxygen of the hydroxamate forms a strong hydrogen bond with the carboxylate oxygen of the catalytic Glu, while the NH of hydroxamate establishes another hydrogen bond with the carbonyl oxygen of Ala; (b SC-44463 inhibitor.

The structure–activity relationship (SAR) studies for a series of hydroxamic acids with a quaternary carbonyl group at R_1 suggested that [13] (Figure 6):

(i) The stoichiometric orientation of the substituent at R1 position is crucial for the activity;
(ii) The phenylpropyl group was established as the best substituent at position R1;
(iii) Hydrophobic substituents at R_2' position and N-metiamides at R_3' position were considered as the most appropriate.

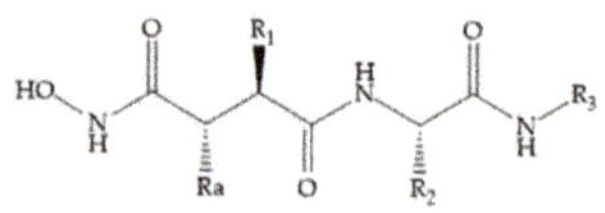

Figure 6. General structure of hydroxamic acid. OH group: catalytic zinc binding group; R_a: α substituent; R1: P_1' substituent group and this group is determinant to selectivity and activity; R_2: P_2' substituent and this substituent can be cyclized with R_a and R_3; R_3: P_3' substituent.

Modification in Ra position (α substituent): a beneficial effect is conferred by lipophilic substituents capable of hydrogen bonding [19]. Analogues of Marimastat have been reported, where the α position is disubstituted by a hydroxyl group and a methyl group [19] (Figure 7a). The X-ray structures of the MMP-3 inhibitor complex showed that there were hydrogen bonds between the hydroxyl group and Ala$_{165}$ [19]. By binding the positions Rα and R$_2$ in a single chain, forming a cyclic inhibitor (Figure 7b), there was a substantial increase in water solubility [19,29,41,42]. This strategy led to the discovery of two inhibitors with similar potency to non-cyclized analogues, SE205 and SC903 [41] (Figure 7c,d).

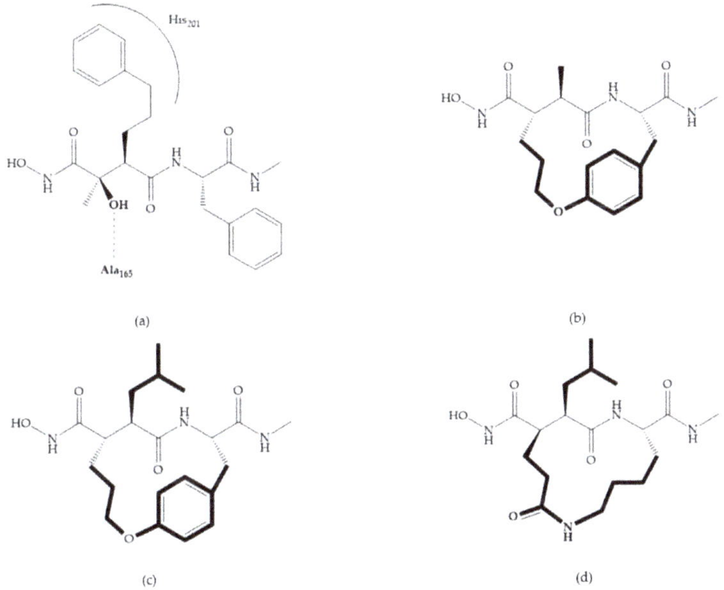

Figure 7. (a) Analogue of Marimastat with the α position disubstituted; (b) analogue of Marimastat with Rα and R$_2$ position connected; (c) SE205; (d) SC903.

The introduction of conformational restrictions through the addition of a three-membered ring between positions α and R$_1$ (Figure 8a) has been reported by Martin et al. [43], and it resulted in reduced inhibition of MMP-9 [43]. However, the introduction of a six-membered ring between these same positions resulted in the inactivity of the compound [19] (Figure 8b).

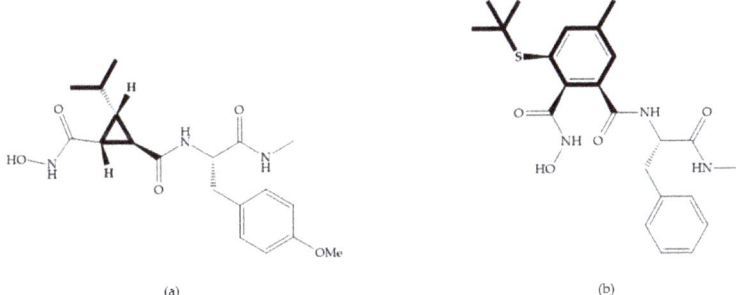

Figure 8. Inhibitors with conformational restrictions between Rα and R$_1$ positions. (a) Inhibitor with three-membered ring; (b) inhibitor with six-membered ring.

Exploring the depth of S$_1$' pocket, bulky groups in Rα position confer selective inhibition for MMP-2, -8, and -9 [29]. An example is the presence of a biphenyl group, which showed higher inhibitory activity against MMP-9 [29].

Modification in R_1 position: the incorporation of long groups in the R_1 position can promote the selectivity of MMPis, since pocket S_1' can undergo conformational changes to accommodate certain substituents [19].

Broadhurst et al. showed that an alkyl chain (C_9) at the R_1 position reduces the inhibition of MMP-1, but maintains the inhibitory activity against MMP-2, -3, and -9 [19] (Figure 9a). For matlystatin derivates in the C_9 chain, R-94138 (Figure 9b) promotes the inhibition against MMP-9 [44]. The succinyl hydroxamates analogues in the C_9 chain promote selectivity for MMP-2, however, a C_{10} chain (Figure 9c) results in MMP-1 inhibition, while a further increase of the chain to C_{16} (Figure 9d) leads to a loss of activity against MMP-1 [19].

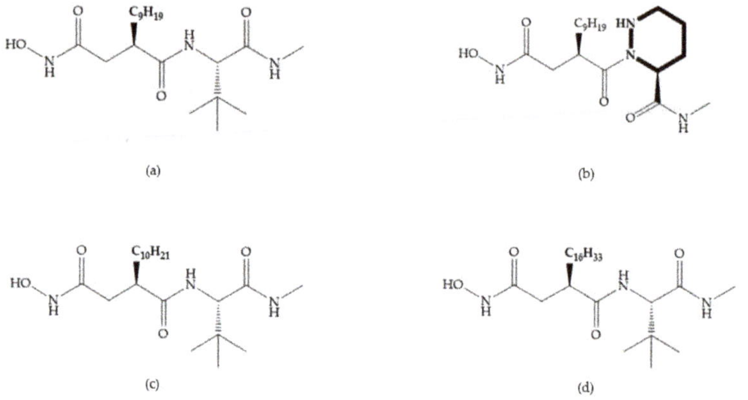

Figure 9. Inhibitors with modification of R_1 position. (a) Inhibitor with alkyl chain. This inhibitor has activity against MMP-2, -3, and -9, but the inhibition of MMP-1 is low; (b) R-94138, Matlystatin derivate. The inhibition of MMP-9 is 10 times higher than analogues with C_8 or C_{10} chains; (c) succinyl hydroxamate analogue with C_{10} chain, which inhibits MMP-1; (d) succinyl hydroxamate analogue with C_{16} chain, which inhibits MMP-1.

Replacement of the R_1-R_2 bond of succinyl hydroxamates acid inhibitors by a sulfonamide bond (Figure 10a) results in substantial loss of inhibitory activity because the hydrogen bond (C=ONH; Figure 10b) with leucine is stronger than the new sulfonyl oxygen bond, due to the pyramidal nature of the sulfonamide [19].

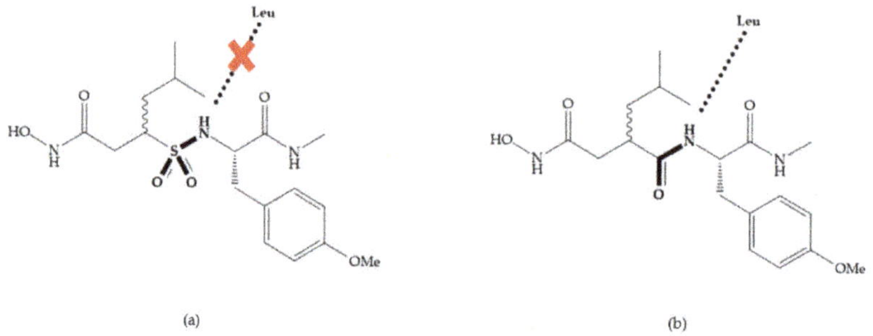

Figure 10. (a) Succinyl hydroxamate acid with a sulphonamide bond. This compound presents low inhibitory activity because of the pyramidal nature of the sulphonamide group. (b) Succinyl hydroxamate acid with carbonyl bond.

Modifications in R_2 position: modifications in the R_2 position led to a modest effect in inhibitory activity, in vitro, and affects the pharmacokinetic properties [29]. Marimastat and Ro31-9790 (Figure 11) have a good oral activity because the bulky tert-butyl group assists the adjacent amide bond during absorption from an aqueous environment to the lipid environment of the cell membrane [45]. The beneficial combination of the tert-butyl group with the α-hydroxyl group increases the water solubility [19,29]. Babine and Bender suggest that the tert butyl as R_2 group leads to less Van der Waals interactions, comparing with other groups [46].

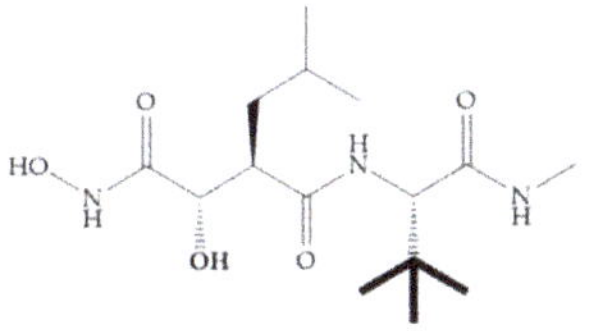

Figure 11. (a) Marimastat. The Ra position is substituted with a hydroxyl group (OH). (b) Ro31-9790. The Ra position has no substituents.

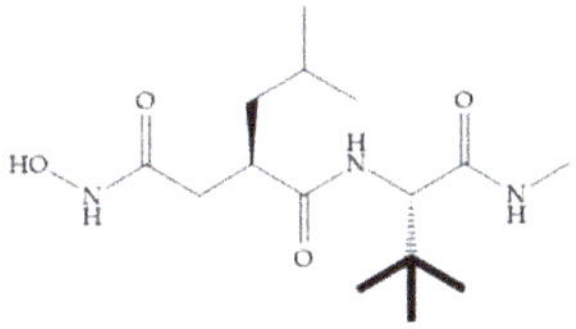

Ikeda et al. described compounds with phenyl R_2 substituents (Figure 12) (KB-R7785), which are active orally, due to the beneficial effect of the R_2 phenyl group on absorption, where the amide shielding and lipophilicity may assist in transepithelial resorption [47]. This inhibitor shows activity against MMP-1 in rats and its effectiveness in arthritis has been demonstrated [47].

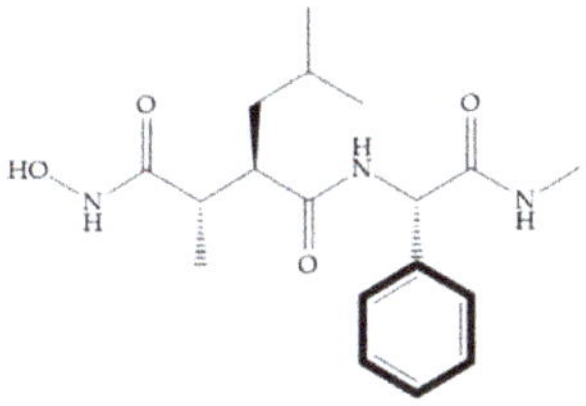

Figure 12. KB-R7785 inhibitor.

Modifications in R_3 position: the S_3' pocket is an open area and several groups can be introduced at the R_3 position [19]. The introduction of the benzhydryl group leads to compounds with selectivity to the MMPs-3 and -7 [19].

4.1.1. Succinyl Hydroxamic Acid-Based Inhibitors

Succinyl hydroxamate derivates can be subdivided to peptide derivatives or non-peptide compounds [48]. The N-acetylcysteine has been reported to affect the tumoral invasion process and metastasis by MMP-2 and -9 inhibition [49]. The L-cysteine-2-phenylethylamide is an effective inhibitor, in which the phenyl group fills the S_1' pocket of MMP-8 [50]. Foley et al. prepared several dipeptides derivatives containing cysteine (**RCO-Cys-AA-NH$_2$**) and concluded [51]:

- The variation of the acyl group and the second amino acid (**AA**) leads to the activity against different MMPs.
- The **R** group interacts with the S_1' pocket.

Batimastat (Table 5) was the first MMPi to enter in clinical trials for cancer as it inhibits MMP-1, -2, -7, and -9, but, due to its poor oral bioavailability, it was superseded by Marimastat [28,29,31] (Table 5), which has an alpha-hydroxyl group increasing the aqueous solubility [29]. Marimastat inhibits the activity of MMP-1, -2, -3, -7, -9, -12, and -13 [31]. However, Marimastat failed in clinical trials due to the absence of a therapeutic effect and the patients treated developed musculoskeletal toxicity (MST) [6,31]. Batimastat, marimastat, and ilomastat are examples of succinyl hydroxamates, which have very analogous structure to that of collagen and inhibit MMPs by bidentate chelation of the Zn^{2+} [2,6,29].

Table 5. Batimastat and Marimastat.

Name	Molecule	α Substituent	Effect
Batimastat	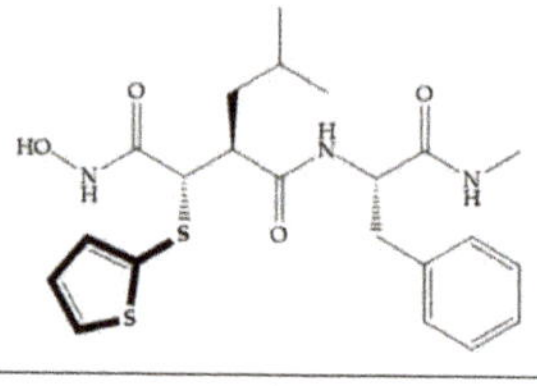	Thienylthiomethylene	Not available orally
Marimastat	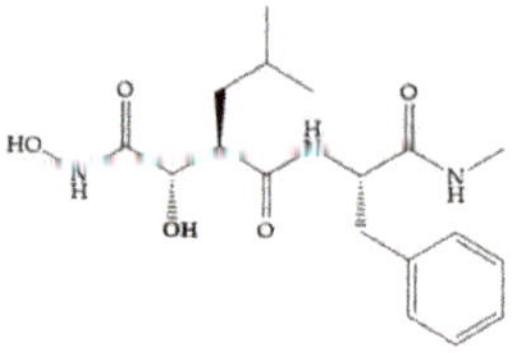	Hydroxyl group (directed to the protein surface, allowing the formation of hydrogen bonds with solvent)	Available orally

Several studies by Jonhson et al. [52] demonstrated that derivatives of succinyl hydroxamic acid (Figure 13a) are more potent for MMP-1 than the corresponding malonyl (Figure 13b) or glutaryl (Figure 13c) derivates.

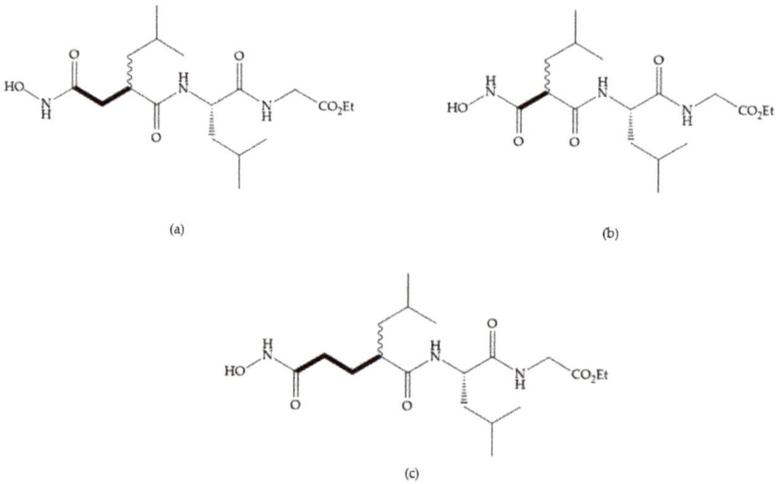

Figure 13. (a) Derivates of succinyl hydroxamic acid; (b) malonyl acid; (c) glutaryl acid.

Marcq et al. [53] developed succinyl hydroxamates derivates selective for MMP-2, by modifications on Ilomastat structure (Figure 14a) to increase the overall hydrophobicity and, consequently, the selectivity [53]. This study resulted in a compound (Figure 14b) with an isobutylidene group of E geometry, which showed a 100-fold greater selectivity for MMP-2 over MMP-3, that is a 70-fold increase compared to Ilomastat [53].

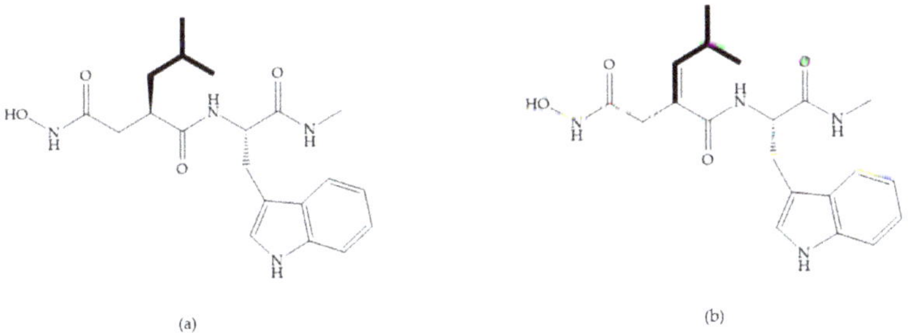

Figure 14. (a) Ilomastat; (b) Ilomastat derivate with isobutylidene group.

Table 6 shows the IC$_{50}$ and Ki values of some succinyl hydroxamic acid-based inhibitors [6,15–19,29,35,37,54,55].

4.1.2. Sulfonamide Hydroxamic Acid-Based Inhibitors

In 1995, Novartis described the CGS-27023A (Figure 15a), a non-peptidic MMP-3 inhibitor, which has good oral availability but did not succeed in clinical trials [56]. The isopropyl group slows down the metabolization of the adjacent hydroxamic acid group and the 3-pyridyl substituent may aid partitioning into the hydrated negatively charged environment of the cartilage [56]. By analysis of the cocrystal structure of this inhibitor and MMP-12, it was possible to conclude that the binding mode between the hydroxamate moiety and the catalytic zinc ion was the same as the binding mode of hydroxamate-based inhibitors [6]. The interaction of CGS-27023A with MMP-3 was possible due to the p-methoxy phenyl substituent occupation of the S$_1$' pocket and the pyridylmethyl and isobutyl groups occupation of the S$_2$' and S$_1$ pockets, respectively [29,56]. The modification of α to form the thioester derivate led to an increase of the inhibition of the deep pocket of the MMPs [29,56] (Figure 15b).

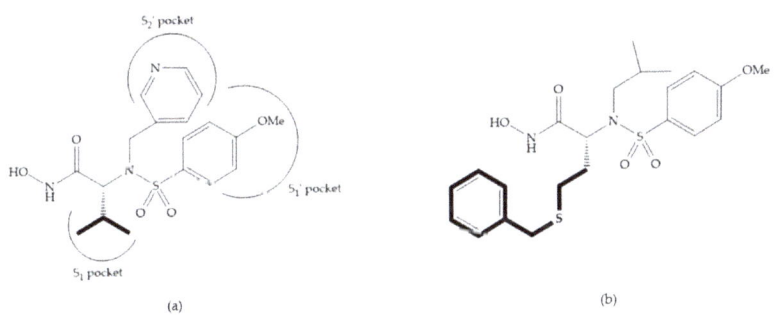

Figure 15. (a) CGS-27023A; (b) thioester derivate of CGS-27023A.

The NNGH (Figure 16a) (N-Isobutyl-N-(4-methoxyphenylsulfonyl)glycyl hydroxamic acid) was the starting point to many potent MMPis and is accommodated in the entry of the S$_1$' pocket, but does not penetrate it [6]. Barta et al. described a series of arylhydroxamate sulphonamides, active against MMP-2 and -13 (Figure 16b) [57]. In this compound, the sulfonyl group formed a single hydrogen bond with Leu$_{160}$ and the piperidine-O-phenyl moiety extends into the S$_1$' pocket by Van der Waals interactions [57]. Noe et al. described a series of 3,3-dimethyl-5-hydroxy pipecolic hydroxamic acid, which possess potent inhibitory activity for MMP-13 [58]. In the first series of compounds, the 3-position of the piperidine ring was explored by the introduction of a polar functionality and it resulted in a compound with excellent activity on MMP-13 (Figure 16c), improved bioavailability, and lower metabolic clearance [58].

Table 6. IC_{50} and K_i values of succinyl hydroxamic acid-based inhibitors.

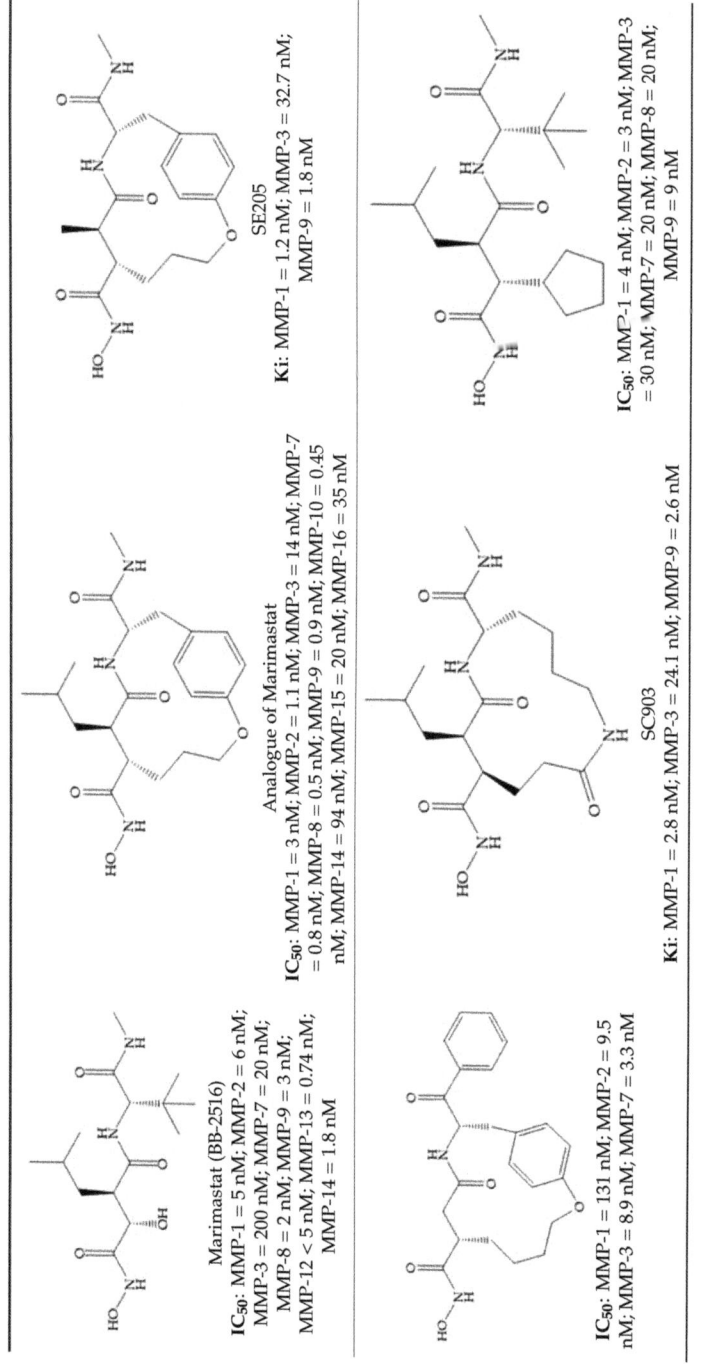

Table 6. Cont.

SC-44463
IC$_{50}$: MMP-1 = 20 nM; MMP-2 = 6 nM; MMP-3 = 30 nM; MMP-7 = 30 nM

BB-16
IC$_{50}$: MMP-1 = 5 nM; MMP-2 = 10 nM; MMP-3 = 40 nM; MMP-7 = 60 nM; MMP-8 = 7 nM

Ro-31-9790
IC$_{50}$: MMP-1 = 10 nM; MMP-2 = 8 nM; MMP-3 = 700 nM; MMP-14 = 1.9 nM

Ro-32-0554
IC$_{50}$: MMP-1 = 0.5 nM; MMP-3 = 9.1 nM; MMP-9 = 4.3 nM

IC$_{50}$: MMP-1 = 10 nM; MMP-2 = 400 nM; MMP-3 = 4.5 μM

Ro-32-3555
K$_i$: MMP-1 = 3 nM; MMP-2 = 154 nM; MMP-3 = 527 nM; MMP-8 = 4 nM; MMP-9 = 59 nM; MMP-13 = 3 nM

Table 6. *Cont.*

IC$_{50}$: MMP-1 = 10 μM	IC$_{50}$: MMP-1 = 29 μM	IC$_{50}$: MMP-1 = 40 nM
K$_i$: MMP-1 = 2 nM; MMP-3 = 3 nM; MMP-9 < 1 nM	Analogue of Marimastat IC$_{50}$: MMP-1 = 1 μM; MMP-2 = 15 nM; MMP-3 = 500 nM; MMP-7 = 10 μM; MMP-8 = 30 nM; MMP-9 = 15 nM	IC$_{50}$: MMP-1 = 9 nM

Table 6. Cont.

Ki: MMP-1 = 1.3 nM; MMP-2 = 1.1 nM; MMP-3 = 187 nM	Ki: MMP-1 = 6.5 nM; MMP-2 = 20 nM; MMP-3 = 240 nM	IC$_{50}$: MMP-1 = 6 nM; MMP-2 = 30 nM; MMP-3 = 40 nM
IC$_{50}$: MMP-1 = 375 nM; MMP-2 < 0.15 nM; MMP-3 = 18 nM; MMP-9 = 1.5 nM	IC$_{50}$: MMP-1 = 20 nM; MMP-2 = 2 nM; MMP-3 = 100 nM; MMP-9 = 2 μM	IC$_{50}$: MMP-2 = 20 nM; MMP-3 = 300 nM; MMP-9 = 1 nM
KB-R7785 IC$_{50}$: MMP-1 = 3 nM; MMP-2 = 7.5 nM; MMP-3 = 1.9 nM; MMP-9 = 3.9 nM	IC$_{50}$: MMP-1 = 5.4 nM; MMP-2 = 8.4 nM; MMP-3 = 2.3 nM; MMP-9 = 5 nM; MMP-14 = 2.3 nM	IC$_{50}$: MMP-1 = 5 nM; MMP-2 = 1 nM; MMP-3 = 15 nM; MMP-9 = 1 nM

Table 6. *Cont.*

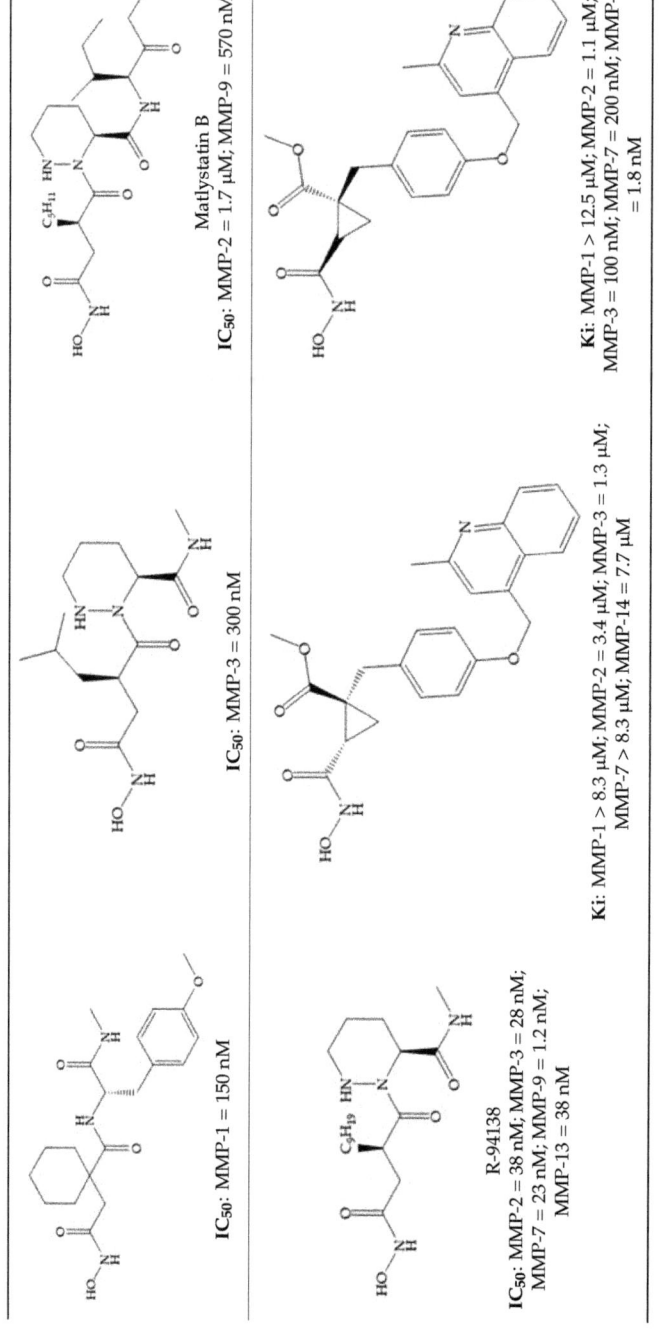

Table 6. *Cont.*

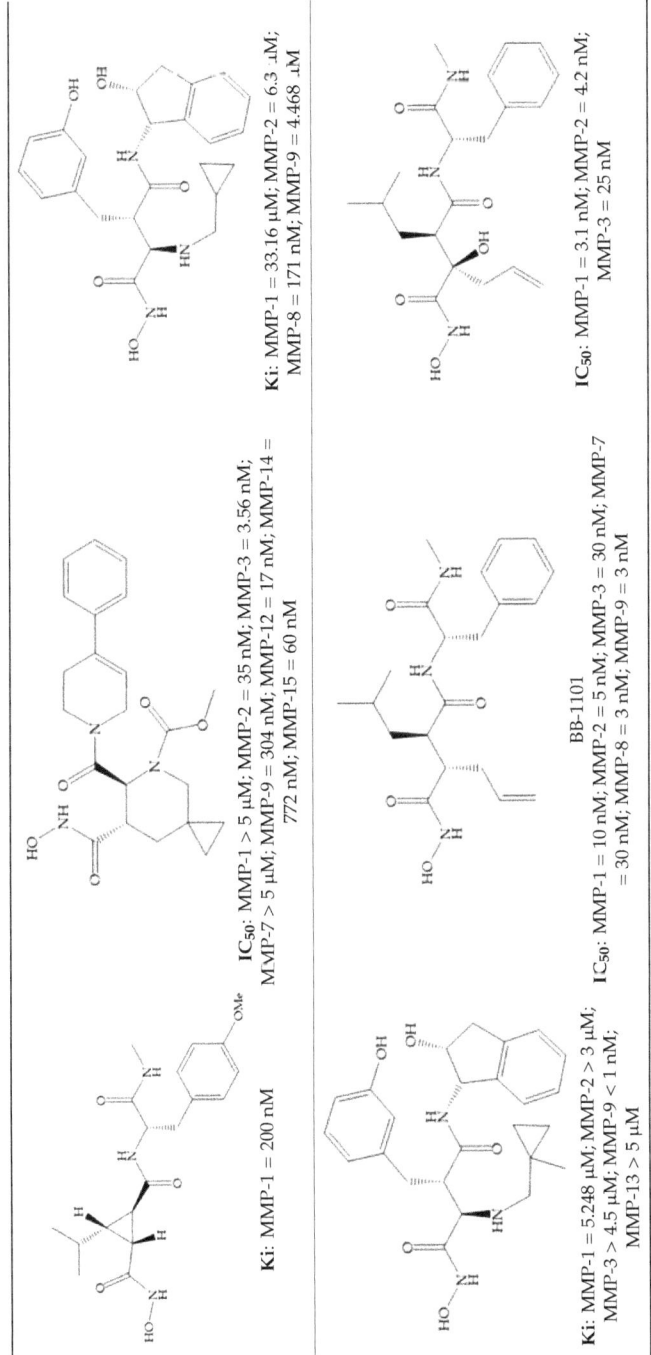

Ki: MMP-1 = 200 nM

IC$_{50}$: MMP-1 > 5 µM; MMP-2 = 35 nM; MMP-3 = 3.56 nM; MMP-7 > 5 µM; MMP-9 = 304 nM; MMP-12 = 17 nM; MMP-14 = 772 nM; MMP-15 = 60 nM

Ki: MMP-1 = 33.16 µM; MMP-2 = 6.3 µM; MMP-8 = 171 nM; MMP-9 = 4.468 µM

Ki: MMP-1 = 5.248 µM; MMP-2 > 3 µM; MMP-3 > 4.5 µM; MMP-9 < 1 nM; MMP-13 > 5 µM

BB-1101
IC$_{50}$: MMP-1 = 10 nM; MMP-2 = 5 nM; MMP-3 = 30 nM; MMP-7 = 30 nM; MMP-8 = 3 nM; MMP-9 = 3 nM

IC$_{50}$: MMP-1 = 3.1 nM; MMP-2 = 4.2 nM; MMP-3 = 25 nM

Table 6. *Cont.*

IC$_{50}$: MMP-1 = 1.1 nM; MMP-2 = 1.1 nM; MMP-3 = 2.3 nM; MMP-7 = 2.2 nM

IC$_{50}$: MMP-1 = 700 nM; MMP-2 = 5 µM; MMP-3 = 2 µM; MMP-9 = 500 nM

OPB-3206

IC$_{50}$: MMP-8 = 300 nM

Batimastat (BB-94)
IC$_{50}$: MMP-1 = 3 nM; MMP-2 = 4 nM; MMP-3 = 20 nM; MMP-7 = 6 nM; MMP-8 = 10 nM; MMP-9 = 1 nM; MMP-13 = 1 nM; MMP-14 = 2.8 nM
Ki: MMP-1 = 10 nM; MMP-2 = 4 nM; MMP-3 = 20 nM; MMP-8 = 10 nM; MMP-9 = 1 nM

Ilomastat (GM6001; Galardin®)
IC$_{50}$: MMP-1 = 0.4 nM; MMP-2 = 0.4 nM; MMP-3 = 0.19 nM; MMP-14 = 5.2 nM
Ki: MMP-1 = 0.4 nM; MMP-2 = 0.39 nM; MMP-3 = 26 nM; MMP-8 = 0.18 nM; MMP-9 = 0.2 nM

Analogue of Ilomastat
IC$_{50}$: MMP-2 = 1.3 nM; MMP-3 = 179 nM

Table 6. *Cont.*

IC$_{50}$: MMP-1 = 3 nM; MMP-3 = 280 nM; MMP-7 = 18 nM	K$_i$: MMP-1 = 3 nM	IC$_{50}$: MMP-1 = 8 µM; MMP-2 = 8 µM; MMP-3 = 3.5 µM
IC$_{50}$: MMP-1 = 3.3 µM; MMP-2 = 32 nM; MMP-3 = 57 nM	IC$_{50}$: MMP-3 = 3.4 µM	IC$_{50}$: MMP-3 = 15 nM
IC$_{50}$: MMP-1 > 50 µM; MMP-2 > 120 µM; MMP-3 = 80 µM; MMP-8 > 120 µM	IC$_{50}$: MMP-2 = 52 µM; MMP-3 = 200 µM; MMP-8 = 1200 µM	IC$_{50}$: MMP-8 = 121 µM

Table 6. Cont.

PKF 242-484
Ki: MMP-1 = 3.6 nM; MMP-2 = 0.1 nM; MMP-3 = 0.9 nM; MMP-9 = 1 nM; MMP-13 = 4.5 nM

CT1746
Ki: MMP-1 = 122 nM; MMP-2 = 0.04 nM; MMP-3 = 10.9 nM; MMP-7 = 136 nM; MMP-9 = 0.17 nM

ONO-4817
IC$_{50}$: MMP-1 = 1600 nM; MMP-9 = 2.1 nM;
Ki: MMP-2 = 0.73 nM; MMP-3 = 42 nM; MMP-7 = 2500 nM; MMP-12 = 0.45 nM; MMP-13 = 1.1 nM

AS 111793#
IC$_{50}$: MMP-1 = 20 nM

MMPI-I
IC$_{50}$: MMP-1 = 1 μM; MMP-3 = 150 μM; MMP-8 = 1 μM; MMP-9 = 30 μM

Table 6. Cont.

IC$_{50}$: MMP-1 = 0.1 nM; MMP-3 = 9 nM; MMP-8 = 0.4 nM; MMP-9 = 0.2 nM

IC$_{50}$: MMP-1 = 30 nM; MMP-2 = 20 nM; MMP-3 = 500 nM; MMP-7 = 200 nM; MMP-8 = 20 nM

K$_i$: MMP-1 = 1450 nM; MMP-3 = 15 nM; MMP-8 = 2 nM; MMP-9 = 3 nM

K$_i$: MMP-1 = 8 nM; MMP-3 = 28 nM; MMP-8 < 2 nM; MMP-9 = 1 nM

IC$_{50}$: MMP-1 = 100 nM; MMP-2 = 0.07 nM; MMP-3 = 3 nM; MMP-7 = 700 nM; MMP-8 = 4 nM; MMP-9 = 1 nM

Table 6. *Cont.*

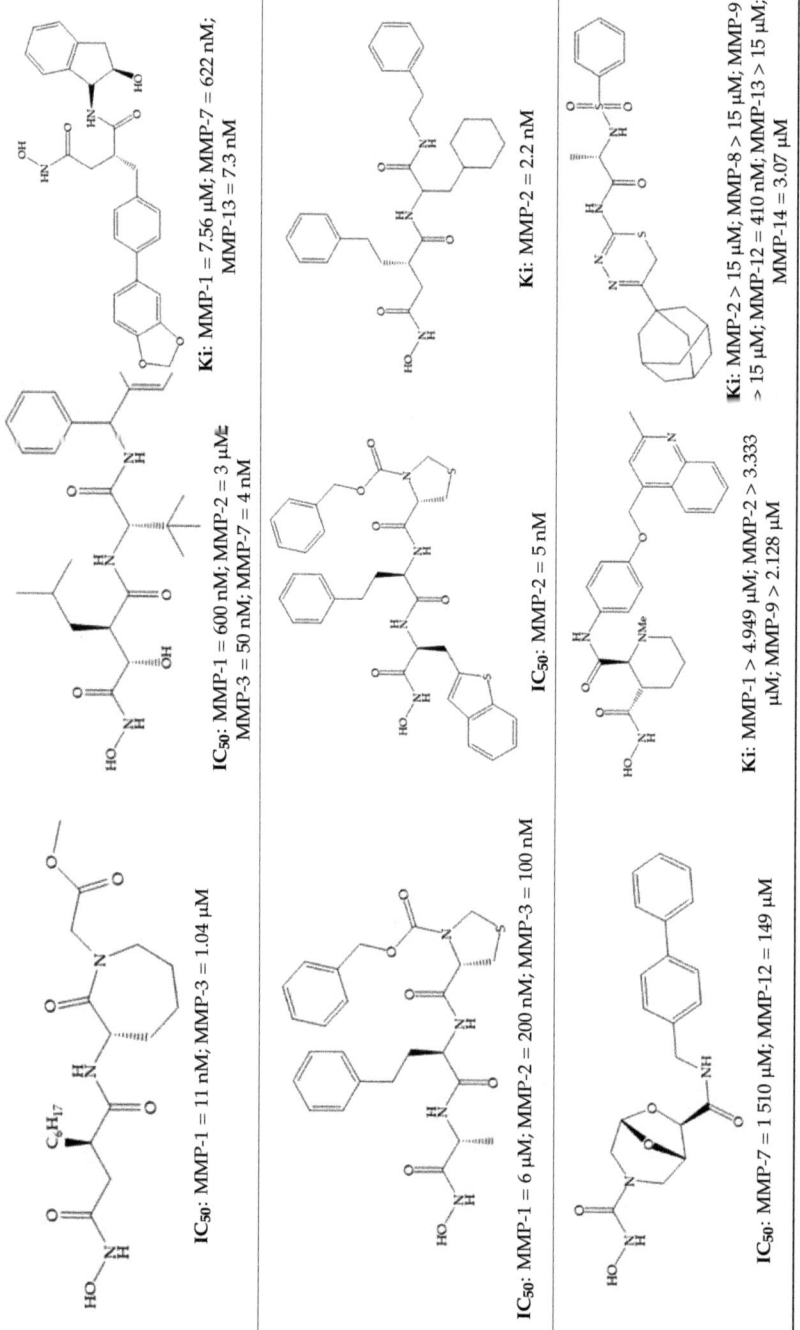

Table 6. *Cont.*

		IC$_{50}$: MMP-1 = 5.9 µM; MMP-2 = 750 nM; MMP-3 = 2.1 nM; MMP-9 = 560 nM; MMP-14 = 930 nM
	IC$_{50}$: MMP-1 = 51 µM; MMP-2 = 1.79 µM; MMP-3 = 5.9 nM; MMP-9 = 840 nM; MMP-13 = 73 nM; MMP-14 = 1.9 µM	
		K$_i$: MMP-1 > 4.946 µM; MMP-2 > 3.333 µM; MMP-3 > 4.501 µM; MMP-7 > 6.368 µM; MMP-8 > 3.058 µM; MMP-9 > 2.128 µM; MMP-10 > 5.346 µM; MMP-12 > 6.023 µM; MMP-13 > 5.025 µM; MMP-14 > 5.290 µM; MMP-15 > 7.088 µM
IC$_{50}$: MMP-1 = 4.6 µM; MMP-2 = 4 nM; MMP-3 = 42 nM; MMP-7 > 10 µM; MMP-9 = 120 nM	K$_i$: MMP-1 > 4.494 µM; MMP-2 > 3.333 µM; MMP-3 = 82 nM; MMP-7 = 25 nM; MMP-8 > 3.1 µM; MMP-9 > 2.128 µM; MMP-13 > 5.025 µM; MMP-14 > 5.290 µM; MMP-15 > 7.088 µM; MMP-16 > 5.554 µM	K$_i$: MMP-1 > 5 µM; MMP-2 > 3 µM; MMP-3 = 762 nM; MMP-8 = 2.05 µM; MMP-9 > 3 µM; MMP-10 > 1.650 µM; MMP-13 > 5 µM; MMP-14 = 163 nM; MMP-15 = 1.7 µM

Table 6. *Cont.*

Ki: MMP-1 = 39 µM; MMP-2 = 2.05 µM; MMP-3 = 141 nM; MMP-7 = 259 nM; MMP-8 = 257 nM; MMP-9 = 10.34 µM; MMP-13 = 1.417 µM; MMP-14 = 15.372 µM; MMP-15 = 3.997 µM; MMP-16 = 1.599 µM

Ki: MMP-1 > 2 µM; MMP-2 > 2 µM; MMP-3 > 2 µM; MMP-7 = 834 nM; MMP-8 = 126 nM; MMP-9 > 2 µM; MMP-10 > 2 µM; MMP-12 > 2 µM; MMP-13 = 653 nM; MMP-14 > 2 µM; MMP-15 > 2 µM; MMP-16 > 2 µM

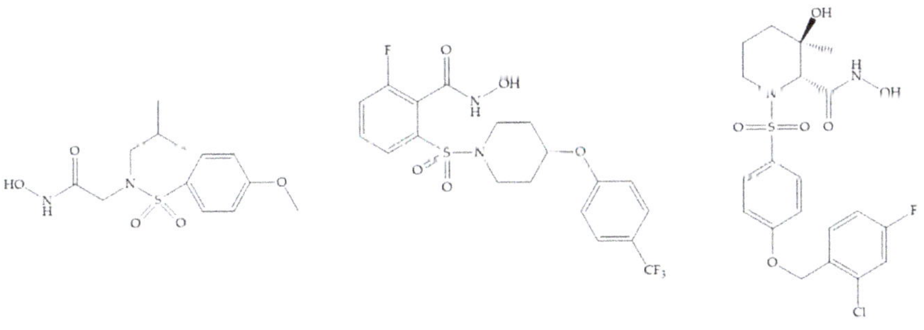

Figure 16. (a) NNGH; (b) arylhydroxamate sulphonamide compound; (c) 3-hydroxy-3-methylpipecolic hydroxamates.

The incorporation of a cyclic quaternary center α led to a strong inhibitory effect against MMP-1, -2, -3, -8, -9, -12, and -13 [29]. The RS-113,456 (Figure 17a) is an inhibitor with better oral bioavailability and metabolic stability compared to the hydroxamate derivates [35]. These two features were improved by shifting the cyclic group to the α-position of the hydroxamic acid (Figure 17b) [29].

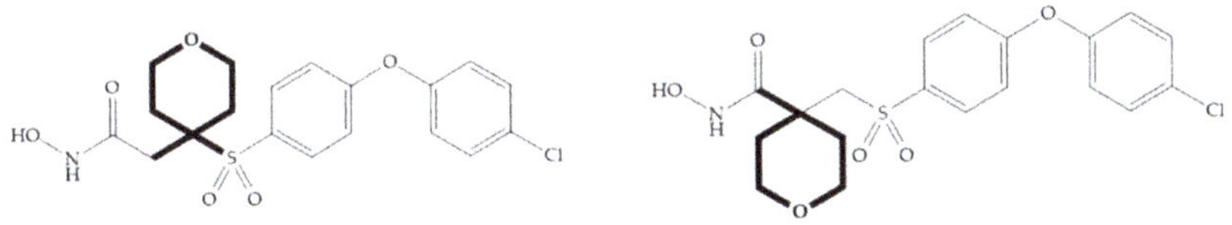

Figure 17. (a) RS-113,456; (b) RS-130,830.

Table 7 shows the IC_{50} and K_i values of some sulfonamide hydroxamic acid-based inhibitors [6,15–19,29,35,37,54,55].

4.1.3. Phosphamides Hydroxamic Acid-Based Inhibitors

The hydroxamic acids based on phosphamides are effective as MMPis due to the electronic environment of the phosphor atom [11]. The replacement of sulphonamide group by phosphinamide group leads to a potent inhibitor of MMP-3 (Figure 18), the collagenases and gelatinases [29]. The interactions between this inhibitor and the MMP-3 are realized by the phosphinamide phenyl group, that accommodates into the S_1' pocket and by the phosphinamide oxygen, which establishes the hydrogen bonds with NH of Leu_{164} and Ala_{165} [29]. However, this group is susceptible to hydrolysis at low pH, limiting the inhibitory activity [29].

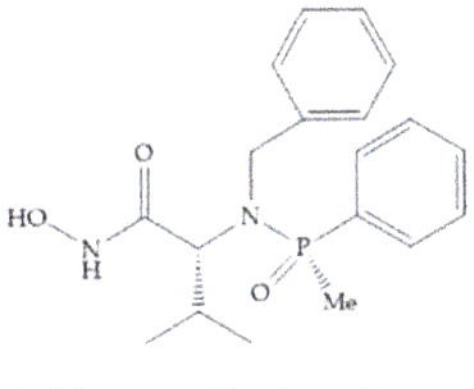

Figure 18. Inhibitor with phosphinamide group.

Table 7. IC_{50} and K_i values of sulfonamide hydroxamic acid-based inhibitors.

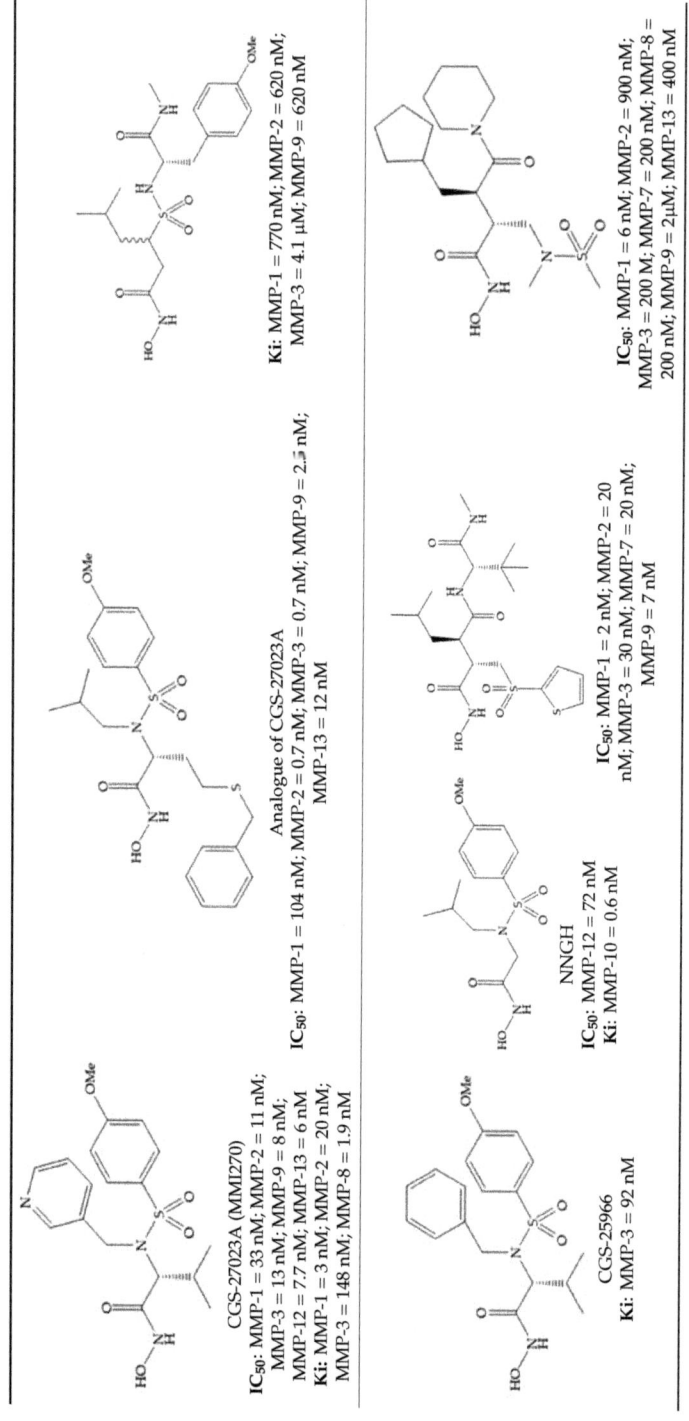

Table 7. *Cont.*

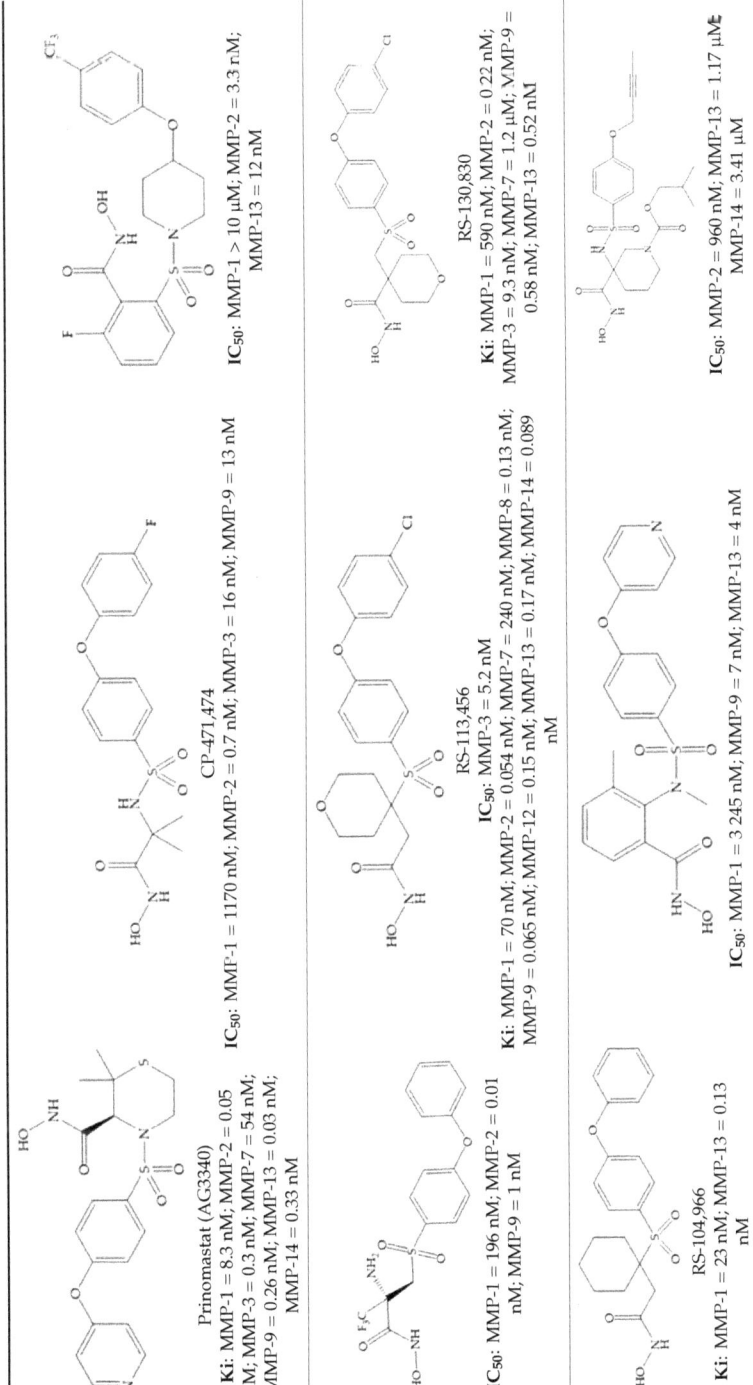

133

Table 7. Cont.

IC$_{50}$: MMP-1 = 763 nM; MMP-9 = 2 nM; MMP-13 = 2 nM

IC$_{50}$: MMP-1 = 841 nM; MMP-9 = 33 nM; MMP-13 = 29 nM

IC$_{50}$: MMP-1 = 920 nM; MMP-13 = 0.95 nM

IC$_{50}$: MMP-1 = 310 nM

IC$_{50}$: MMP-1 = 346 μM; MMP-9 = 24 μM

Ro-32-7315
IC$_{50}$: MMP-1 = 500 nM; MMP-2 = 250 nM; MMP-3 = 210 nM; MMP-7 = 310 nM; MMP-9 = 100 nM; MMP-12 = 11 nM; MMP-13 = 110 nM

MMP-8 inhibitor I
IC$_{50}$: MMP-8 = 4 nM

Table 7. *Cont.*

PGE-4410186
IC$_{50}$: MMP-1 = 24 nM; MMP-3 = 18.4 nM; MMP-7 = 30 nM; MMP-9 = 2.7 nM

IC$_{50}$: MMP-1 = 1.05 nM; MMP-9 = 5 nM; MMP-13 = 113 nM

MMP-9 inhibitor I

K$_i$: MMP-1 = 1.085 µM; MMP-2 = 1 nM; MMP-9 = 10 nM; MMP-13 = 3 nM

MMPI-II (MMP-2/MMP-9 inhibitor II)
IC$_{50}$: MMP-1 = 970 nM; MMP-2 = 17 nM; MMP-3 > 1000 nM; MMP-7 = 800 nM; MMP-9 = 30 nM; MMP-14 = 17 nM

IC$_{50}$: MMP-1 > 50 µM; MMP-2 = 12 nM; MMP-3 = 4.5 µM; MMP-7 > 50 µM; MMP-9 = 200 nM

IC$_{50}$: MMP-1 = 147 nM; MMP-2 = 0.09 nM; MMP-3 = 50 nM; MMP-7 > 1 µM; MMP-8 = 1.6 nM; MMP-9 = 6.7 nM; MMP-14 = 9.8 nM

Table 7. *Cont.*

Ki: MMP-1 = 2 µM; MMP-2 = 10 nM; MMP-3 = 500 nM

IC₅₀: MMP-1 = 200 nM; MMP-9 = 0.43 nM

IC₅₀: MMP-1 = 2.471 µM; MMP-7 = 961 nM; MMP-8 = 35 nM; MMP-9 = 777 nM; MMP-13 = 96 nM; MMP-14 = 582 nM

IC₅₀: MMP-1 = 37.3 µM; MMP-2 = 664 nM; MMP-9 = 5.5 µM; MMP-13 = 2.277 µM; MMP-14 = 24 µM

IC₅₀: MMP-1 = 8.78 µM; MMP-2 = 355 nM; MMP-9 = 1.67 µM; MMP-13 = 230 nM; MMP-14 = 4.71 µM

Ki: *S* enantiomer) MMP-3 = 19 nM (*R* enantiomer) MMP-3 = 36 nM

IC₅₀: MMP-1 = 2.268 µM; MMP-9 = 152 nM; MMP-13 = 18 nM

IC₅₀: MMP-1 = 14 µM; MMP-2 = 529 nM; MMP-3 = 1 nM; MMP-9 = 2.42 µM; MMP-14 = 20.1 µM

All hydroxamate-based inhibitors are very potent and they inhibit MMPs at low concentrations [18]. On the other hand, the hydroxamate acids have poor oral bioavailability, inhibit multiple MMPs, and cause side effects [2,17,27,28,35]. Additionally, this functional group may be metabolized via dehydroxylation or may be cleaved by endopeptidases and releasing hydroxylamine, can be hydrolyzed to carboxylic acids or reduced to O-glucuronyl or O-sulfate, leading to decreased effective inhibitor concentration and reducing its potency in vivo [18,27,28,35].

Table 8 shows the IC_{50} and Ki values of some phosphamides hydroxamic acid-based inhibitor [6,15–19,29,35,37,54,55].

Table 8. IC_{50} and Ki values of phosphamides hydroxamic acid-based inhibitors.

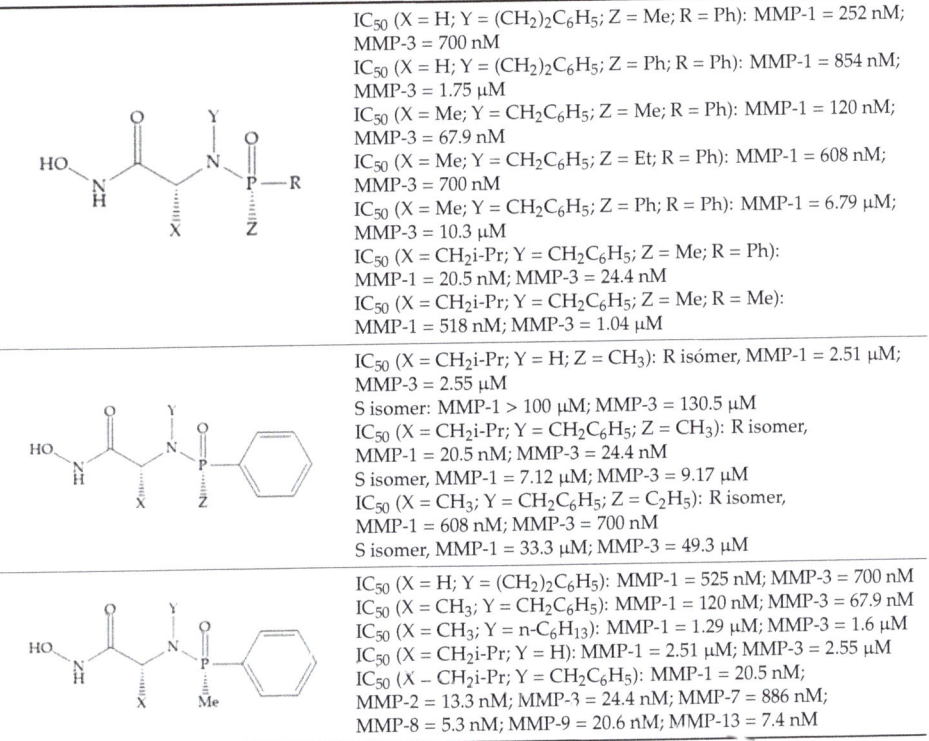

Structure	IC_{50} values
(top structure)	IC_{50} (X = H; Y = (CH$_2$)$_2$C$_6$H$_5$; Z = Me; R = Ph): MMP-1 = 252 nM; MMP-3 = 700 nM IC_{50} (X = H; Y = (CH$_2$)$_2$C$_6$H$_5$; Z = Ph; R = Ph): MMP-1 = 854 nM; MMP-3 = 1.75 µM IC_{50} (X = Me; Y = CH$_2$C$_6$H$_5$; Z = Me; R = Ph): MMP-1 = 120 nM; MMP-3 = 67.9 nM IC_{50} (X = Me; Y = CH$_2$C$_6$H$_5$; Z = Et; R = Ph): MMP-1 = 608 nM; MMP-3 = 700 nM IC_{50} (X = Me; Y = CH$_2$C$_6$H$_5$; Z = Ph; R = Ph): MMP-1 = 6.79 µM; MMP-3 = 10.3 µM IC_{50} (X = CH$_2$i-Pr; Y = CH$_2$C$_6$H$_5$; Z = Me; R = Ph): MMP-1 = 20.5 nM; MMP-3 = 24.4 nM IC_{50} (X = CH$_2$i-Pr; Y = CH$_2$C$_6$H$_5$; Z = Me; R = Me): MMP-1 = 518 nM; MMP-3 = 1.04 µM
(middle structure)	IC_{50} (X = CH$_2$i-Pr; Y = H; Z = CH$_3$): R isómer, MMP-1 = 2.51 µM; MMP-3 = 2.55 µM S isomer: MMP-1 > 100 µM; MMP-3 = 130.5 µM IC_{50} (X = CH$_2$i-Pr; Y = CH$_2$C$_6$H$_5$; Z = CH$_3$): R isomer, MMP-1 = 20.5 nM; MMP-3 = 24.4 nM S isomer, MMP-1 = 7.12 µM; MMP-3 = 9.17 µM IC_{50} (X = CH$_3$; Y = CH$_2$C$_6$H$_5$; Z = C$_2$H$_5$): R isomer, MMP-1 = 608 nM; MMP-3 = 700 nM S isomer, MMP-1 = 33.3 µM; MMP-3 = 49.3 µM
(bottom structure)	IC_{50} (X = H; Y = (CH$_2$)$_2$C$_6$H$_5$): MMP-1 = 525 nM; MMP-3 = 700 nM IC_{50} (X = CH$_3$; Y = CH$_2$C$_6$H$_5$): MMP-1 = 120 nM; MMP-3 = 67.9 nM IC_{50} (X = CH$_3$; Y = n-C$_6$H$_{13}$): MMP-1 = 1.29 µM; MMP-3 = 1.6 µM IC_{50} (X = CH$_2$i-Pr; Y = H): MMP-1 = 2.51 µM; MMP-3 = 2.55 µM IC_{50} (X – CH$_2$i-Pr; Y = CH$_2$C$_6$H$_5$): MMP-1 = 20.5 nM; MMP-2 = 13.3 nM; MMP-3 = 24.4 nM; MMP-7 = 886 nM; MMP-8 = 5.3 nM; MMP-9 = 20.6 nM; MMP-13 = 7.4 nM

4.2. Non-Hydroxamate-Based Inhibitors

The side effects caused by hydroxamate-based inhibitors, due to the lack of selectivity and in vivo lability, have been fostering the development of new compounds with alternative ZBGs [5,6,11,16,17,27–29]. The second generation of MMPis (1999–2003 [16]) was designed with a wide variety of peptidomimetic and non-peptidomimetic structures with higher selectivity and exploiting the deep S_1' pocket present in some MMPs [6,15,16,18,59–61]. These compounds include carboxylic acids, sulfonylhydrazides, thiols, aminomethyl benzimidazole, phosphorous-based, nitrogen-based and heterocycles bidentate chelators, and can be monodentade, bidentade, and tridentade chelates [2,6,18,28,29].

The non-hydroxamate-based inhibitors open up a wide spectrum of affinities for the zinc ion from the catalytic site and new opportunities for targeting and inhibiting the active center [18,28]. They have weak Zn^{2+} chelating ability and the rates of severe side effects, such as the musculoskeletal syndrome (MSS) decreased dramatically compared with the hydroxamate inhibitors [28].

4.2.1. Thiolates-Based Inhibitors

The ability of the monodentate binding of thiols to zinc ion in proenzymes has served as inspiration for the design of several MMPis [5,29]. The potency of thiol inhibitors is intermediate between that of hydroxamate- and carboxylate- based inhibitors [29]. The first example of inhibitor thiol-based for MMP-1 is a bipeptidic analogue, where the incorporation of a thiol group as α substituent leads to improvement of activity (Figure 19a) [19]. Derivates with "linker" substituent between P_1-P_1' positions show a total loss of activity (Figure 19b) [19,62]. On the contrary incorporation of a methyl carboxylate group leads to a significant increase in activity (Figure 19c) [19]. The increased activity of these compounds may be a consequence of beneficial interactions between S_1, the carbonyl ester, and the thiol group, participating in the bidentate coordination of the zinc [19].

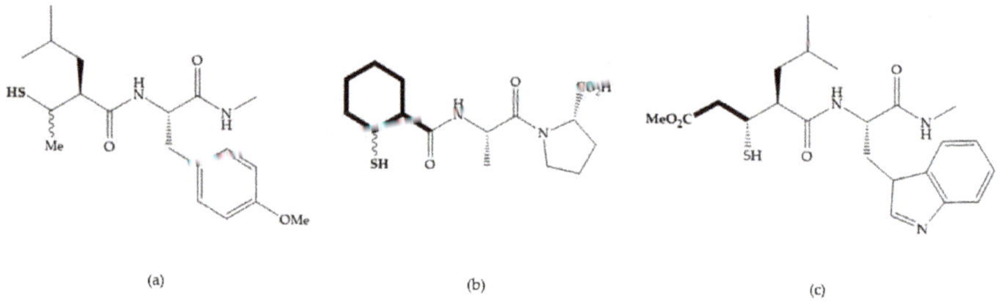

Figure 19. (a) Thiol-based inhibitor with the thiol group as α-substituent. The stoichiometric is S when the thiol group is present. In its absence, the compound with R stoichiometric is more active than the S analogue; (b) thiol-based inhibitor with "linker" substituent; (c) thiol-based inhibitor with methyl carboxylate group.

Montana et al. have identified a series of inhibitors with mercaptoacyl, obtaining moderate inhibitors (Figure 20a) against a wide variety of enzymes with a deep pocket shown to be orally active in mouse models with arthritis [63]. The thiol and acyl carbonyl groups could cooperate in binding to the zinc of the active site [63]. Warshasky et al. have produced a variety of compounds in the Montana series, in which the amide nitrogen P_2' is linked to the group P_1' (Figure 20b) [19].

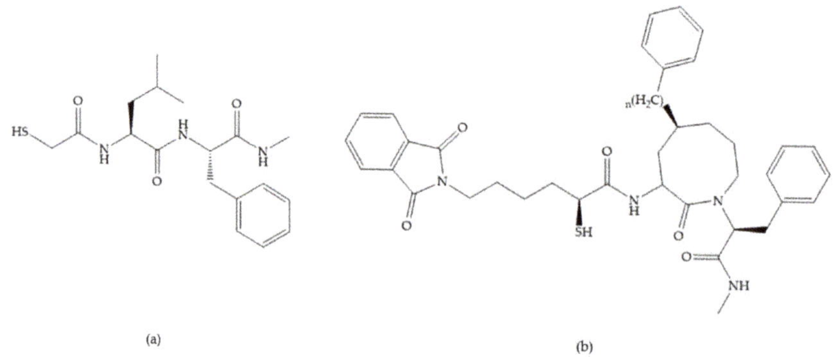

Figure 20. (a) Inhibitor with mercaptoacyl, where the thiol and acyl carbonyl groups could cooperate in binding to the zinc ion. (b) Variant of Montana compounds. n = 0, the compound does not have activity against MMPs-2, 3, and -12. n = 1, the compound has low activity against MMP-3.

The β-mercaptoacilamide represented in Figure 21 is active against the MMP-9 in vitro and exhibits oral activity in rats [19]. The 4-alcoxy substituent of cyclohexane group improved the activity against all MMPs [19]. Replacement of the 4-ethoxy substituent with 4-propyloxy leads to a significant reduction in MMP-1 activity and improves selectivity for MMP-3 [19]. The equivalent cyclopentyl compounds are inactive [19]. The mercaptoamide is unstable in solution hence, to overcome this issue, Campbell and Levin have prepared a series of mercaptoalcohols and mercaptoketones inhibitors [64]. The mercaptoalcohols have exhibited modest activity against MMP-1, -3, and -9, while the equivalent mercaptoketones could be optimized to active broad-spectrum inhibitors [64].

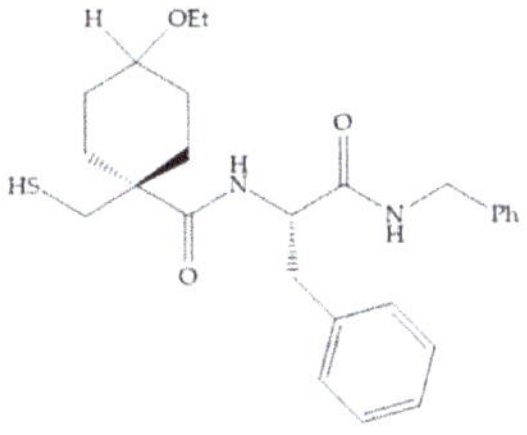

Figure 21. β-mercaptoacilamide inhibitor.

In 2005, Hurst et al. [65] reported a series of mercaptosulphides inhibitors that targeted MMP-1 [65]. The structure–activity relationship indicates that the five-membered ring increases the stability of the inhibitor compared to the linear structure, which can be quickly oxidized and lose its potency [65].

Table 9 shows the IC_{50} and Ki values of some thiolates-based inhibitors [6,15–19,29,35,37,54,55].

4.2.2. Carboxylates-Based Inhibitors

The carboxylic inhibitors are synthetic precursors of the more popular hydroxamates yet they are weaker zinc (II) ligands than hydroxamates [17,27] and monodentate chelate [27]. Carboxylic acid is present in several MMPis that contain large lipophilic groups, such as biphenyls, since they fit in the S_1' pocket [5,6]. These ZBGs are particularly appreciated for their high stability in vivo and their great positive effects on solubility, bioavailability, and selective properties [5,17]. The hydroxamate-based inhibitors are more potent in physiological conditions than carboxylate inhibitors, due to differences in acidity constants [29]. The carboxylate inhibitors bind more tightly to MMPs at low pH, while hydroxamate-based ones have a wider range of pH from 5 to 8 [29]. Fray et al. [66] compared the inhibition profiles of hydroxamates and carboxylic inhibitors (Figure 21a) and observed that the substitution of a carboxylate by a hydroxamate causes a 10-fold increase in potency of the inhibitor towards MMP-3 but decreases the selectivity against MMP-1, -2, -9, and -14 [66]. This effect is attributed to the fact that the strong zinc (II) affinity to the hydroxamic acid group is the main determinant of the binding energy, while in carboxylates this energy relies to a bigger extent on specific interactions with the specific pockets [66].

Hagmann et al. [67] described a series with N-carboxyalkyl group substituents, which presented inhibition for MMP-1, -2, and -3 [67] (Figure 21b). However, the substitution of the phenethyl group, in P_1' position, for a linear alkyl chain removes the inhibitory activity for MMP-1 but it does not affect the activity for MMP-2 and -3 [67]. A similar effect was achieved by the 4-substitution of the phenyl ring of the phenethyl group with a small linear alkyl group [67] (Figure 22b). A similar range of P3' esters has been identified with "phthalamidobutyl" (Figure 22b), increasing activity against MMP-3 and further increasing selectivity [67].

Table 9. IC$_{50}$ and Ki values of thiolates-based inhibitors.

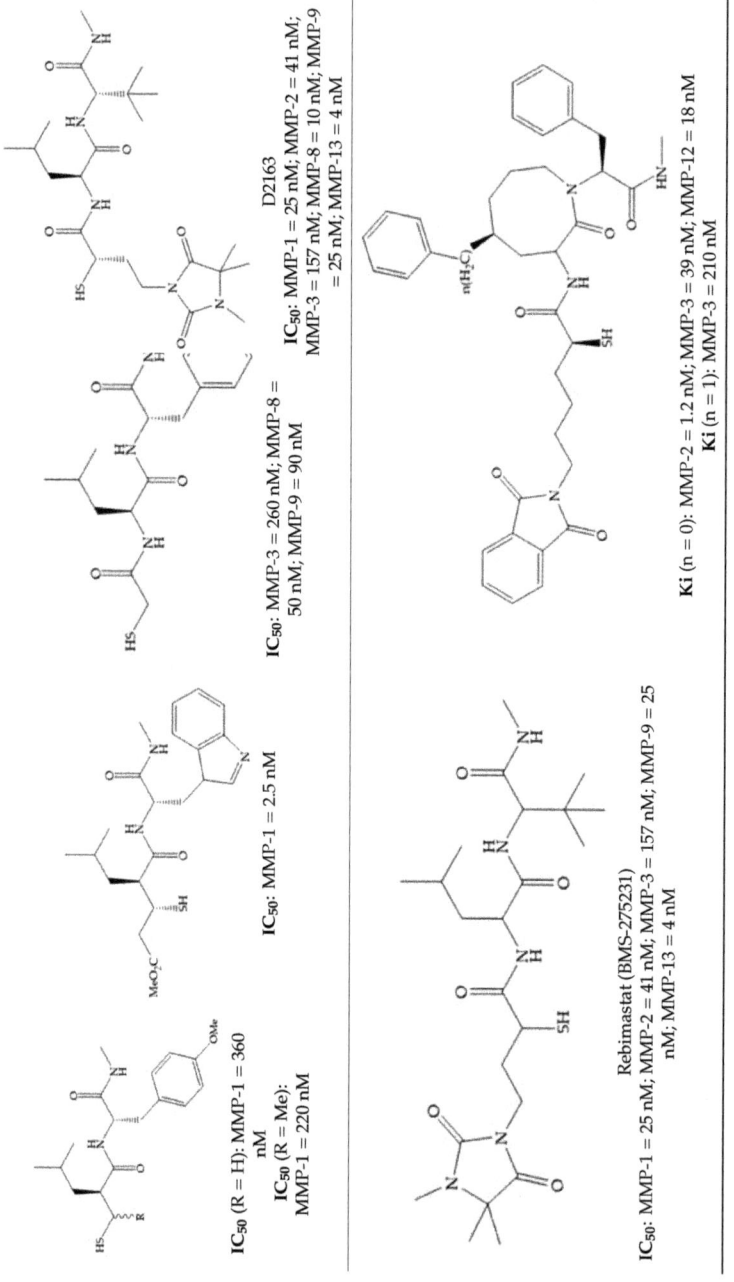

Table 9. Cont.

IC$_{50}$: MMP-3 = 45 nM; MMP-8 = 3 nM; MMP-9 = 5 nM

Ki: MMP-1 = 49 nM; MMP-2 = 1.1 nM; MMP-3 = 470 nM; MMP-7 = 40 nM; MMP-9 = 0.57 nM; MMP-14 = 24 nM

Ki: MMP-8 = 1.2 μM

IC$_{50}$ (X = CH): MMP-1 = 30 nM
IC$_{50}$ (X = N): MMP-1 > 100 μM

IC$_{50}$: MMP-3 = 2.5 μM

IC$_{50}$: MMP-3 = 600 nM

IC$_{50}$: MMP-1 = 890 nM; MMP-3 = 4.6 μM; MMP-9 = 4.5 μM

IC$_{50}$: MMP-1 = 15 nM; MMP-3 = 16 nM; MMP-9 = 0.3 nM

IC$_{50}$: MMP-1 > 10 μM; MMP-3 = 36 nM; MMP-9 = 20 nM

Table 9. Cont.

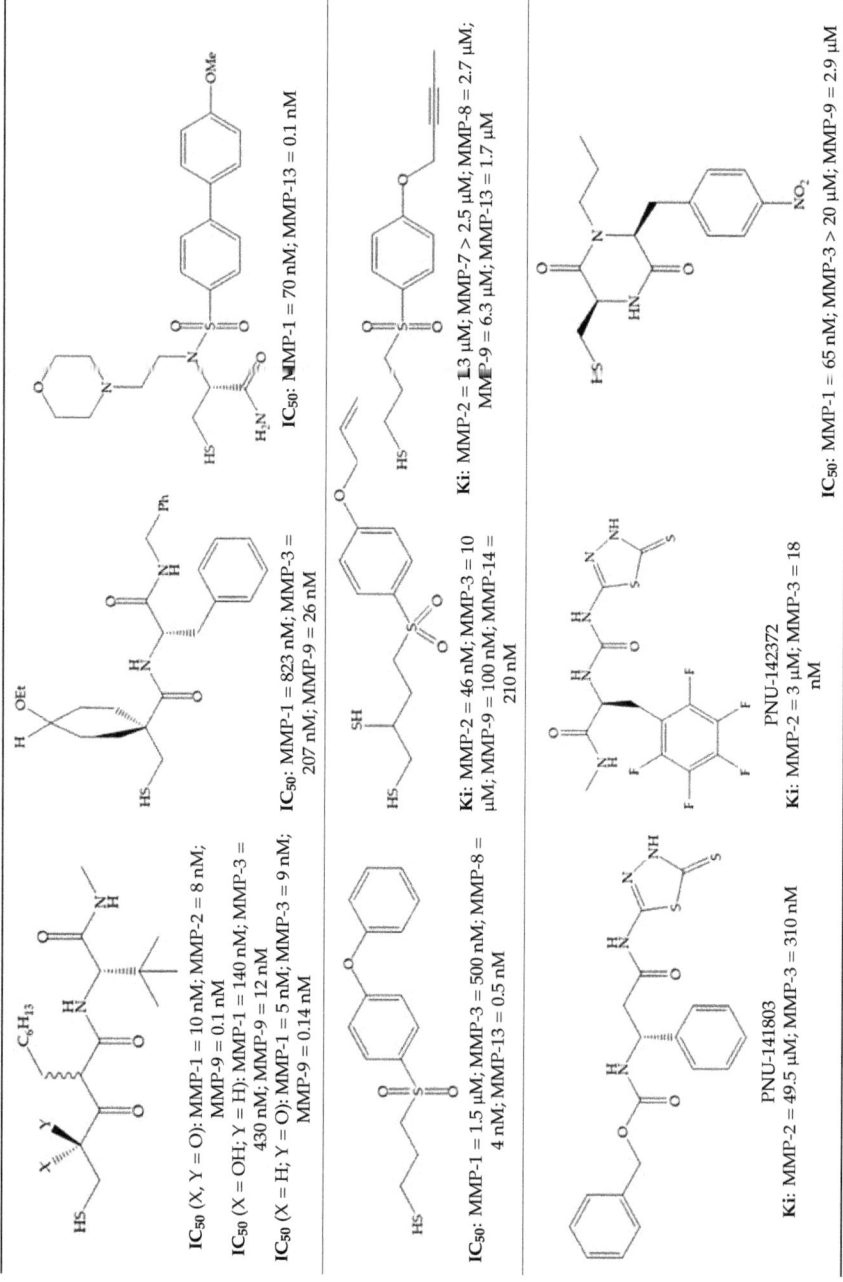

Table 9. *Cont.*

IC$_{50}$: MMP-1 = 15 µM

Ki: MMP-1 = 11 µM; MMP-2 = 50 nM; MMP-14 = 590 nM

CP-271485
IC$_{50}$: MMP-9 = 5.1 µM; MMP-12 > 100 µM

Ki: MMP-2 = 16 nM; MMP-3 = 3.6 µM; MMP-7 = 295 µM; MMP-9 = 180 nM; MMP-14 = 900 nM

SB-3CT
Ki: MMP-1 = 206 µM; MMP-2 = 14 nM; MMP-3 = 15 µM; MMP-7 = 96 µM; MMP-9 = 600 nM

Ki: MMP-1 = 5.4 µM; MMP-2 = 110 nM; MMP-3 = 12.2 µM; MMP-7 = 39 nM; MMP-9 = 130 nM; MMP-14 = 680 nM

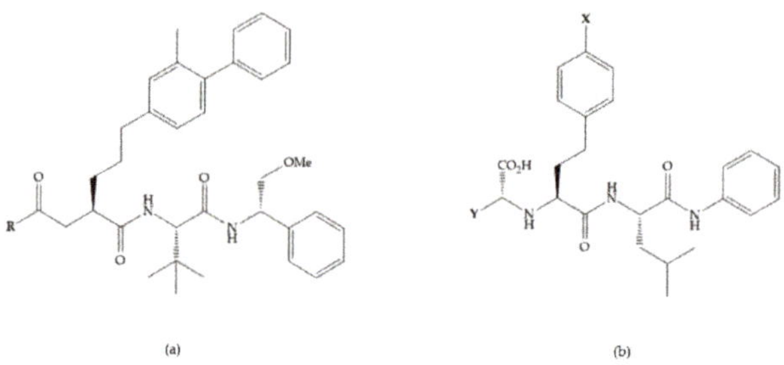

Figure 22. (a) Fray et al. inhibitors. R = NH(OH), hydroxamate-based inhibitor. R = OH, carboxylate-based inhibitor. (b) Hagmann inhibitors. If X = H and Y = Me the compound presents inhibition to MMP-1, -2, and -3. When X = C_4H_9 and Y = Me, the inhibitor has a similar effect to the previous one. The inhibitor with X = H and Y = Phthbutyl (phthalamidibutyl) shows activity against MMP-3.

The interaction of the P_1' biphenyl substituent with pocket S_1' is an important factor contributing to the binding of the inhibitor [19]. The X-ray structure of the acyclic compound with MMP-3 revealed an important interaction between the phenyl terminal of the biphenyl group and the side chain of histidine (His_{224}) [19]. The carboxylic acids derived from "D-valine" have a selective inhibition for MMP-2 and -3 [19]. The 4-substitution of the biphenyl ring helped to increase potency compared to the unsubstituted analogue and also helped to improve the pharmacokinetic properties [19].

With the aim of development inhibitors with high selectivity for a single MMP, Wyeth published, in 2005, a series of biphenyl compounds with carboxylates sulphonamides (Figure 23a). These compounds were tested for the treatment of osteoarthritis and indeed presented selectivity against MMP-13 [18]. Wyeth research developed a series of carboxylic acids-based inhibitors, which were potent and selective against MMP-13, with the carboxylate function connected to a benzofuran via a biphenyl sulphonamide spacer (Figure 23b) [16]. The presence of a bulky substituent in the benzofuran 4-position resulted in a compound 100-fold more selective for MMP-13 over MMP-2 [16].

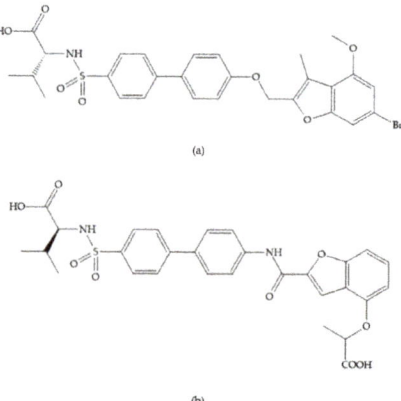

Figure 23. (a) Inhibitor of Wyeth with carboxylate sulphonamide; (b) inhibitor of Wyeth with the carboxylate function connected to a bezofuran via biphenyl sulphonamide spacer.

Tanomastat (Bayer) inhibits MMP-2, -3, -9, and -13 but not MMP-1 [6,29]. This inhibitor participated in clinical trials, proving tolerable and no serious MSS, but the efficacy was negative in small-cell lung cancer because the median overall survival of patients treated did not increase [6,29].

Table 10 shows the IC_{50} and Ki values of some carboxylates-based inhibitors [6,15–19,29,35,37,54,55].

Table 10. IC$_{50}$ and Ki values of carboxylates-based inhibitors.

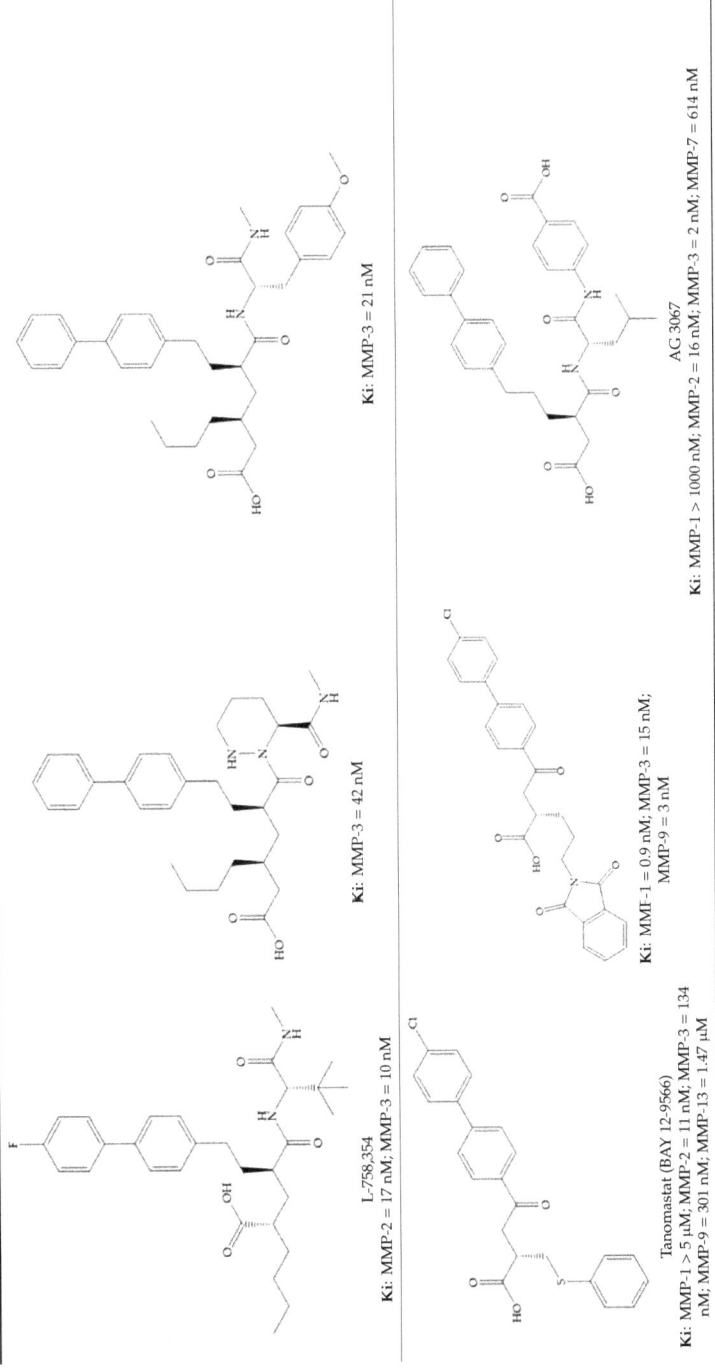

Table 10. *Cont.*

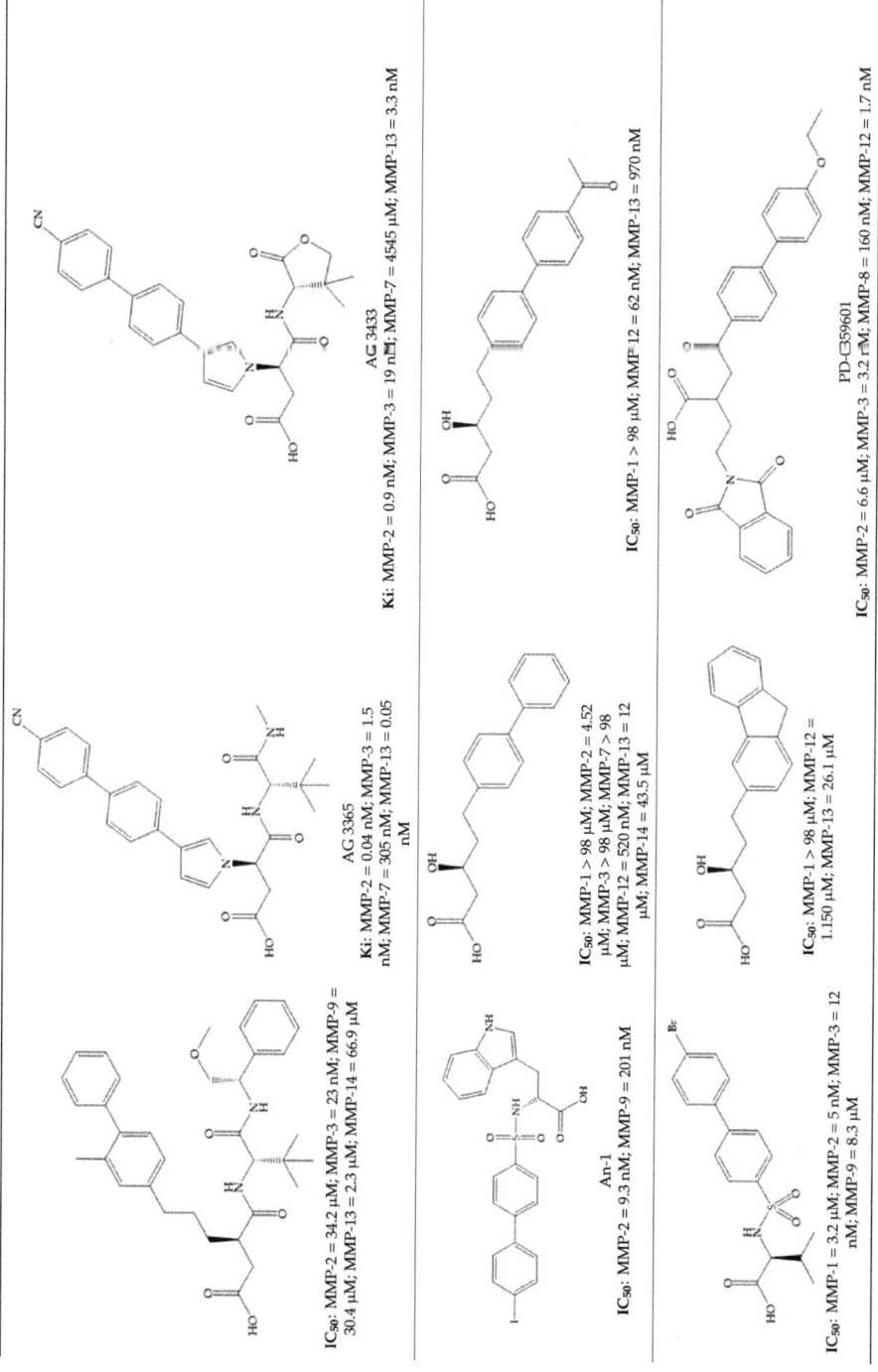

Table 10. *Cont.*

IC$_{50}$: MMP-9 = 91 nM
K$_i$: MMP-1 = 20 nM; MMP-3 = 91 nM; MMP-9 = 91 nM

IC$_{50}$ (X = NH): MMP-1 = 90 nM
IC$_{50}$ (X = CH$_2$): MMP-1 = 380 nM

IC$_{50}$: MMP-1 > 400 µM; MMP-2 = 132 nM; MMP-3 = 81 nM; MMP-7 = 1.1 µM; MMP-8 = 42 nM; MMP-9 > 7 µM; MMP-13 = 1.8 nM; MMP-14 = 5 µM

IC$_{50}$: MMP-13 = 6.72 nM

PF-00356231
IC$_{50}$: MMP-2 > 100 µM; MMP-3 = 390 nM; MMP-8 = 1.7 µM; MMP-9 = 980 nM; MMP-12 = 14 nM; MMP-13 = 270 nM

MMP 408
IC$_{50}$: MMP-1 > 6 µM; MMP-3 = 351 nM; MMP-7 > 6 µM; MMP-9 = 1.3 µM; MMP-12 = 2 nM; MMP-13 = 120 nM; MMP-14 = 1.1 µM

IC$_{50}$: MMP-3 = 50 nM

Table 10. *Cont.*

Ki (X = H; Y = Me): MMP-1 > 10 μM; MMP-2 > 1.06 μM; MMP-3 = 3.88 μM; MMP-7 = 2.01 μM; MMP-8 = 410 nM; MMP-9 > 10 μM; MMP-12 = 1 nM; MMP-13 = 684 nM; MMP-14 = 3.01 μM

Ki: MMP-1 = 127 nM; MMP-3 = 5.819 μM; MMP- = 671 nM; MMP-9 = 2.232 μM; MMP-12 = 2.5 nM; MMP-13 = 501 nM; MMP-14 = 968 nM

Ki (X = H; Y = Me): MMP-1 = 760 nM; MMP-2 = 200 nM; MMP-3 = 470 nM
Ki (X = C₄H₉; Y = Me): MMP-1 = 5.9 μM; MMP-2 = 3.5 nM; MMP-3 = 18 nM
Ki (X = H; Y = Phthbutyl): MMP-1 = 720 nM; MMP-2 = 86 nM; MM-3 = 8 nM

Ki (Y = [H2]-Phthbutyl): MMP-1 > 10 μM; MMP-2 = 6 nM; MMP-3 = 0.36 nM
Ki (Y = Me): MMP-1 > 10 μM; MMP-2 = 310 nM; MMP-3 = 58 nM

Ki: MMP-1 > 25 μM; MMP-2 > 25 μM; MMP-3 > 25 μM; MMP-7 > 25 μM; MMP-8 > 25 μM; MMP-9 > 25 μM; MMP-12 > 25 μM; MMP-13 = 4.4 nM; MMP-14 > 25 μM; MMP-15 > 25 μM; MMP-16 > 25 μM; MMP-24 > 25 μM; MMP-25 > 25 μM; MMP-26 > 25 μM

Table 10. *Cont.*

IC$_{50}$: MMP-1 > 1000 nM; MMP-2 = 19 nM; MMP-3 > 1000 nM; MMP-7 > 1000 nM; MMP-9 = 32 nM

Ki: MMP-8 = 205 nM; MMP-12 = 3.3 nM; MMP-13 = 18 nM; MMP-14 = 1.054 μM

Ki: MMP-1 = 67 μM; MMP-2 = 192 nM; MMP-3 = 40 nM; MMP-7 = 626 nM; MMP-8 = 271 nM; MMP-9 = 1 265 μM; MMP-11 = 18.4 μM; MMP-12 = 0.19 nM; MMP-13 = 49 nM; MMP-14 = 140 nM

Ki: MMP-2 = 57 nM; MMP-3 = 2.164 μM; MMP-8 = 5.3 nM; MMP-13 = 338 nM

Ki: MMP-1 = 2.5 μM; MMP-2 = 8.1 μM; MMP-3 = 13.5 μM; MMP-8 = 17 nM; MMP-9 = 6.6 μM

4.2.3. Phosphorus-Based Inhibitors

The capacity of the phosphoric group to reproduce the gem-diol intermediate during peptide hydrolysis was explored with different structures to obtain potent MMPis [5]. The phosphorus-based of the peptide-analogous inhibitors can be phosphonates/phosphonic acids, phosphoramidates, phosphonamidates, and phosphinates/phosphinic peptides [27]. The phosphinic acid (PO(OH)-CH$_2$) mimics the transition state obtained in substrate degradation, where each oxygen atom can coordinate both the catalytic zinc and the catalytic Glu [6,19,27]. The phosphinic acids are monodentate chelates [27]. In contrast to hydroxamate compounds, the phosphinic compounds interact with both the primed and unprimed side of the catalytic site [17,27,35] due to the placement of the ZBG in the middle of the scaffold and not at its N- or C-terminal, as in the cases of hydroxamate and carboxylate inhibitors [17]. Another advantage of phosphinic acids is the improved metabolic stability compared with hydroxamate acids [27].

The effectiveness of phosphoric acid inhibitors has been studied and it has been found that the three pockets unprimed are connected to obtain the maximum performance [19]. The S_1-S_2 pockets can be exploited using aromatic groups [19,68], that is why Reiter et al. prepared compounds with 4-benzyl (Figure 24) as a substituent to fill S_2 pocket. They found that in the absence of this substituent or its replacement by small aliphatic or cyclohexyl methyl groups led to a loss of activity [19,68].

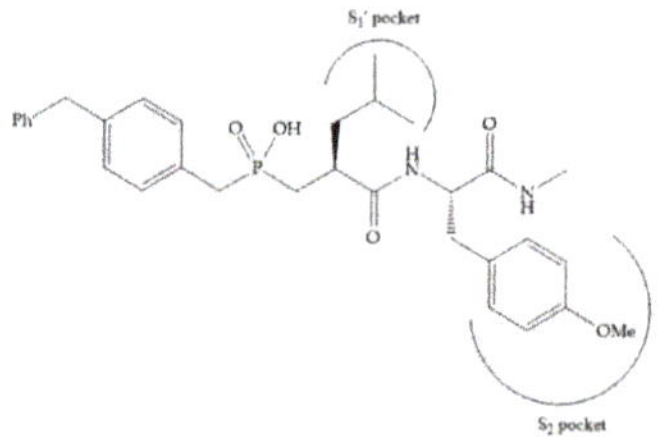

Figure 24. Compound prepared by Reiter et al., with a 4-benzyl substituent. The 4-benzyl group fills the S_2 pocket and if the benzyl group was omitted or replaced by a small aliphatic or cyclohexyl methyl group, the activity is lost. The isobuthyl group fills the S_1' pocket in a manner similar to other substrate-like inhibitors.

Matziari et al. [69] synthesized a series of phosphinic pseudopeptides bearing long P_1' side chains, compounds that contain groups at the *ortho*-position of the phenyl ring and are selective for MMP-11 by the interaction of these groups with residues located at the entrance of the S_1' cavity [69]. These results suggest that the development of compounds able to probe the entrance of the S_1' cavity might represent an alternative strategy to gain selectivity [69].

Other phosphorus-based ZBGs are the carbamoyl phosphates, in which the two oxygens form a five membered ring with the zinc ion [18]. The negative charge of these inhibitors prevents their penetration into the cell and restrain them for extracellular space, contributing to low cytotoxicity [18]. Pochetti et al. [70] described a compound with high affinity to MMP-8 (Ki = 0.6 nM) but inhibits also MMP-2 (Ki = 5 nM) and MMP-3 (Ki = 40 nM) (Figure 25). The R enantiomer is more potent (1000 time more) than the S enantiomer (Ki = 0.7 µM) [70].

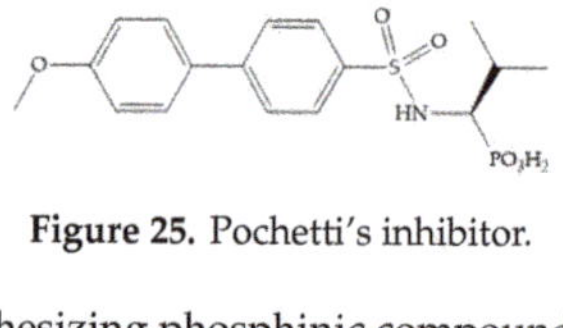

Figure 25. Pochetti's inhibitor.

The classical approach to synthesizing phosphinic compounds limits the full exploitation of this class of compounds for development of highly selective inhibitors of MMPS [35].

Table 11 shows the IC$_{50}$ and Ki values of some phosphorus-based inhibitors [6,15–19,29,35,37,54,55].

Table 11. IC$_{50}$ and Ki values of phosphorus-based inhibitors.

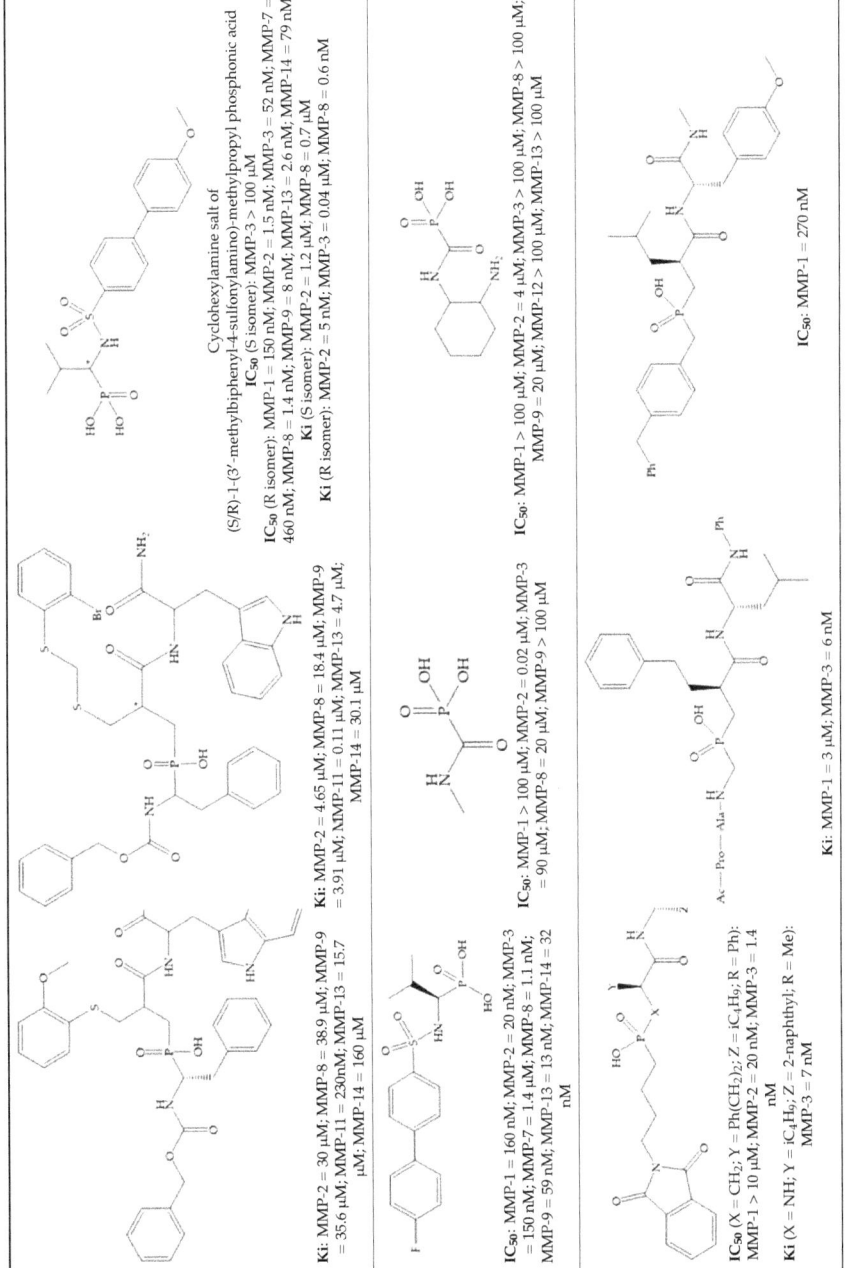

Table 11. Cont.

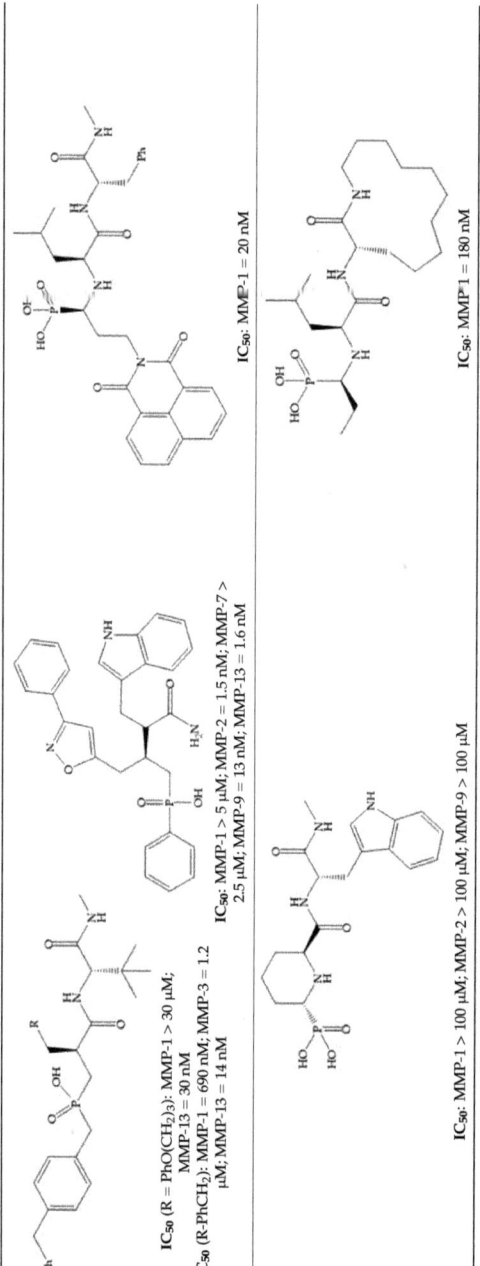

4.2.4. Nitrogen-Based Inhibitors

The nitrogen-based inhibitors have a binding preference to late transition metals and improved selectivity to zinc-dependent enzymes like MMPs [2]. The nitrogen-based inhibitors are studied by the Food and Drug Administration (FDA) and its metabolic availability and bioavailability are well described [2,18]. This ZBG type binds to Zn^{2+} using the nitrogen atom and the carbonyl oxygen adjacent to nitrogen, which favors the formation of an enol because it is established by two hydrogen bonds [18].

The pyrimidine-2,4,6-trione inhibitors were published in 2001 by Hoffman-LaRoche. These compounds show relative specificity to gelatinases and potential usefulness as anticancer drugs [2]. The derivatization of position 5 of this compound promotes access to S_1' and S_2' pockets [18]. In development of osteoarthritis drugs, the pyrimidine-2,4,6-trione inhibitors have been optimized to inhibit MMP-13 [2].

4.2.5. Heterocyclic Bidentate-Based Inhibitors

Heterocyclic bidentate ZBGs have better biostability and higher catalytic zinc ion binding capacity than hydroxamic acids, due to ligand rigidity [2]. Compared heterocycles bidentate and acetohydroxamic acid, the first are more potent to inhibit MMP-1, -2, and -3 and show low toxicity in cell viability assays [2].

Pyrones are biocompatible and they present good aqueous solubility [16]. The arylic portion was added to fit the MMP-3 hydrophobic S_1' pocket, resulting in the compounds more potent than the corresponding hydroxamate-based inhibitors [16].

Table 12 shows the IC_{50} and Ki values of some heterocyclic bidentate-based inhibitors [6,15–19,29,35,37,54,55].

4.2.6. Tetracyclines-Based Inhibitors

Tetracyclines are antibiotics that can chelate zinc and calcium ions and inhibit MMP activity [2,16,29]. Chemically modified tetracyclines (CMT) are preferred over conventional tetracyclines because they reach higher plasma levels for prolonged periods, consequently require less frequent administration, cause less gastrointestinal side effects, and have promising anti-proliferative and anti-metastatic activity [2,16,29]. The CMT binds to pro- or active MMPs, disrupt the native conformation of the protein, and leave the enzymes inactive [29]. In the search for new anticancer agents, the first series of CMT was obtained by removal of the dimethylamino group from the carbon-4 position, resulting in a compound without antimicrobial activity but with anticollagenolytic activity, in vitro and in vivo [16]. Preclinical studies demonstrated that CMT can inhibit gelatinases, stromelysins, collagenases, and MT-MMPs, by downregulating the expression of gelatinases, reducing the production of pro-enzymes and inhibiting the activation of pro-gelatinases and pro-collagenases [16,29].

Doxycycline (Figure 26a) is a semi-synthetic tetracycline that inhibits MMP-2, -9, -7, and -8 and is the only compound approved as an MMP inhibitor for the treatment of periodontitis [2,6]. The COL-3 (Figure 26b) showed specificity for MMP-2, -9, and -14, by decrease trypsinogen-2 and inducible nitric oxide (iNO) production, which are regulators of MMP activity [16]. Although COL-3 is currently being evaluated in clinical phase II trials, it showed poor solubility and stability [16].

4.2.7. Mechanism-Based Inhibitors

The mechanism-based inhibitors coordinate with catalytic zinc ion, in a monodentate mode, allowing the nucleophilic attack by a conserved glutamic residue on the active site and forming a covalent bond [2,17]. This attack causes a conformational change in the catalytic site environment [17] preventing dissociation of the inhibitor and decreasing the rate of catalytic turnover and the amount of inhibitor needed to saturate the enzyme [2].

Table 12. IC$_{50}$ and Ki values of heterocyclic bidentate-based inhibitors.

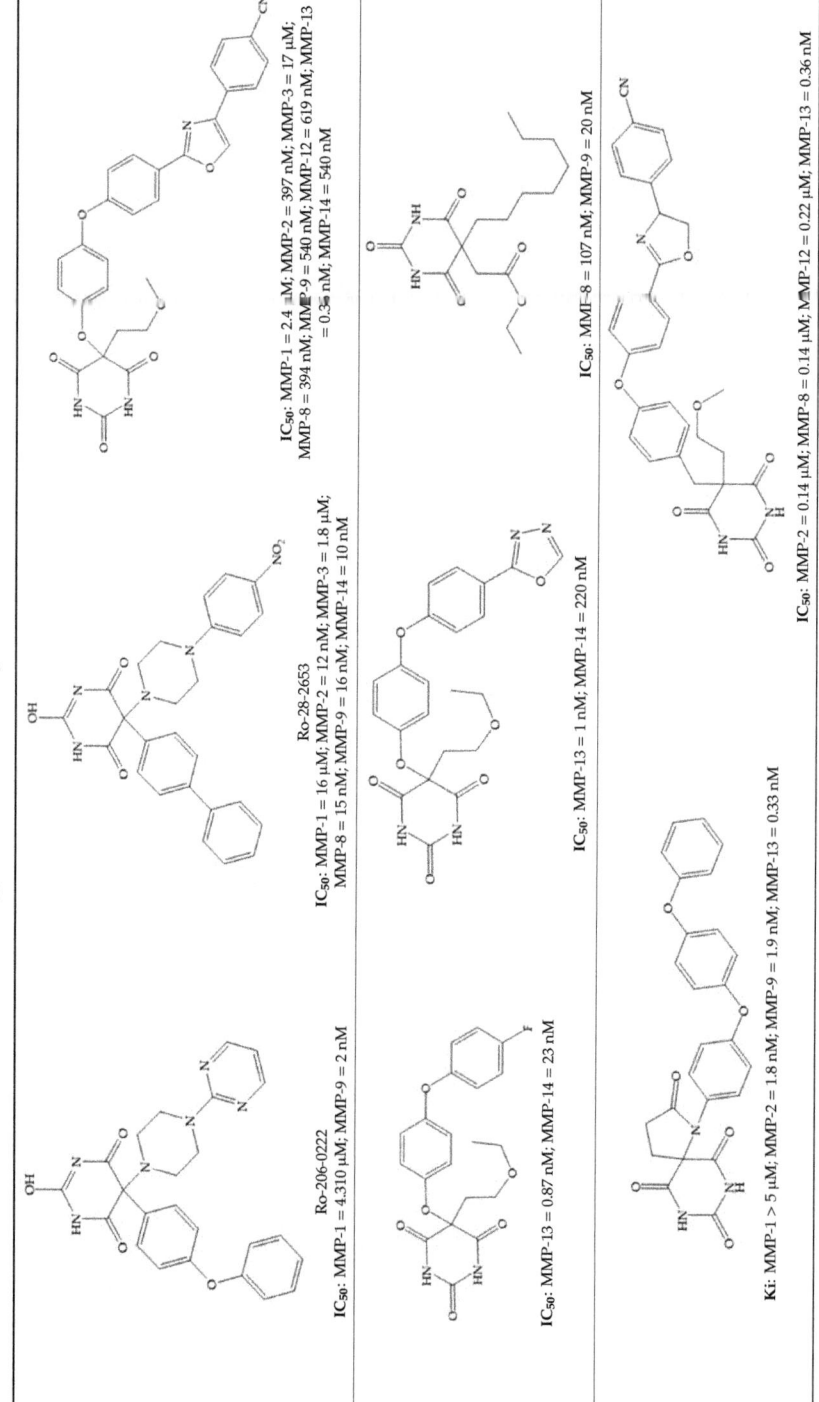

Table 12. *Cont.*

Ki: MMP-2 = 2.17 µM; MMP-3 > 4.50 µM; MMP-7 > 6.37 µM; MMP-12 = 1.02 µM	GW-3333 IC₅₀: MMP-1 = 19 µM; MMP-3 = 20 nM; MMP-9 = 16 nM	S-3304 IC₅₀: MMP-2 = 2 nM; MMP-9 = 10 nM
AZD-126 IC₅₀: MMP-9 = 4.5 nM; MMP-12 = 6.1 nM	IC₅₀: MMP-1 > 50 µM; MMP-2 = 610 nM; MMP-3 = 10 nM	IC₅₀: MMP-1 > 50 µM; MMP-2 > 50 µM; MMP-3 = 19 nM
IC₅₀: MMP-1 > 50 µM; MMP-2 = 4.4 µM; MMP-3 = 77 nM; MMP-7 > 50 µM; MMP-8 = 245 nM; MMP-9 = 32.3 µM; MMP-12 = 85 rM; MMP-13 = 6.6 µM	IC₅₀: MMP-1 > 50 µM; MMP-2 = 9.3 µM; MMP-3 = 0.24 µM; MMP-7 > 50 µM; MMP-8 = 64 nM; MMP-9 > 50 µM; MMP-12 = 22 nM; MMP-13 = 20.6 µM	IC₅₀: MMP-1 > 50 µM; MMP-2 = 16.5 µM; MMP-3 = 41.7 µM; MMP-7 > 50 µM; MMP-8 = 3.8 µM; MMP-9 > 50 µM; MMP-12 = 1.2 µM; MMP-13 = 16.5 µM

Table 12. *Cont.*

IC$_{50}$: MMP-1 > 50 µM; MMP-2 = 7.6 µM; MMP-3 > 50 µM; MMP-7 > 50 µM; MMP-8 = 5.0 µM; MMP-9 > 50 µM; MMP-12 = 6.7 µM; MMP-13 = 6.7 µM

IC$_{50}$: MMP-1 > 50 µM; MMP-2 = 0.92 µM; MMP-3 = 0.56 µM; MMP-7 > 50 µM; MMP-8 = 86 nM; MMP-9 = 27.1 µM; MMP-12 = 18 nM; MMP-13 = 4.1 µM

IC$_{50}$: MMP-1 > 400 µM; MMP-2 = 135 nM; MMP-3 = 81 nM; MMP-7 = 1.1 µM; MMP-8 = 42 nM; MMP-9 > 7 µM; MMP-13 = 1.8 nM; MMP-14 = 5 µM

IC$_{50}$: MMP-1 = 14 µM; MMP-2 = 529 nM; MMP-3 = 1 nM; MMP-9 = 2.42 µM; MMP-14 = 20.1 µM

Ki: MMP-1 > 500 µM; MMP-9 = 6 µM

IC$_{50}$: MMP-1 > 1 µM; MMP-2 = 5 nM; MMP-3 = 56 nM; MMP-9 = 2.4 nM; MMP-12 = 2.5 nM

IC$_{50}$: MMP-1 > 10 µM; MMP-7 > 10 µM; MMP-9 > 10 µM; MMP-13 = 12 nM; MMP-14 > 10 µM

IC$_{50}$: MMP-1 = 30 nM; MMP-2 = 9.8 nM; MMP-3 = 1.7 nM; MMP-7 = 475 nM; MMP-9 = 3 nM; MMP-14 = 17 nM

IC$_{50}$: MMP-1 > 100 µM; MMP-2 > 100 µM; MMP-3 > 100 µM; MMP-7 > 100 µM; MMP-8 > 100 µM; MMP-9 > 100 µM; MMP-12 > 100 µM; MMP-13 > 100 µM; MMP-14 > 100 µM

Table 12. *Cont.*

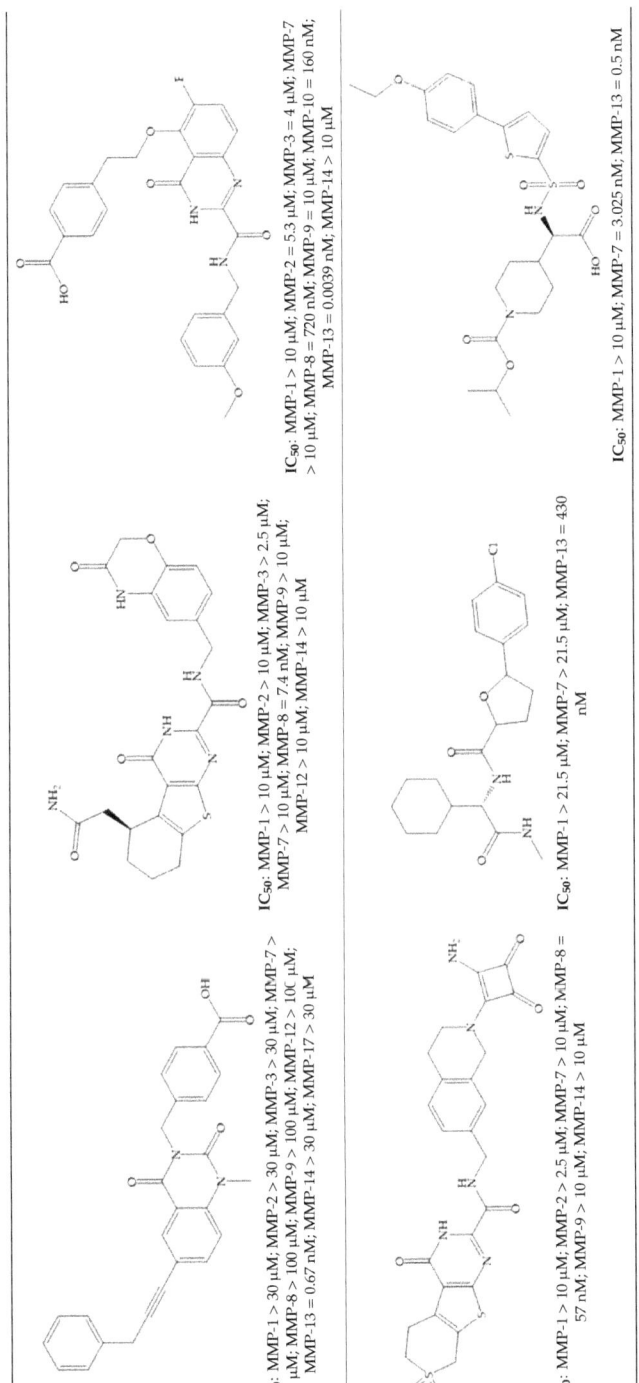

Table 12. *Cont.*

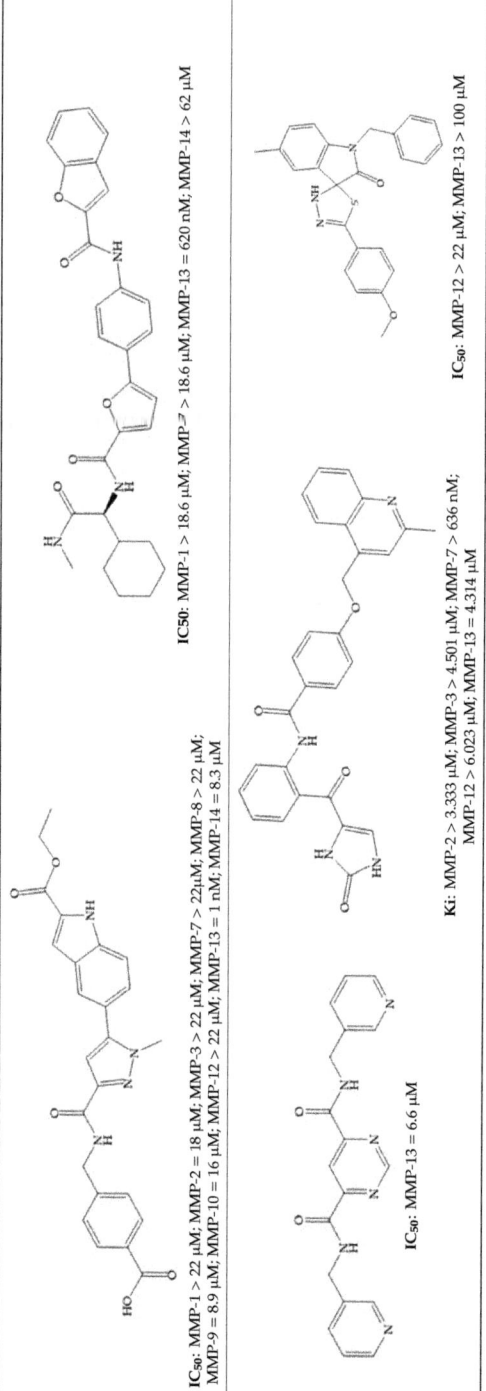

IC$_{50}$: MMP-1 > 22 µM; MMP-2 = 18 µM; MMP-3 > 22 µM; MMP-7 > 22µM; MMP-8 > 22 µM; MMP-9 = 8.9 µM; MMP-10 = 16 µM; MMP-12 > 22 µM; MMP-13 = 1 nM; MMP-14 = 8.3 µM

IC$_{50}$: MMP-1 > 18.6 µM; MMP-7 > 18.6 µM; MMP-13 = 620 nM; MMP-14 > 62 µM

IC$_{50}$: MMP-13 = 6.6 µM

K$_i$: MMP-2 > 3.333 µM; MMP-3 > 4.501 µM; MMP-7 > 636 nM; MMP-12 > 6.023 µM; MMP-13 = 4.314 µM

IC$_{50}$: MMP-12 > 22 µM; MMP-13 > 100 µM

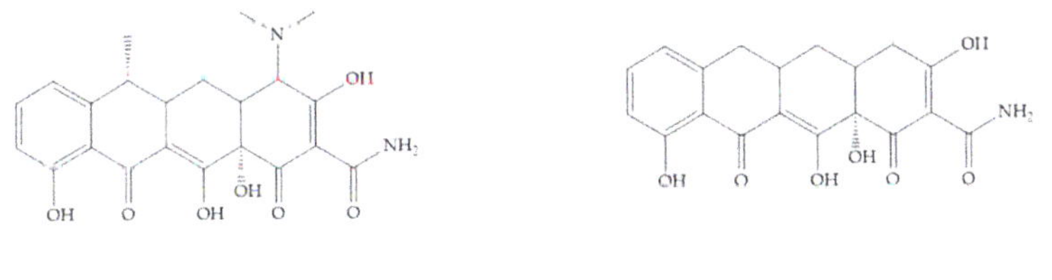

Figure 26. (a) Doxycycline; (b) COL-3.

Table 13 shows the IC$_{50}$ values of some tetracyclines-based inhibitors [6,15–19,29,35,37,54,55,71].

Table 13. IC$_{50}$ values of tetracyclines-based inhibitors.

Structure	IC$_{50}$ values
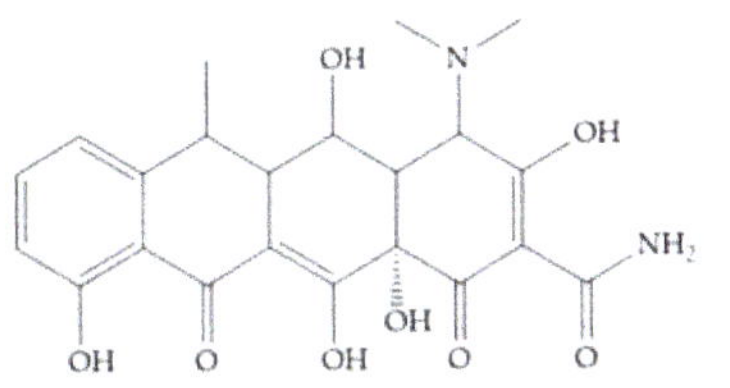 Doxycycline	IC$_{50}$: MMP-1 > 400 µM; MMP-7 = 28 µM; MMP-3 = 30 µM; MMP-13 = 2 µM
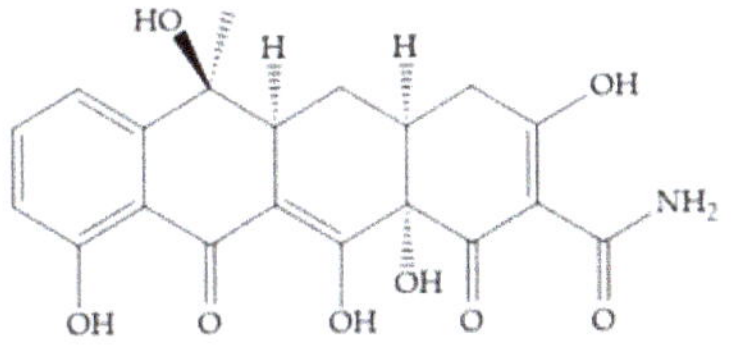 CMT-1	IC$_{50}$: MMP-8 = 30 µM; MMP-13 = 1 µM
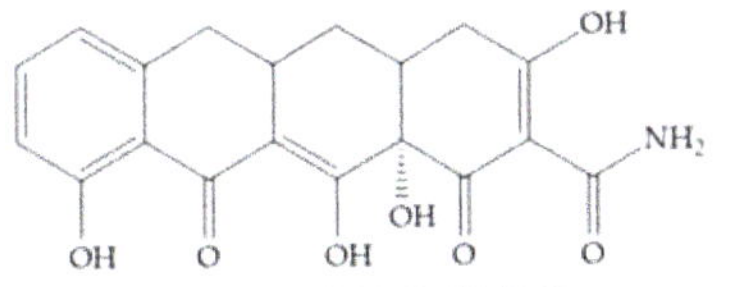 Matastat (COL-3; CMT-3)	IC$_{50}$: MMP-1 = 34 µg·mL^{-1}; MMP-8 = 48 µg·mL^{-1}; MMP-13 = 0.3 µg·mL^{-1}
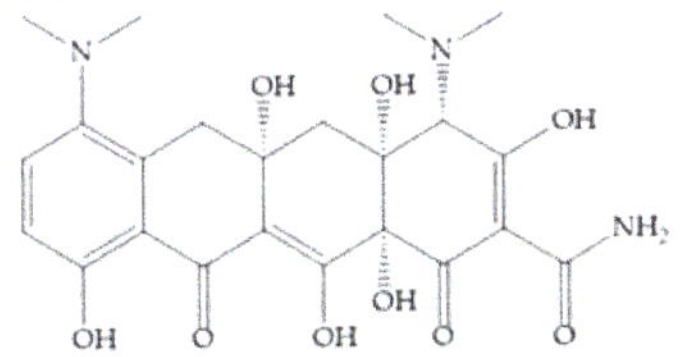 Minocycline	IC$_{50}$: MMP-9 = 272 µM

In 2000, Mobashery et al. [72] were the first to report this novel type of MMPi that blocks gelatinases with a unique mechanistic mode [72]. The thiirane inhibitor showed a mechanism-based, slow-binding inhibition for MMP-2 and MMP-9 [72]. Bernardo et al. [73] also reported a slow-binding thiirane-containing inhibitor, (Figure 27), selective for MMP-2 and -9, where the sulfur group coordinates with the catalytic zinc ion, activates the thiirane group to interact with the active site glutamate, by nucleophilic attack causing a loss of activity [73]. These inhibitors are the first example of a suicide-inhibitor of MMPs [73].

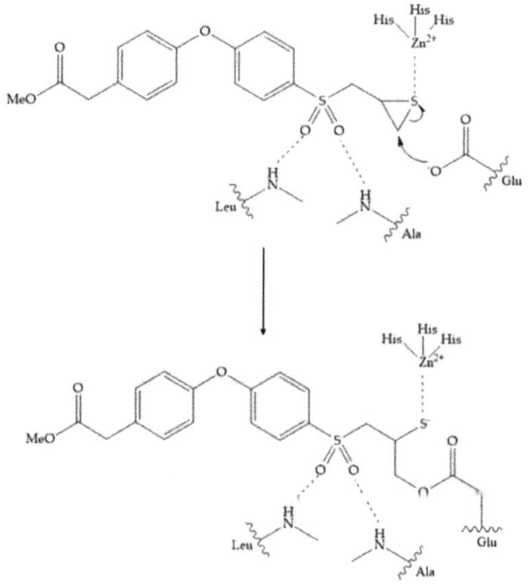

Figure 27. Inhibitor developed by Bernardo el al. The sulfur group coordinates with the catalytic zinc ion and the activation of the thiirane group happened with interactions between the active site glutamate, by nucleophilic attack.

Thiirane-based ND-322 is a small molecule selective to MMP-2/MT1-MMP [2]. This inhibitor has been shown to reduce melanoma cell growth, migration, and invasion, and to delay metastatic dissemination [2].

SB-3CT is a selective inhibitor of MMP-2 and -9 [2]. The inhibition mechanism is similar to a "suicide inhibitor" in which a functional group is activated, leading to covalent modification of the active site [2]. SB-3CT also shows slow-binding kinetics with MMP-2, -3, and -9, contributing to slow dissociation of the MMP-inhibitor complex, but it is a reversible inhibitor which differentiates it from the truly irreversible suicide inhibitors [2]. O SB-3CT has potential benefits in brain damage caused by cerebral ischemia and has anti-cancer effects in T-cells lymphoma and prostate cancer models [2].

4.3. Catalytic Domain (Non-Zinc Binding) Inhibitors

The catalytic domain of MMPs contains other regions that can be exploited [17]. The first 3D-structure of the complex MMP-1 (catalytic domain)-synthetic inhibitor was reported in 1994 by Glaxo researchers [35]. Thereafter, other complexes have been studied and it was found that the S_1' pockets have different depths among MMPS and this difference has been utilized in developing selective MMPis [28,35].

Stockman and Finel optimized two distinct series of MMP-3 inhibitors: PNU-141803 (amide, Figure 28a) and PNU-142372 (urea, Figure 28b) [19]. The connection between MMP-3 and PNU-142372 shows that the aromatic ring from the inhibitor extends to the S_3 pocket (hydrophobic) and the thiadiazole sulfur group interacts with the catalytic zinc [19]. Moreover, the two nitrogen atoms form hydrogen bonds with Ala_{164} and Glu_{202} residues [19]. The alkylation of nitrogen atom or its replacement for carbon leads to the removal activity [19]. The replacement of a tyrosine for a serine within the S_3 pocket (present in MMP-1) leads to the removal of inhibitory activity and explains the absence of activity against collagenases [19].

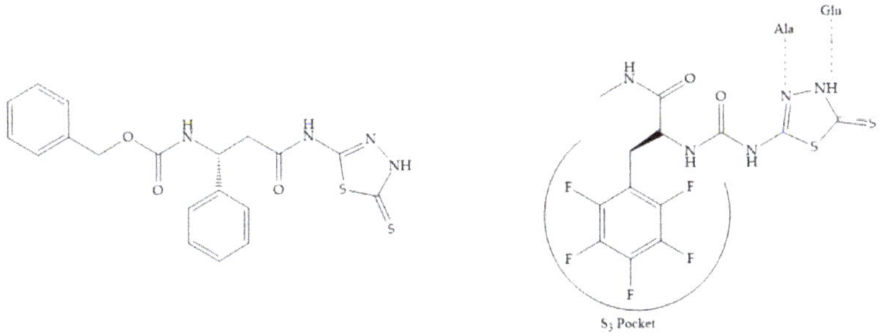

(a) (b)

Figure 28. (a) PNU-141803; (b) PNU-142372.

Sanofi-Aventis developed a compound (Figure 29) for MMP-13 (IC_{50} = 6.6 µM), with very high selectivity [6]. This compound binds deeply to the S_1' pocket and to a side pocket that has not been identified for other MMPs [6]. The pyridyl moiety is towards to the entrance of the S_1' pocket, without interacting with the catalytic Zn(II) ion and the oxygen atoms neither from the amide (peptidic) bonds of the main chain (between Thr_{245} and Thr_{247}) nor from hydroxyl group from the Thr_{247} side chain in the S_1' pocket [6].

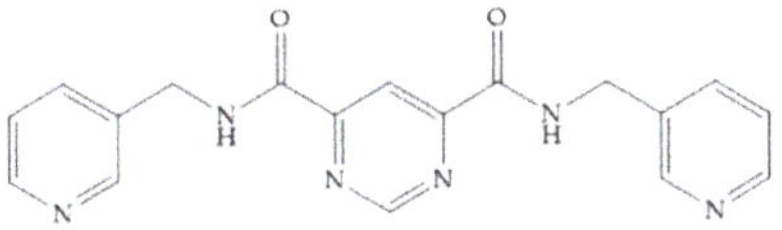

Figure 29. Sanofi-Aventis compound.

Many natural compounds have been shown to possess selective inhibition [28]. Wang et al. identified 19 potential MMPis from 4000 natural compounds isolated from medicinal plants [28]. The caffeates and flavonoids were found to be selective inhibitors against MMP-2 and -9, by occupying the S_1' and S_3 pockets [28].

The marine natural products are another pharmacological resource and include derivates from algae, sponges, and cartilages [28]. Some examples are Neovastat, Dieckol, and Ageladine A and they manifest anti-angiogenic, anti-proliferative, and anti-tumor effects [28].

Although the natural MMPis are more biocompatible and less toxic, they have disadvantages such as the effective dosages are in micromolar scale, which is thousands of times higher than synthetic inhibitors and are difficult to patent, making the pharmacological companies and investors reluctant to sponsor large-scale clinical trials [28].

4.4. Allosteric and Exosite Inhibitors

The catalytic zinc ion is common in all MMPs, therefore, if interactions of the substrates with this ion are minimized this would improve the inhibitor selectivity [2]. The hemopexin-like domain can move relatively to the catalytic domain and allosterically manipulate enzymatic activity by conformation deformation [28]. The allosteric drugs have a non-competitive inhibition mode [16,28], they bind and lock the MMP active site, forcing it to take less favorable conformation for substrate binding [2,16], avoiding off-target inhibition [28] and preventing the occurrence of side effects [28]. Exosite inhibitors are another alternative for selective MMPis since these inhibitors bind to alternative sites of MMPs [16,28].

Remacle et al. reported NSC405020, a small molecule that binds selectively to the hemopexin-like domain of MMP-14 [28]. This molecule inhibits the MMP-14 homodimerization and the interaction between the hemopexin-like domain and catalytic domain, preventing the type I collagen degradation [28].

Dufour et al. developed a peptide targeting the MMP-9 hemopexin-like domain, which blocks MMP-9 dimer formation and cell migration [28]. Scannevin et al. identified a highly selective compound (JNJ0966), which binds to the MMP-9 pro-peptide domain, inhibiting its activation, but not affecting the activity of MMP-1, -2, and -14 [28].

Xu et al. synthesized a peptide which inhibits the hydrolysis of type I and IV collagen by MMP-2, through binding to its collagen binding domain [28].

4.5. Antibody-Based Inhibitors

Antibodies are selective and have high affinity to MMP [27]. Clinical trials utilizing antibodies have provided evidence that selective MMP inhibitors do not induce MSS [27]. The therapeutic potential of anti-MMP antibodies has yet to be realized [27]. The antibodies may also undergo proteolysis, may be removed from circulation rapidly, and are costly [27].

Antibodies are large Y-sharped proteins which bind to an antigen via the fragment antigen-binding (Fab variable region) [28]. Monoclonal antibodies are highly specific, and they have affinity to MMPs [2,29]. The hemopexin domain can be a potential target for MMPs antibodies [2].

REGA-3G12 and REGA-2D9 are antibodies specific to MMP-9 [2,27,28] but not MMP-2 [28]. The inhibition mode of the REGA-3G12 involves the catalytic domain, the N-terminal region Trp_{116}-Lys_{214} [28], and not the catalytic zinc ion or the fibronectin region [2]. The AB0041 and AB0046 are monoclonal anti-MMP-9 antibodies, which showed inhibition to tumor growth and metastasis in a model of colorectal carcinoma [27].

Andecaliximab (GS-5745), the humanized version of AD0041 [27], is a highly selective antibody and exerts allosteric control over tumor growth and metastasis in a colorectal carcinoma model (IC_{50} = 0.148 nM) [28]. This antibody is the only inhibitor that has undergone clinical trials [27,28] and it inhibits the pro-MMP-9 activation and inhibits non-competitively the MMP-9 activity [27].

DX-2400 is an antibody isolated from phage and it targets MMP-14 and the MMP-14-pro-MMP-2 complex, decreasing MMP activity [28]. DX-2400 inhibits the metastasis in a breast cancer xenograft mouse model [27]. However, the LAM-2/15 is the only selective inhibitor that inhibits MMP-14 catalytic activity, but not the pro-MMP-2 activation or MMP-14 dimerization [28]. The 9E8 is another antibody targeting MMP-14 which does not affect the catalytic activity of MMP-14 but inhibits the pro-MMP-2 activation [28].

Human scFv-Fc antibody E3 is bound to the catalytic domain of MMP-14 and inhibits type I collagen binding [27]. Human antibody Fab libraries were synthetized and the peptide G sequence (Phe-Ser-Ile-Ala-His-Glu) was incorporated resulting in Fab 1F8 antibody inhibitor, which inhibits the catalytic domain of MMP-14 [27].

Antibodies can also inhibit a specific activation of an MMP [27]. For example, the mAb 9E8 inhibits the MMP-14 activation of proMMP-2 but not the catalytic activities of MMP-14 [27]. The antibody $LOOP_{AB}$ also inhibits the MMP-14 activation of pro-MMP-2 but not collagenolysis activity of MMP-14 [27]. There are antibodies that reduce the MMP expression [71].

5. Why Do MMP is Fail?

MMI inhibitor side effects are predominantly related to off-target metal chelation [74]. The majority of MMPis used clinically are hydroxamic acid derivates with low selectivity [74] hence, they can inhibit other proteinases [28]. The most frequent side effects observed in MMPis clinical trials is the musculoskeletal syndrome (MSS) [17,28], which manifested as pain and immobility in the joints, arthralgias, contractures in the hands, and an overall reduced quality of life [14,15,74], leading to MMPis failing in the last phases of clinical trials [14]. Several studies indicate that the development of MSS is related to dose and time, with slightly different kinetic for the different MMPis, and the development of MSS is an indicator of successful MMPis [14,74]. The MMP inhibitors focused on chelating the catalytic zinc ion have poor selectivity and resulted in MSS and gastrointestinal disorders [27]. However, the exact causes of MSS remains unknown [74], but can be related to a simultaneous inhibition of several MMPs [6,17,27].

Analysis of the expression of a target protein shows its presence at high levels when a disease is manifested or at low levels or absence in a healthy state [74]. However, these studies do not determine if a particular protein is directly associated with the disease process or if it is involved in ancillary event [74]. Studies of genetic manipulation in mouse as animal models determine the roles of MMPs in various pathological processes [74]. However, there are caveats in the use of animal models [74]:

- The observed effects can be a consequence of the manipulated absence of MMP, being a compensation mechanism;
- The mouse models are unable to replicate the complexity of any human disease. The mouse models serve to recreate specific processes or sets of processes but not the physiological changes that occur in humans.

6. Conclusions

Due to the side effects rising from the lack of selectivity and from the insufficient knowledge about the role of each MMP in the different pathological processes, none of the designed synthetic MMP inhibitors have yet passed the clinical trials and reached the market [6,27]. The poor performance of MMP inhibitors in clinical trials has globally been attributed to [27]:

- Inhibition of other metalloenzymes;
- Lack of specificity within the MMP family;
- Poor pharmacokinetics;
- Dose-limiting side effects/toxicity;
- In vivo instability;
- Low oral availability/inability to assess inhibition efficacy.

In 1988, the first inhibitor was synthesized but after nearly 30 years, only one drug, Periostat®, doxycycline hydrate, had obtained approval from the FDA for the treatment of periodontal disease [6,16,17,27,28]. This inhibitor exhibited also therapeutic effects in treating aortic aneurysm, multiple sclerosis, as well as Type II diabetes [28].

Funding: This research was funded by A MOLECULAR VIEW OF DENTAL RESTORATION, grant number PTDC/SAU-BMA/122444/2010 and by MOLECULAR DESIGN FOR DENTAL RESTAURATION, grant number SAICT-POL/24288/2016. The work was supported by the Associate Laboratory for Green Chemistry-LAQV FCT/MCTES (UIDB/50006/2020), and Applied Molecular Biosciences Unit-UCIBIO FCT/MCTES (UID/Multi/04378/2019), which are financed by national funds.

Conflicts of Interest: The authors declare no conflict of interest.

References

1. Cui, N.; Hu, M.; Khalil, R.A. Biochemical and Biological Attributes of Matrix Metalloproteinases. *Prog. Mol. Biol. Transl. Sci.* **2017**, *147*, 1–73. [CrossRef] [PubMed]
2. Liu, J.; Khalil, R.A. Matrix Metalloproteinase Inhibitors as Investigational and Therapeutic Tools in Unrestrained Tissue Remodeling and Pathological Disorders. *Prog. Mol. Biol. Transl. Sci.* **2017**, *148*, 355–420. [CrossRef] [PubMed]
3. Klein, T.; Bischoff, R. Physiology and pathophysiology of matrix metalloproteases. *Amino Acids* **2011**, *41*, 271–290. [CrossRef] [PubMed]
4. Maskos, K. Crystal structures of MMPs in complex with physiological and pharmacological inhibitors. *Biochimie* **2005**, *87*, 249–263. [CrossRef]
5. Cerofolini, L.; Fragai, M.; Luchinat, C. Mechanism and Inhibition of Matrix Metalloproteinases. *Curr. Med. Chem.* **2019**, *26*, 2609–2633. [CrossRef]

6. Fischer, T.; Senn, N.; Riedl, R. Design and Structural Evolution of Matrix Metalloproteinase Inhibitors. *Chemistry* **2019**, *25*, 7960–7980. [CrossRef]
7. Nagase, H.; Visse, R.; Murphy, G. Structure and function of matrix metalloproteinases and TIMPs. *Cardiovasc. Res.* **2006**, *69*, 562–573. [CrossRef]
8. Amălinei, C.; Căruntu, I.D.; Bălan, R.A. Biology of metalloproteinases. *Rom. J. Morphol. Embryol.* **2007**, *48*, 323–334.
9. Visse, R.; Nagase, H. Matrix metalloproteinases and tissue inhibitors of metalloproteinases: Structure, function, and biochemistry. *Circ. Res.* **2003**, *92*, 827–839. [CrossRef]
10. Tallant, C.; Marrero, A.; Gomis-Rüth, F.X. Matrix metalloproteinases: Fold and function of their catalytic domains. *Biochim. Biophys. Acta* **2010**, *1803*, 20–28. [CrossRef]
11. Verma, R.P.; Hansch, C. Matrix metalloproteinases (MMPs): Chemical-biological functions and (Q)SARs. *Bioorg. Med. Chem.* **2007**, *15*, 2223–2268. [CrossRef] [PubMed]
12. Murphy, G.; Nagase, H. Progress in matrix metalloproteinase research. *Mol. Asp. Med.* **2008**, *29*, 290–308. [CrossRef] [PubMed]
13. Mannello, F.; Medda, V. Nuclear localization of matrix metalloproteinases. *Prog. Histochem. Cytochem.* **2012**, *47*, 27–58. [CrossRef] [PubMed]
14. Rangasamy, L.; Geronimo, B.D.; Ortín, I.; Coderch, C.; Zapico, J.M.; Ramos, A.; de Pascual-Teresa, B. Molecular Imaging Probes Based on Matrix Metalloproteinase Inhibitors (MMPIs). *Molecules* **2019**, *24*, 2982. [CrossRef]
15. Vandenbroucke, R.E.; Dejonckheere, E.; Libert, C. A therapeutic role for matrix metalloproteinase inhibitors in lung diseases? *Eur. Respir. J.* **2011**, *38*, 1200–1214. [CrossRef] [PubMed]
16. Nuti, E.; Tuccinardi, T.; Rossello, A. Matrix metalloproteinase inhibitors: New challenges in the era of post broad-spectrum inhibitors. *Curr. Pharm. Des.* **2007**, *13*, 2087–2100. [CrossRef]
17. Georgiadis, D.; Yiotakis, A. Specific targeting of metzincin family members with small-molecules inhibitors: Progress toward a multifarious challenge. *Bioorg. Med. Chem.* **2008**, 8781–8794. [CrossRef]
18. Jacobsen, J.A.; Major Jourden, J.L.; Miller, M.T.; Cohen, S.M. To bind zinc or not to bind zinc: An examination of innovative approaches to improved metalloproteinase inhibition. *Biochim. Biophys. Acta* **2010**, *1803*, 72–94. [CrossRef]
19. Whittaker, M.; Floyd, C.D.; Brown, P.; Gearing, A.J. Design and therapeutic application of matrix metalloproteinase inhibitors. *Chem. Rev.* **1999**, *99*, 2735–2776. [CrossRef]
20. Tokuhara, C.K.; Santesso, M.R.; Oliveira, G.S.N.; Ventura, T.M.D.S.; Doyama, J.T.; Zambuzzi, W.F.; Oliveira, R.C. Updating the role of matrix metalloproteinases in mineralized tissue and related diseases. *J. Appl. Oral Sci.* **2019**, *27*, e20180596. [CrossRef]
21. Liu, Y.; Tjäderhane, L.; Bresch, L.; Mazzoni, A.; Li, N.; Mao, J.; Pashley, D.H.; Tay, F.R. Limitations in Bonding to Dentin and Experimental Strategies to Prevent Bond Degradation. *J. Dent. Res.* **2011**, *90*, 953–968. [CrossRef] [PubMed]
22. Young, D.; Das, N.; Anowai, A.; Dufour, A. Matrix Metalloproteases as Influencers of the Cells' Social Media. *Int. J. Mol. Sci.* **2019**, *20*, 3847. [CrossRef] [PubMed]
23. Kwan, J.A.; Schulze, C.J.; Wang, W.; Leon, H.; Sariahmetoglu, M.; Sung, M.; Sawicka, J.; Sims, D.E.; Sawicki, G.; Schulz, R. Matrix metalloproteinase-2 (MMP-2) is present in the nucleus of cardiac myocytes and is capable of cleaving poly (ADP-ribose) polymerase (PARP) in vitro. *Faseb J.* **2004**, *18*, 690–692. [CrossRef]
24. Cauwe, B.; Van den Steen, P.E.; Opdenakker, G. The biochemical, biological, and pathological kaleidoscope of cell surface substrates processed by matrix metalloproteinases. *Crit. Rev. Biochem. Mol. Biol.* **2007**, *42*, 113–185. [CrossRef]
25. Cauwe, B.; Opdenakker, G. Intracellular substrate cleavage: A novel dimension in the biochemistry, biology and pathology of matrix metalloproteinases. *Crit Rev. Biochem. Mol. Biol.* **2010**, *45*, 351–423. [CrossRef]
26. Jobin, P.G.; Butler, G.S.; Overall, C.M. New intracellular activities of matrix metalloproteinases shine in the moonlight. *Biochim Biophys Acta Mol. Cell Res.* **2017**, *1864*, 2043–2055. [CrossRef]
27. Fields, G.B. The Rebirth of Matrix Metalloproteinase Inhibitors: Moving Beyond the Dogma. *Cells* **2019**, *8*, 984. [CrossRef]
28. Li, K.; Tay, F.R.; Yiu, C.K.Y. The past, present and future perspectives of matrix metalloproteinase inhibitors. *Pharmacol. Ther.* **2020**, *207*, 107465. [CrossRef]

29. Hu, J.; Van den Steen, P.E.; Sang, Q.X.; Opdenakker, G. Matrix metalloproteinase inhibitors as therapy for inflammatory and vascular diseases. *Nat. Rev. Drug Discov.* **2007**, *6*, 480–498. [CrossRef] [PubMed]
30. Murphy, G. Tissue inhibitors of metalloproteinases. *Genome Biol.* **2011**, *12*, 233. [CrossRef]
31. Folgueras, A.R.; Pendás, A.M.; Sánchez, L.M.; López-Otín, C. Matrix metalloproteinases in cancer: From new functions to improved inhibition strategies. *Int. J. Dev. Biol* **2004**, *48*, 411–424. [CrossRef] [PubMed]
32. Maskos, K.; Bode, W. Structural basis of matrix metalloproteinases and tissue inhibitors of metalloproteinases. *Mol. Biotechnol.* **2003**, *25*, 241–266. [CrossRef]
33. Arbeláez, L.F.; Bergmann, U.; Tuuttila, A.; Shanbhag, V.P.; Stigbrand, T. Interaction of matrix metalloproteinases-2 and -9 with pregnancy zone protein and alpha2-macroglobulin. *Arch. Biochem. Biophys.* **1997**, *347*, 62–68. [CrossRef] [PubMed]
34. Serifova, X.; Ugarte-Berzal, E.; Opdenakker, G.; Vandooren, J. Homotrimeric MMP-9 is an active hitchhiker on alpha-2-macroglobulin partially escaping protease inhibition and internalization through LRP-1. *Cell Mol. Life Sci.* **2019**. [CrossRef]
35. Cuniasse, P.; Devel, L.; Makaritis, A.; Beau, F.; Georgiadis, D.; Matziari, M.; Yiotakis, A.; Dive, V. Future challenges facing the development of specific active-site-directed synthetic inhibitors of MMPs. *Biochimie* **2005**, *87*, 393–402. [CrossRef]
36. Castelhano, A.L.; Billedeau, R.; Dewdney, N.; Donnelly, S.; Horne, S.; Kurz, L.J.; Liak, T.J.; Martin, R.; Uppington, R.; Yuan, Z.; et al. Novel indolactam-based inhibitors of matrix metalloproteinases. *Bioorg. Med. Chem. Lett.* **1995**, *5*, 1415–1420. [CrossRef]
37. Gimeno, A.; Beltrán-Debón, R.; Mulero, M.; Pujadas, G.; Garcia-Vallvé, S. Understanding the variability of the S1' pocket to improve matrix metalloproteinase inhibitor selectivity profiles. *Drug Discov. Today* **2019**, *1*, 38–57. [CrossRef]
38. Moore, W.M.; Spilburg, C.A. Peptide hydroxamic acids inhibit skin collagenase. *Biochem. Biophys. Res. Commun.* **1986**, *136*, 390–395. [CrossRef]
39. Moore, W.M.; Spilburg, C.A. Purification of human collagenases with a hydroxamic acid affinity column. *Biochemistry* **1986**, *25*, 5189–5195. [CrossRef]
40. Reich, R.; Thompson, E.W.; Iwamoto, Y.; Martin, G.R.; Deason, J.R.; Fuller, G.C.; Miskin, R. Effects of inhibitors of plasminogen activator, serine proteinases, and collagenase IV on the invasion of basement membranes by metastatic cells. *Cancer Res.* **1988**, *48*, 3307–3312.
41. Xue, C.B.; He, X.; Roderick, J.; DeGrado, W.F.; Cherney, R.J.; Hardman, K.D.; Nelson, D.J.; Copeland, R.A.; Jaffee, B.D.; Decicco, C.P. Design and synthesis of cyclic inhibitors of matrix metalloproteinases and TNF-alpha production. *J. Med. Chem.* **1998**, *41*, 1745–1748. [CrossRef] [PubMed]
42. Steinman, D.H.; Curtin, M.L.; Garland, R.B.; Davidsen, S.K.; Heyman, H.R.; Holms, J.H.; Albert, D.H.; Magoc, T.J.; Nagy, I.B.; Marcotte, P.A.; et al. The design, synthesis, and structure-activity relationships of a series of macrocyclic MMP inhibitors. *Bioorg. Med. Chem. Lett.* **1998**, *8*, 2087–2092. [CrossRef]
43. Martin, S.F.; Oalmann, C.J.; Liras, S. Cyclopropanes as conformationally restricted peptide isosteres. Design and synthesis of novel collagenase inhibitors. *Tetrahedron* **1993**, *49*, 3521–3532. [CrossRef]
44. Tamaki, K.; Tanzawa, K.; Kurihara, S.; Oikawa, T.; Monma, S.; Shimada, K.; Sugimura, Y. Synthesis and structure-activity relationships of gelatinase inhibitors derived from matlystatins. *Chem. Pharm. Bull. (Tokyo)* **1995**, *43*, 1883–1893. [CrossRef] [PubMed]
45. Conradi, R.A.; Hilgers, A.R.; Ho, N.F.; Burton, P.S. The influence of peptide structure on transport across Caco-2 cells. *Pharm Res.* **1991**, *8*, 1453–1460. [CrossRef] [PubMed]
46. Babine, R.E.; Bender, S.L. Molecular Recognition of Proteinminus signLigand Complexes: Applications to Drug Design. *Chem. Rev.* **1997**, *97*, 1359–1472. [CrossRef]
47. Hirayama, R.; Yamamoto, M.; Tsukida, T.; Matsuo, K.; Obata, Y.; Sakamoto, F.; Ikeda, S. Synthesis and biological evaluation of orally active matrix metalloproteinase inhibitors. *Bioorg. Med. Chem.* **1997**, *5*, 765–778. [CrossRef]
48. Graf von Roedern, E.; Grams, F.; Brandstetter, H.; Moroder, L. Design and synthesis of malonic acid-based inhibitors of human neutrophil collagenase (MMP8). *J. Med. Chem.* **1998**, *41*, 339–345. [CrossRef]
49. Albini, A.; D'Agostini, F.; Giunciuglio, D.; Paglieri, I.; Balansky, R.; De Flora, S. Inhibition of invasion, gelatinase activity, tumor take and metastasis of malignant cells by N-acetylcysteine. *Int. J. Cancer* **1995**, *61*, 121–129. [CrossRef]

50. Müller, J.C.; von Roedern, E.G.; Grams, F.; Nagase, H.; Moroder, L. Non-peptidic cysteine derivatives as inhibitors of matrix metalloproteinases. *Biol Chem* **1997**, *378*, 1475–1480. [CrossRef]
51. Foley, M.A.; Hassman, A.S.; Drewry, D.H.; Greer, D.G.; Wagner, C.D.; Feldman, P.L.; Berman, J.; Bickett, D.M.; McGeehan, G.M.; Lambert, M.H.; et al. Rapid synthesis of novel dipeptide inhibitors of human collagenase and gelatinase using solid phase chemistry. *Bioorg. Med. Chem. Lett.* **1996**, *6*, 223–243. [CrossRef]
52. Johnson, W.H.; Roberts, N.A.; Borkakoti, N. Collagenase inhibitors: Their design and potential therapeutic use. *J. Enzym. Inhib.* **1987**, *2*, 1–22. [CrossRef] [PubMed]
53. Valérie, M.; Mirand, C.; Decarme, M.; Emonard, H.; Hornebeck, W. MMPs inhibitors: New succinylhydroxamates with selective inhibition of MMP-2 over MMP-3. *Bioorg. Med. Chem. Lett.* **2003**, *13*, 2843–2846. [CrossRef]
54. Pikul, S.; McDow Dunham, K.L.; Almstead, N.G.; De, B.; Natchus, M.G.; Anastasio, M.V.; McPhail, S.J.; Snider, C.E.; Taiwo, Y.O.; Chen, L.; et al. Design and synthesis of phosphinamide-based hydroxamic acids as inhibitors of matrix metalloproteinases. *J. Med. Chem.* **1999**, *42*, 87–94. [CrossRef] [PubMed]
55. Aureli, L.; Gioia, M.; Cerbara, I.; Monaco, S.; Fasciglione, G.F.; Marini, S.; Ascenzi, P.; Topai, A.; Coletta, M. Structural bases for substrate and inhibitor recognition by matrix metalloproteinases. *Curr. Med. Chem.* **2008**, *15*, 2192–2222. [CrossRef] [PubMed]
56. MacPherson, L.J.; Bayburt, E.K.; Capparelli, M.P.; Carroll, B.J.; Goldstein, R.; Justice, M.R.; Zhu, L.; Hu, S.; Melton, R.; Fryer, L.; et al. Discovery of CGS 27023A, a Non-Peptidic, Potent, and Orally Active Stromelysin Inhibitor That Blocks Cartilage Degradation in Rabbits. *J. Med. Chem.* **1997**, *40*, 2525–2532. [CrossRef] [PubMed]
57. Barta, T.E.; Becker, D.P.; Bedell, L.J.; De Crescenzo, G.A.; McDonald, J.J.; Munie, G.E.; Rao, S.; Shieh, H.S.; Stegeman, R.; Stevens, A.M.; et al. Synthesis and activity of selective MMP inhibitors with an aryl backbone. *Bioorg. Med. Chem. Lett.* **2000**, *10*, 2815–2817. [CrossRef]
58. Noe, M.C.; Natarajan, V.; Snow, S.L.; Mitchell, P.G.; Lopresti-Morrow, L.; Reeves, L.M.; Yocum, S.A.; Carty, T.J.; Barberia, J.A.; Sweeney, F.J.; et al. Discovery of 3,3-dimethyl-5-hydroxypipecolic hydroxamate-based inhibitors of aggrecanase and MMP-13. *Bioorg. Med. Chem. Lett.* **2005**, *15*, 2808–2811. [CrossRef]
59. Hu, J.; Fiten, P.; Van den Steen, P.E.; Chaltin, P.; Opdenakker, G. Simulation of evolution-selected propeptide by high-throughput selection of a peptidomimetic inhibitor on a capillary DNA sequencer platform. *Anal. Chem.* **2005**, *77*, 2116–2124. [CrossRef]
60. Hu, J.; Dubois, V.; Chaltin, P.; Fiten, P.; Dillen, C.; Van den Steen, P.E.; Opdenakker, G. Inhibition of lethal endotoxin shock with an L-pyridylalanine containing metalloproteinase inhibitor selected by high-throughput screening of a new peptide library. *Comb. Chem. High. Throughput Screen* **2006**, *9*, 599–611. [CrossRef]
61. Bhowmick, M.; Tokmina-Roszyk, D.; Onwuha-Ekpete, L.; Harmon, K.; Robichaud, T.; Fuerst, R.; Stawikowska, R.; Steffensen, B.; Roush, W.; Wong, H.R.; et al. Second Generation Triple-Helical Peptide Inhibitors of Matrix Metalloproteinases. *J. Med. Chem.* **2017**, *60*, 3814–3827. [CrossRef] [PubMed]
62. Beszant, B.; Bird, J.; Gaster, L.M.; Harper, G.P.; Hughes, I.; Karran, E.H.; Markwell, R.E.; Miles-Williams, A.J.; Smith, S.A. Synthesis of novel modified dipeptide inhibitors of human collagenase: Beta-mercapto carboxylic acid derivatives. *J. Med. Chem.* **1993**, *36*, 4030–4039. [CrossRef] [PubMed]
63. Baxter, A.D.; Bird, J.; Bhogal, R.; Massil, T.; Minton, K.J.; Montana, J.; Owen, D.A. A novel series of matrix metalloproteinase inhibitors for the treatment of inflammatory disorders. *Bioorg. Med. Chem. Lett.* **1997**, *7*, 897–902. [CrossRef]
64. Campbell, D.A.; Xiao, X.Y.; Harris, D.; Ida, S.; Mortezaei, R.; Ngu, K.; Shi, L.; Tien, D.; Wang, Y.; Navre, M.; et al. Malonyl alpha-mercaptoketones and alpha-mercaptoalcohols, a new class of matrix metalloproteinase inhibitors. *Bioorg. Med. Chem. Lett.* **1998**, *8*, 1157–1162. [CrossRef]
65. Hurst, D.R.; Schwartz, M.A.; Jin, Y.; Ghaffari, M.A.; Kozarekar, P.; Cao, J.; Sang, Q.X. Inhibition of enzyme activity of and cell-mediated substrate cleavage by membrane type 1 matrix metalloproteinase by newly developed mercaptosulphide inhibitors. *Biochem. J.* **2005**, *392*, 527–536. [CrossRef] [PubMed]
66. Fray, M.J.; Dickinson, R.P.; Huggins, J.P.; Occleston, N.L. A potent, selective inhibitor of matrix metalloproteinase-3 for the topical treatment of chronic dermal ulcers. *J. Med. Chem.* **2003**, *46*, 3514–3525. [CrossRef]
67. Chapman, K.T.; Kopka, I.E.; Durette, P.L.; Esser, C.K.; Lanza, T.J.; Izquierdo-Martin, M.; Niedzwiecki, L.; Chang, B.; Harrison, R.K.; Kuo, D.W. Inhibition of matrix metalloproteinases by *N*-carboxyalkyl peptides. *J. Med. Chem.* **1993**, *36*, 4293–4301. [CrossRef]

68. Reiter, L.A.; Rizzi, J.P.; Pandit, J.; Lasut, M.J.; McGahee, S.M.; Parikh, V.D.; Blake, J.F.; Danley, D.E.; Laird, E.R.; Lopez-Anaya, A.; et al. Inhibition of MMP-1 and MMP-13 with phosphinic acids that exploit binding in the S2 pocket. *Bioorg. Med. Chem. Lett.* **1999**, *9*, 127–132. [CrossRef]
69. Matziari, M.; Beau, F.; Cuniasse, P.; Dive, V.; Yiotakis, A. Evaluation of P1′-diversified phosphinic peptides leads to the development of highly selective inhibitors of MMP-11. *J. Med. Chem.* **2004**, *47*, 325–336. [CrossRef]
70. Pochetti, G.; Gavuzzo, E.; Campestre, C.; Agamennone, M.; Tortorella, P.; Consalvi, V.; Gallina, C.; Hiller, O.; Tschesche, H.; Tucker, P.A.; et al. Structural insight into the stereoselective inhibition of MMP-8 by enantiomeric sulfonamide phosphonates. *J. Med. Chem.* **2006**, *49*, 923–931. [CrossRef]
71. Vandooren, J.; Knoops, S.; Aldinucci Buzzo, J.L.; Boon, L.; Martens, E.; Opdenakker, G.; Kolaczkowska, E. Differential inhibition of activity, activation and gene expression of MMP-9 in THP-1 cells by azithromycin and minocycline versus bortezomib: A comparative study. *PLoS ONE* **2017**, *12*, e0174853. [CrossRef] [PubMed]
72. Ikejiri, M.; Bernardo, M.M.; Bonfil, R.D.; Toth, M.; Chang, M.; Fridman, R.; Mobashery, S. Potent mechanism-based inhibitors for matrix metalloproteinases. *J. Biol. Chem.* **2005**, *280*, 33992–34002. [CrossRef] [PubMed]
73. Bernardo, M.M.; Brown, S.; Li, Z.H.; Fridman, R.; Mobashery, S. Design, synthesis, and characterization of potent, slow-binding inhibitors that are selective for gelatinases. *J. Biol. Chem.* **2002**, *277*, 11201–11207. [CrossRef]
74. Fingleton, B. MMPs as therapeutic targets–still a viable option? *Semin. Cell Dev. Biol.* **2008**, *19*, 61–68. [CrossRef] [PubMed]

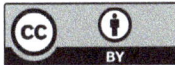

© 2020 by the authors. Licensee MDPI, Basel, Switzerland. This article is an open access article distributed under the terms and conditions of the Creative Commons Attribution (CC BY) license (http://creativecommons.org/licenses/by/4.0/).

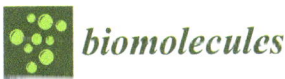

Review

The Many Faces of Matrix Metalloproteinase-7 in Kidney Diseases

Zhao Liu [1], Roderick J. Tan [2] and Youhua Liu [1,3,*]

[1] State Key Laboratory of Organ Failure Research, National Clinical Research Center of Kidney Disease, Nanfang Hospital, Southern Medical University, Guangzhou 510515, China; lz0103@i.smu.edu.cn
[2] Renal-Electrolyte Division, Department of Medicine, University of Pittsburgh School of Medicine, Pittsburgh, PA 15261, USA; tanrj@upmc.edu
[3] Department of Pathology, University of Pittsburgh School of Medicine, Pittsburgh, PA 15261, USA
* Correspondence: yhliu@pitt.edu

Received: 1 May 2020; Accepted: 22 June 2020; Published: 25 June 2020

Abstract: Matrix metalloproteinase-7 (MMP-7) is a secreted zinc-dependent endopeptidase that is implicated in regulating kidney homeostasis and diseases. MMP-7 is produced as an inactive zymogen, and proteolytic cleavage is required for its activation. MMP-7 is barely expressed in normal adult kidney but upregulated in acute kidney injury (AKI) and chronic kidney disease (CKD). The expression of MMP-7 is transcriptionally regulated by Wnt/β-catenin and other cues. As a secreted protein, MMP-7 is present and increased in the urine of patients, and its levels serve as a noninvasive biomarker for predicting AKI prognosis and monitoring CKD progression. Apart from degrading components of the extracellular matrix, MMP-7 also cleaves a wide range of substrates, such as E-cadherin, Fas ligand, and nephrin. As such, it plays an essential role in regulating many cellular processes, such as cell proliferation, apoptosis, epithelial-mesenchymal transition, and podocyte injury. The function of MMP-7 in kidney diseases is complex and context-dependent. It protects against AKI by priming tubular cells for survival and regeneration but promotes kidney fibrosis and CKD progression. MMP-7 also impairs podocyte integrity and induces proteinuria. In this review, we summarized recent advances in our understanding of the regulation, role, and mechanisms of MMP-7 in the pathogenesis of kidney diseases. We also discussed the potential of MMP-7 as a biomarker and therapeutic target in a clinical setting.

Keywords: matrix metalloproteinase-7; fibrosis; proteinuria; acute kidney injury; chronic kidney disease; apoptosis

---

1. Introduction

Matrix metalloproteinase-7 (MMP-7), also known as matrilysin-1, is one of the smallest secreted proteases of the MMP family, which consists of more than 20 structurally-related zinc-dependent endopeptidases with broad substrate specificity [1,2]. Collectively, MMPs degrade virtually all kinds of extracellular matrix (ECM) proteins and contribute to their turnover and remodeling. Furthermore, MMPs can also cleave many non-ECM substrates, making them a critical player in a wide variety of physiologic and pathologic processes, such as cell proliferation and apoptosis, endothelial cell function, inflammation, and tumor metastasis and invasion [3,4].

Extensive studies have shown that many MMPs are implicated in regulating kidney development and the pathogenesis of kidney diseases. Dysregulation of MMPs has been described in a wide variety of kidney disorders, including acute kidney injury (AKI), chronic kidney disease (CKD), diabetic kidney disease (DKD), glomerulonephritis, and inherited kidney diseases. Over the last two decades, due to the availability of MMP knockout models and specific pharmacological inhibitors, the role of MMPs, particularly MMP-2 and MMP-9, in regulating the development and progression of kidney diseases have been extensively investigated. The detailed discussion of these MMPs in kidney pathology as well as in non-renal diseases is beyond the scope of the present paper, and the interested readers are referred to several comprehensive reviews on this topic [1,2,5]. Instead, the focus of this review is on MMP-7 in kidney diseases.

MMP-7 was first discovered in the rat uterus [6]. Structurally, MMP-7 comprises a pro-peptide domain and a catalytic domain. While it was formerly believed to cleave only ECM proteins, the evidence is emerging that MMP-7 also degrades a variety of non-ECM substrates, such as nephrin, E-cadherin, Fas ligand (FasL), pro-MMP-2, and pro-MMP-9 [7–10]. As such, MMP-7 is able to regulate a diverse array of biological processes, such as podocyte dysfunction, epithelial to mesenchymal transition (EMT), cell proliferation, and apoptosis [11,12]. It should be stressed that many actions of MMP-7 in the kidney are highly specific and unique. For instance, only MMP-7, but neither MMP-2 nor MMP-9, can cleave podocyte slit diaphragm protein nephrin and cause proteinuria [7]. In this context, it is conceivable that MMP-7 may be more important than other MMPs to the pathogenesis of kidney diseases.

In the past several years, significant progress has been made in our understanding of the biology of MMP-7 in kidney diseases. Numerous novel substrates of MMP-7 have been identified, enabling us to better comprehend the exact role of MMP-7 in the pathogenesis of kidney disorders. Mounting evidence suggests that urinary MMP-7 (uMMP-7) can be utilized as a noninvasive biomarker for predicting AKI prognosis and monitoring CKD progression in patients [13–15]. In this review, we discussed the expression, regulation, novel substrates, and mechanisms of MMP-7 in various kidney diseases.

2. MMP-7 Structure, Activation, and Regulation

The human *MMP-7* gene is located on chromosome 11 q22.3. The cDNA of *MMP-7* encodes a protein containing 267 amino acids. Structurally, MMP-7 only consists of a pro-peptide domain and a catalytic domain (Figure 1A), which separates it from most other MMPs that contain an additional hinge region and a hemopexin-like domain [1,2,16]. The crystal structure of MMP-7 containing the two domains aforementioned is shown in Figure 1B.

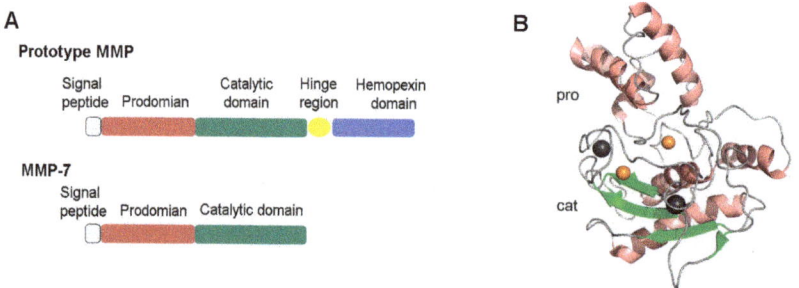

Figure 1. Structure of proMMP-7. (**A**) Full-length proMMP7 only consists of two domains: a pro-peptide domain (pro) and a catalytic domain (cat), which separates it from the prototype of MMPs. (**B**) The pro-peptide domain consists of three α-chains and connecting loops. The catalytic domain contains two zinc ions, two copper ions, and a ball-like structure consisting of three α-helices, five β-sheets, and multiple loops [16]. The image was prepared from Protein Data bank entries 2MZE (proMMP-7) using the PyMol (http://www.pymol.org). MMP, matrix metalloproteinase.

MMP-7 protein is produced and secreted as an inactive zymogen, which is maintained by a conserved cysteine residue that interacts with the zinc in the active site, rendering the protease inactive [16]. Disruption of this so-called cysteine switch is required for activation and can occur via proteolytic cleavage by many proteases, including trypsin, plasmin, or even other MMPs [17]. To generate a functional MMP-7 from the zymogen, the pro-peptide domain is proteolytically degraded in a stepwise manner [18]. The latent form of MMP-7 is a 28 kDa protein. After removing an approximately 9 kDa sequence from the pro-peptide domain, the resultant 19 kDa peptide represents the active and functional endopeptidase. MMP-7 is also bound by two calcium ions, which plays an important role in stabilizing the secondary structure of the protein.

The activity of MMP-7 is regulated by a family of naturally occurring endogenous inhibitors known as tissue inhibitors of metalloproteinases (TIMPs). There are four known TIMPs; however, it remains elusive which TIMP has the greatest specificity for MMP-7. There are also potent inhibitors of MMP-7, such as MMP inhibitor II, that can reversibly block MMP-7 activity. However, the selectivity of these inhibitors for MMP-7 is uncertain, as they often inhibit, to a lesser degree, other MMPs as well. One of the challenges in the field is to develop potent and selective inhibitors that are specific for a given MMP.

The expression of MMP-7 is transcriptionally regulated by different cues, particularly the Wnt/β-catenin and transforming growth factor-β (TGF-β). The promoter of the human *MMP-7* gene contains a TATA box, an activator protein 1 (AP-1) site, and T cell factor (TCF)-binding elements. The AP-1 binding site is essential for mediating MMP-7 expression in response to growth factors, oncogenes, and phorbol ester, while the TCF-binding elements are responsible for mediating MMP-7 induction by Wnt/β-catenin. As TGF-β is known to activate β-catenin signaling [19], it remains elusive whether TGF-β controls MMP-7 expression directly or via β-catenin indirectly.

3. MMP-7 Expression in the Kidney

MMP-7 is commonly expressed in epithelial cells, including the liver, the ductal epithelium of exocrine glands in the skin, salivary glands, and pancreas, and the glandular epithelium of the intestine and reproductive organ and breast. Under normal physiologic conditions, adult kidney exhibits little MMP-7 expression [12,18,20]. Consistent with this notion, mice with global knockout of *MMP-7* are phenotypically normal, without any renal abnormality [12]. These data suggest that MMP-7 is dispensable for kidney structure and function in basal physiologic conditions.

The expression of MMP-7 is, however, induced in a wide variety of kidney diseases, including AKI, CKD, glomerular disease, inherited kidney disease, and renal cell carcinoma [11,21–24], suggesting that MMP-7 induction is a common feature of the kidney after various injuries. The expression and localization of MMP-7 protein in various kidney disorders are summarized in Table 1.

3.1. Animal Models

MMP-7 is markedly induced after AKI. In experimental animal models of AKI induced by ischemia-reperfusion injury (IRI), cisplatin, or folic acid, both mRNA and protein levels of MMP-7 are upregulated [11]. Following IRI, MMP-7 protein is mainly expressed and localized in the renal tubular epithelium, particularly in the S3 segment of proximal tubules, the epicenter of kidney injury in this model [11]. These results indicate a spatial correlation of MMP-7 induction with tubular injury and repair and regeneration. At this stage, the exact cues for triggering MMP-7 induction in AKI in vivo remain ambiguous, but it is most likely related to activation of Wnt/β-catenin signaling. In vitro studies show that human kidney proximal tubular cells (HKC-8) increase MMP-7 expression upon stimulation of Wnt/β-catenin, whereas inhibition of Wnt/β-catenin by small molecule inhibitor ICG-001 negates MMP-7 induction [21].

Induction of MMP-7 is a common finding in a wide variety of CKD characterized by renal fibrosis. MMP-7 expression is increased in renal tubular epithelia in the mouse model of unilateral ureteral obstruction (UUO) [21]. Similar results are obtained in adriamycin nephropathy, a model of focal and segmental glomerulosclerosis (FSGS). Immunohistochemical staining reveals that MMP-7 expression and Wnt/β-catenin activation are closely correlated in both UUO and adriamycin nephropathy [21]. This result is compatible with the findings in tumors that MMP-7 transcript overlaps with the accumulation of β-catenin protein [25,26]. Therefore, it is conceivable that MMP-7 expression in CKD is causatively linked to the activation of Wnt/β-catenin signaling.

Table 1. Expression of matrix metalloproteinase-7 (MMP-7) in kidney diseases.

Disease	Location	Expression	Ref.
Animal models			
Ischemia–reperfusion -induced AKI [1]	Renal tubular epithelia	Increase	[11]
Folic acid-induced AKI	Renal tubular epithelia	Increase	[11,23]
Cisplatin-induced AKI	Renal tubular epithelia	Increase	[11]
UUO [2]	Renal tubular epithelia, interstitial cells	Increase	[12,21]
Human kidney diseases			
FSGS [3]	Renal tubular epithelia, interstitial cells, podocytes	Increase	[12,21]
Lupus nephritis	Renal tubular epithelia	Increase	[27]
Membranous nephritis	Renal tubular epithelia	Increase	[12]
Autosomal dominant polycystic kidney disease	Epithelial cells lining cysts, atrophic tubules	Increase	[23]
Diabetic nephropathy	Renal tubular epithelia, interstitial cells	Increase	[12,21]
Hydronephrosis	Cells lining dilated and atrophic tubules	Increase	[23]
Thrombotic microangiopathy	Renal tubular epithelia	Increase	[12]
IgA nephropathy	Renal tubular epithelia, infiltrated inflammatory cells	Increase	[12,21]
Acute renal allograft rejection	Renal tubular epithelia	No change	[28]
Chronic allograft nephropathy	Renal tubular epithelia	Increase	[29]
Amyloid light-chain amyloidosis	Glomerulus, tubular interstitium, vasculatures	Increase	[30]
Light chain deposition disease	Glomerulus, tubular interstitium, vasculatures	No change	[30]
Renal cell carcinoma	Cancer cells and endothelial cells	Increase	[22]

[1] Acute kidney injury. [2] Unilateral ureteral obstruction. [3] Focal segmental glomerulosclerosis.

3.2. Human Kidney Biopsies

Consistent with animal studies, the induction of MMP-7 expression is also evident in the kidney from patients with various renal disorders. For instance, in the kidney biopsies of patients with an autosomal dominant polycystic kidney disease, MMP-7 staining is observed in tubular epithelial lining cysts and atrophic tubules [23]. In the specimens of patients with hydronephrosis, MMP-7 is detected in dilated and atrophic renal tubules [31].

Kidney tissues from patients with IgA nephropathy (IgAN) show positive MMP-7 staining in renal tubular epithelia, fluids in the tubular lumen, and glomerular podocytes [12,21]. The RNA sequencing data from IgAN patients also show a significant increase in the mRNA expression of MMP-7 in the kidneys [32]. MMP-7 protein is increased in both tubular epithelial cells and the tubulointerstitial compartment of human diabetic kidneys [12,33]. Similarly, renal biopsy specimen analysis reveals MMP-7 induction in lupus nephritis and chronic allograft nephropathy [27,29]. Induction of MMP-7 expression has also been observed in the kidneys of patients with FSGS [12,21].

3.3. Mechanism of MMP-7 Regulation In Vivo

As to the cues responsible for MMP-7 induction in vivo, many studies have pointed to Wnt/β-catenin signaling, which is activated in virtually every kind of nephropathy [21,34,35]. When Wnt ligands bind to their receptors, β-catenin is stabilized and subsequently translocates into the nucleus for binding to the TCF/lymphoid enhancer-binding factor to regulate the transcription of its target genes, including MMP-7 [34,36,37]. Bioinformatics analysis reveals the presence of putative TCF-binding sites in the promoter region of the *MMP-7* gene [21]. Chromatin immunoprecipitation confirms that β-catenin activation promotes the binding of TCF to the *MMP-7* gene promoter, resulting in the expression of MMP-7 in kidney tubular epithelial cells [21].

There is also a correlation between MMP-7 and TGF-β in vivo, suggesting that TGF-β may play a role in mediating MMP-7 expression. Both TGF-β1 and MMP-7 are upregulated in streptozotocin-induced diabetic nephropathy rats. Sirtuin 1 (Sirt1) deacetylates Smad4 and inhibits the expression of MMP-7, indicating that the over-activation of TGF-β is related to the excessive acetylation of Smad4, which, in turn, causes MMP-7 induction [38,39]. Along these lines, resveratrol increases the expression of Sirt1, which inhibits MMP-7 and ultimately alleviates renal injury and fibrosis. Furthermore, TGF-β may indirectly augment MMP-7 by activating canonical Wnt signaling [19]. TGF-β also inhibits Dickkopf-1, an antagonist of Wnt, and potentiates the activity of β-catenin, thereby activating Wnt/β-catenin signaling [40,41]. Of interest, a study shows that MMP-7 can further induce TGF-β production via an MMP-7/Syndecan-1/TGF-β autocrine loop [42,43].

4. MMP-7 As a Biomarker for Kidney Diseases

Early identification and diagnosis are of importance in slowing the progression of kidney disease and preventing its complications [44]. Serum creatinine and blood urea nitrogen (BUN), two widely used markers for the diagnosis of kidney failure, increase only in the advanced stage of nephropathy. Consequently, kidney diseases are usually diagnosed at a later stage, and the implementation of therapeutic interventions is usually delayed. Therefore, there is an urgent need to develop novel biomarkers for early detection and prognostic assessment of kidney disorders [45]. MMP-7 is upregulated in various kidney diseases, and its protein is predominantly distributed in the apical region of tubular epithelial cells and is detected in the fluids present in the tubular lumen [12,21], suggesting that this protein could be secreted to the urine. Therefore, the level of uMMP-7 can be used as a potential non-invasive biomarker of kidney disease.

4.1. uMMP-7 Predicts the Risk of AKI

AKI is a relatively common disorder among hospitalized patients, occurring in more than 20% of all hospitalizations in large academic hospitals [46]. AKI causes approximately 2 million deaths each year worldwide. Current diagnostic criteria for AKI require changes in serum creatinine and urine output, which are not sensitive and represent delayed markers. Estimated glomerular filtration rate (eGFR) must decline by approximately 50% before any changes in serum creatinine can be detected [47,48]. Therefore, a sensitive and robust biomarker to predict the risk of AKI and its associated outcomes in patients is urgently needed. Over the past decades, there are tremendous efforts in the nephrology community to discover and validate potential biomarkers for AKI. Several biomarkers, such as kidney injury molecule-1 (Kim-1), neutrophil gelatinase-associated lipocalin (NGAL), and TIMP-2/insulin-like growth factor-binding protein-7 (IGFBP7), have been identified. Although some of them are applied to the clinic, they have various limitations.

There are two prospective cohort studies showing uMMP-7 as a valuable predictor of severe AKI after cardiac surgery [13,49]. In a prospective, multicenter, two-stage cohort study with 721 patients undergoing cardiac surgery, compared with the lowest quartile, a postoperative uMMP-7 level of 22.6 μg/g creatinine in children represents a >36-fold risk of severe AKI, whereas a postoperative uMMP-7 level of >15.2 μg/g creatinine in adults indicates a 17-fold risk of severe AKI [13]. In terms of predicting prognosis, higher uMMP-7 levels shortly after cardiac surgery are associated with an increased risk of acute dialysis or in-hospital deaths among children and adults, as well as longer duration of intensive care unit and hospital stays [13]. uMMP-7 outperforms other biomarkers, including urinary interleukin-18, NGAL, urinary angiotensinogen, albumin-to-creatinine ratio, and TIMP2/IGFBP7 [50–53], and the area under the receiver operating characteristic curve (AUC) of uMMP-7 is the largest for predicting severe AKI [13]. Of particular interest, uMMP-7 level peaks at 4 h after surgery, whereas the rise in serum creatinine occurs after 24 h in patients [13]. This is of clinical significance because it allows much earlier identification of the patients who have a high risk of developing AKI than serum creatinine. Therefore, uMMP-7 could be a valuable and robust biomarker for predicting the AKI after cardiac surgery. More studies are needed to replicate the results in larger and more diverse populations and in different settings of AKI.

4.2. uMMP-7 As a Biomarker of CKD Progression

Kidney fibrosis is a common outcome of virtually all CKDs [54,55], which is characterized by excessive accumulation and deposition of ECM, leading to tissue scarring. Measuring the extent of renal fibrosis is essential for determining the prognosis of renal outcomes, monitoring CKD progression, and evaluating the therapeutic efficacy of new treatments [55]. Currently, renal fibrosis is assessed only via percutaneous renal biopsy [55,56]. It is necessary to find non-invasive surrogate biomarkers for evaluating the development and progression of kidney fibrosis. Because activation of Wnt/β-catenin is a common feature of fibrotic CKD [57–60], one would speculate that the activity of renal Wnt/β-catenin signaling parallels the severity of renal fibrosis. Because the uMMP-7 level reflects the activity of renal Wnt/β-catenin [21], it is then reasonable to measure uMMP-7 to estimate the extent of kidney fibrosis.

In patients with CKD, uMMP-7 levels are found to positively correlate with renal fibrosis scores and have an inverse association with the renal function [12]. Therefore, uMMP-7 levels may serve as a noninvasive biomarker for kidney fibrosis and a predictor for CKD outcomes, as well as monitor the dynamic of fibrosis progression. Consistent with the findings in the kidney, MMP-7 also affects liver and lung fibrosis after a chronic injury. MMP-7 is upregulated in biliary atresia-associated liver fibrosis, and its expression is considered the best strategy to distinguish between cirrhosis and pre-cirrhosis stages [61,62]. Elevated MMP-7 levels are also detected in the peripheral blood of patients with human idiopathic pulmonary fibrosis (IPF) and may be used as a biomarker for predicting disease progression and death [63–66]. Serum MMP-7 levels are also increased in IPF patients with severe obstructive sleep apnea [67]. It should be pointed out that uMMP-7 is much more robust than serum MMP-7 in predicting kidney injury, as it is mainly produced from the injured tubular epithelium and expressed apically in CKD. In this context, uMMP-7 is particularly suitable for assessing the severity of fibrosis in the kidney, compared to other organs.

The feasibility and validity of uMMP-7 as a biomarker to predict CKD progression are recently supported by a prospective cohort study for uMMP-7 to serve as a predictor for IgAN progression [15]. The course of IgAN is highly variable and heterogeneous. The clinical manifestations range from benign asymptomatic microscopic hematuria to severe hypertension and progressive CKD, and renal pathological appearances range from normal to different degrees of mesangial cell proliferation [68]. At present, the final diagnosis of IgAN mainly relies on renal biopsy [68]. On the basis of a histological assessment, variables including mesangial hypercellularity (M), endocapillary hypercellularity (E), segmental glomerulosclerosis (S) and tubular atrophy and interstitial fibrosis (T) give rise to MEST score and provide valuable information to prognostication of IgAN [69]. The lack of sensitive and specific surrogate indicators for long-term outcomes makes it challenging to improve treatment options [70]. A recent prospective observational cohort study shows that the level of uMMP-7 may serve as an independent and powerful predictor for IgAN progression, even for those patients who are still in the early stages of IgAN, as defined by an eGFR of $\geq$ 60 mL/min/1.73 m^2 [15]. High levels (> 3.9 μg/g of creatinine) of uMMP-7 increase the risk of IgAN progression by 2.7 times in an adjusted analysis [15]. Several earlier studies have suggested numerous possible biomarkers in serum or urine for predicting IgAN progressions, such as galactose-deficient IgA1, auto-antibodies against Gd-IgA1, fibroblast growth factor 23, angiotensinogen, epidermal growth factor, and Kim-1 [71–77]. Measurement of uMMP-7 level outperforms each of these biomarkers in risk prediction and improves the risk predictive power of a MEST score [15]. Some retrospective follow-up studies also show that an increase in serum MMP-7 levels is associated with a high risk of poor renal outcome and renal fibrosis [74]. In addition, uMMP-7 is also identified to serve as an independent predictor of tissue remodeling and renal interstitial fibrosis in children with CKD [78]. Another study shows that among people with type 2 diabetes and proteinuric DKD, uMMP-7 concentration is strongly associated with disease progression and subsequent mortality [14]. Taken together, these findings indicate that uMMP-7 may hold promise as a noninvasive biomarker for kidney fibrosis and CKD progression.

5. Roles of MMP-7 in Kidney Diseases

Thanks to the availability of MMP-7 knockout mice, we now have a better understanding of the role of MMP-7 in the pathogenesis of kidney diseases. Although the specific action of MMP-7 in different nephropathy models has not been fully clarified, numerous studies have discovered discrete roles of MMP-7 in renal pathophysiology in different settings. Furthermore, the role of MMP-7 may also evolve with different disease types or the time course of kidney disorders. For instance, MMP-7 may be reparative in the early stages of AKI, whereas it may be detrimental as the disease progresses. Table 2 summarizes the roles of MMP-7 in various kidney diseases.

Table 2. Roles of MMP-7 in kidney diseases.

Disease	Role of MMP-7	Ref.
AKI [1]	Protecting against AKI by priming tubular cells for proliferation and survival	[11]
UUO [2]	Promoting renal fibrosis by activating partial EMT and β-catenin	[12]
Proteinuric CKD [3]	Increasing urinary albumin excretion by impairing the glomerular filtration barrier	[7]
Diabetic nephropathy	Initiating diabetic nephropathy by expanding glomerular mesangium and thickening glomerular basement membrane	[79]
Chronic allograft nephropathy	MMPs, including MMP-7, contribute to the deregulation of extracellular matrix remodeling and possibly EMT.	[29]
Light chain deposition disease	The decrease of MMPs, including MMP-7, leads to the accumulation of tenascin and extracellular matrix	[30]
Amyloid light-chain amyloidosis	The increase of MMPs, including MMP-7, leads to the reduction of extracellular matrix	[30]
Renal cell carcinoma	Affecting tumor progression by regulating invasion and angiogenesis	[22]

[1] Acute kidney injury. [2] Unilateral ureteral obstruction. [3] Chronic kidney disease.

5.1. MMP-7 Protects Against AKI

MMP-7 is induced specifically in renal tubular epithelium after AKI, a condition characterized by the death of tubular cells and the infiltration of inflammatory cells to the kidney [80–82]. In AKI patients after cardiac surgery, uMMP-7 levels increase rapidly and peak at 4 h, suggesting MMP-7 induction is an early event [13]. Using MMP-7$^{-/-}$ null mice, a recent study shows that MMP-7 has a renal protective effect against AKI as it alleviates injury by reducing the number of dead tubular cells, promoting the proliferation of tubular cells, and suppressing inflammation [11]. Compared with wild-type controls, MMP-7$^{-/-}$ mice display higher mortality, elevated serum creatinine, and more severe histologic lesions after IRI or cisplatin. These changes are accompanied by more prominent tubular cell death and interstitial inflammation in MMP-7$^{-/-}$ kidneys. In a rescue experiment, injection of exogenous MMP-7 protects against kidney injury in MMP-7$^{-/-}$ mice after IRI, confirming a renal protective action of MMP-7. Of note, MMP-7 may only play a protective role in the early stages of AKI because the long-term activation of MMP-7 leads to kidney fibrosis [12].

5.2. MMP-7 Promotes Kidney Fibrosis and CKD Progression

CKD is characterized by excessive ECM accumulation and interstitial fibroblast activation [54,83–85]. Given its proteolytic potential to degrade ECM proteins, MMP-7 was originally thought to be anti-fibrotic. Surprisingly, it is found that MMP-7 plays a critical role in the development of fibrotic CKD [12]. In mice, the genetic ablation of MMP-7 reduces the fibrotic lesions and ECM accumulation induced by UUO. Knockout of *MMP-7* also preserves E-cadherin protein and inhibits the de novo expression of vimentin in renal tubules of obstructed kidneys, suggesting that MMP-7 may promote EMT in vivo. Although the role of EMT in renal fibrosis remains controversial, partial EMT is an indispensable part of renal fibrosis [57,86]. Along these lines, it appears that MMP-7 plays an important role in the onset and progression of renal fibrosis by impairing the integrity of renal tubular epithelium and causing partial EMT [12]. Loss of E-cadherin mediated by MMP-7 leads to β-catenin liberation and nuclear translocation, which facilitates CKD progression [57,87]. Of note, MMP-7-mediated β-catenin liberation further induces MMP-7 expression, creating a vicious cycle [12]. Furthermore, TGF-β is known to induce MMP-7 expression, consistent with their role in promoting EMT and kidney fibrosis [38,39]. More studies are needed to confirm the detrimental role of MMP-7 in other models of CKD.

5.3. MMP-7 Induces Podocyte Dysfunction and Proteinuria

In glomerular diseases, MMP-7 is specifically induced in glomerular podocytes of the diseased kidney, implying its potential role in regulating podocyte injury and proteinuria. Indeed, a recent study shows that the infusion of MMP-7 protein or injection of *MMP-7* expression vector induces transient proteinuria in normal mice [7], suggesting that MMP-7 can trigger podocyte injury and impair the glomerular filtration barrier. Furthermore, MMP-7$^{-/-}$ mice are protected against proteinuria and glomerular injury induced by either angiotensin II or adriamycin [7]. Consistent with this finding, incubation of isolated glomeruli with MMP-7 ex vivo increases glomerular permeability and causes foot process effacement. These observations illustrate that MMP-7 impairs glomerular filtration and causes proteinuria in vivo.

CKD progression is characterized by increasingly widespread lesions in different compartments of the kidney parenchyma. There is ample evidence to suggest that the progression of the primary glomerular disease can trigger tubular injury and interstitial fibrosis, but whether tubular injury affects the function of the glomerulus remains ambiguous [88]. Recently, using conditional knockout mice with tubule-specific ablation of β-catenin, we discovered that tubule-derived MMP-7 is a pathological mediator of glomerular damage [7]. MMP-7 is secreted as a soluble protein from the tubules to the glomeruli and mediates the impairment of slit diaphragm integrity, leading to podocyte dysfunction and increased proteinuria [7]. This suggests that MMP-7 is the key mediator of tubular-to-glomerular crosstalk that promotes proteinuria and CKD progression.

6. Mechanisms and Novel Targets of MMP-7 in Kidney Diseases

The diverse actions of MMP-7 in kidney diseases are presumably mediated by its ability to cleave different substrates. As the primary role of activated MMP-7 is to break down ECM components, MMP-7 is well known to degrade macromolecules, including casein, type I, II, IV, and V gelatins, fibronectin, and proteoglycan [2,89]. Recent findings reveal, however, that MMP-7 is also capable of degrading a multitude of non-ECM substrates, such as FasL, E-cadherin, nephrin, and proMMP-2 and -9 [8–10,12]. These novel actions of MMP-7 play a crucial role in mediating its diverse functions in the pathogenesis of kidney disorders. Figure 2 illustrates the mechanisms of MMP-7 action in kidney disease.

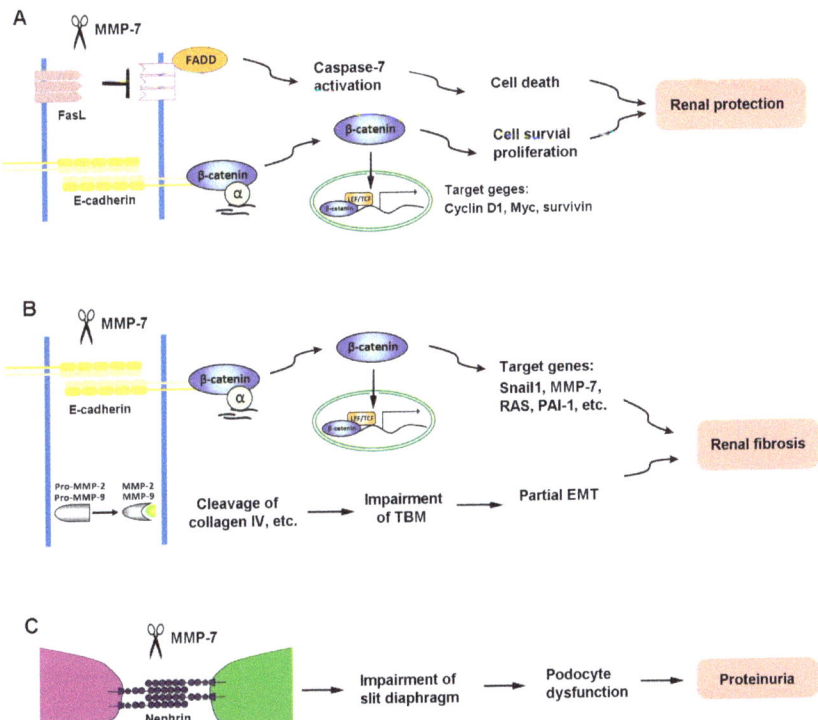

Figure 2. The mechanisms of MMP-7 action in kidney disease. (**A**) In renal tubular epithelial cells, MMP-7 promotes cell proliferation and reduces cell death by degrading E-cadherin and FasL, respectively, and finally plays a role in protecting the kidney during acute kidney injury (AKI). (**B**) However, MMP-7 also degrades E-cadherin and activates proMMP-2 and -9, leading to renal fibrosis. (**C**) In podocytes, MMP-7-mediated degradation of nephrin impairs the integrity of the slit diaphragm, which subsequently causes an increase in proteinuria and eventually leads to renal fibrosis.

6.1. FasL

There are two signaling pathways leading to apoptosis: the intrinsic pathway and extrinsic pathway [90–92]. The FasL plays a central role in the death receptor-dependent extrinsic apoptosis pathway [93]. Dependent upon different pathological conditions and different cells, MMP-7 shows a bi-directional effect on the induction or degradation of FasL, which plays distinct roles in regulating cell survival/death in different settings. MMP-7 degrades FasL to decrease the apoptosis of renal tubular cells through FasL/Fas-associated death domain (FADD)/caspase-7 activation, which is one of the mechanisms underlying MMP-7 protection of kidney tubular cells against death in the early stage of AKI [11] (Figure 2). Consistently, MMP-7-induced cleavage of the membrane-bound FasL also plays a role in the process of pulmonary fibrosis [94].

Studies also show that MMP-7 affects the fate of renal interstitial fibroblasts in the opposite way. MMP-7 is shown to induce the expression of FasL in cultured fibroblasts, which promotes fibroblast apoptosis and facilitates its resolution after kidney repair following AKI [95]. This observation is supported by studies conducted on cancer cells, which also shows that MMP-7 induces the expression of FasL and subsequently activates the extrinsic apoptotic pathway [10,96]. Furthermore, MMP-7 enhances the staurosporine-mediated intrinsic apoptosis pathway [97,98], leading to fibroblast apoptosis [95]. In this regard, MMP-7-induced fibroblast apoptosis requires the synergistic action of both the intrinsic and extrinsic pathways. At this stage, the mechanism by which MMP-7 induces FasL expression remains to be determined. It is likely that MMP-7 cleaves and activates an unidentified intermediate molecule, which, in turn, induces FasL expression.

6.2. E-Cadherin

E-cadherin, a classical member of the cadherin superfamily, is an epithelial marker that plays an important role in maintaining the integrity of tubular epithelial cells and cell–cell adhesion [99]. It is a calcium-dependent cell–cell adhesion receptor composed of five extracellular cadherin repeats, a transmembrane region, and a highly conserved cytoplasmic tail. MMP-7 is capable of degrading E-cadherin via ectodomain shedding. It has been shown that MMP-7 affects both CKD and AKI by cleaving E-cadherin [8,100]. Loss of E-cadherin impairs the integrity of tubular epithelial cells, which is recognized as the initial step of partial EMT, a process that is essential for tubular atrophy and kidney fibrosis [101,102]. Because E-cadherin and β-catenin associate with each other in a cellular adhesion complex [99,103], the cleavage of E-cadherin would result in the dissociation of the E-cadherin/β-catenin complex, leading to β-catenin liberation (Figure 2). In essence, MMP-7 can induce kidney fibrosis by activating β-catenin in the absence of Wnt ligands [12]. Notably, such β-catenin release caused by MMP-7-mediated degradation of E-cadherin is also found in mouse prostate cancer cells [104].

The liberation of β catenin caused by MMP-7-mediated degradation of E-cadherin provides a rational explanation for why MMP-7 promotes renal fibrosis. The exact same pathway, however, is beneficial and plays a protective role against AKI (Figure 2). E-cadherin maintains tight cell–cell adhesion among tubular epithelia [105]. The ability of MMP-7 to degrade E-cadherin disrupts epithelial cell contact inhibition [106] and leads to cell proliferation [107–109]. E-cadherin degradation also leads to β-catenin liberation and downstream signaling. In vitro experiments have confirmed that proliferation-related proteins, such as proliferating cell nuclear antigen (PCNA) and c-Fos, are increased in isolated renal tubules cultured with mitogen-rich serum and MMP-7, compared with serum alone [11]. In short, by cleaving E-cadherin and releasing β-catenin, MMP-7 creates an environment conducive to cell proliferation and protects renal tubules against AKI [11]. However, loss of cell contact inhibition can also trigger EMT and lead to a profibrotic phenotype after the acute injury has resolved. Therefore, MMP-7 induction could be beneficial in the early phase of kidney injury but not in the late stage of chronic kidney disorders. The balance of beneficial versus detrimental effects may rely upon the time point at which MMP-7 activation occurs.

6.3. Nephrin

Nephrin is a key component of the slit diaphragm, which connects adjacent podocyte foot processes and plays a fundamental role in glomerular filtration [110]. We recently demonstrated that nephrin is a specific and direct substrate of MMP-7 [7] (Figure 2). MMP-7 is shown to degrade nephrin in cultured glomeruli, cultured cells, and cell-free systems, which is dependent on its proteolytic activity. Such action of MMP-7 on nephrin degradation is rapid, starting as early as 5 min after incubation. Furthermore, the action of MMP-7 on nephrin appears direct, cleaving purified recombinant nephrin protein in a cell-free system. It should be stressed that the action of MMP-7 is specific, as other MMPs, such as MMP-2 and MMP-9, are unable to degrade nephrin in the same conditions. These findings not only identify nephrin as a novel substrate of MMP-7 but also offer a mechanistic insight into the role of MMP-7 in the development of proteinuria and glomerular lesions [7]. Therefore, MMP-7-mediated cleavage of nephrin impairs slit diaphragm integrity to promote podocyte injury and proteinuria.

6.4. Pro-MMP-2 and -9

MMP-7 also promotes renal fibrosis by proteolytically activating MMP-2 and MMP-9 from their latent zymogen forms. In an in vitro experiment, it has been shown that MMP-7 activates pro-MMP-2 by propeptide removal [111]. Earlier studies in tumor cells also show that MMP-7 is a potential activator of pro-MMP-2 [112], through competitively binding to the TIMP-2 from MMP-2/TIMP-2 complexes, leading to the release of functional MMP-2 [113,114]. Because MMP-2 can convert pro-MMP-9 into MMP-9, it is conceivable that MMP-7 can activate MMP-9 by generating active MMP-2 in both direct and indirect ways [113–115]. At present, some studies show that MMP-2 and MMP-9 play an important role in the onset and progression of CKD via degrading type IV collagen, promoting partial EMT and mediating a complex interaction with various cytokines [116,117]. Therefore, MMP-7 could promote kidney fibrosis and CKD progression by activating MMP-2 and MMP-9.

7. Conclusion and Perspectives

Over the last several years, our understanding of MMP-7 in the pathogenesis of kidney disease has dramatically improved. MMP-7 is upregulated in AKI, CKD, and glomerular diseases and is predominantly localized in renal tubular epithelia. Recent findings on novel substrates of MMP-7, such as nephrin, have shed new light on its role and mechanisms of action in a wide variety of kidney diseases. By cleaving E-cadherin and FasL, MMP-7 protects the kidney from AKI by priming renal tubular cells for survival and proliferation. The same MMP-7-mediated degradation of E-cadherin in CKD setting, however, promotes tubular EMT and activates β-catenin in a Wnt-independent fashion, leading to kidney fibrosis. MMP-7 can directly degrade nephrin, resulting in podocyte dysfunction and proteinuria. Several clinical cohort studies suggest that uMMP-7 levels may be used as a noninvasive biomarker for predicting AKI prognosis and monitoring CKD progression in patients.

Although the present studies have provided invaluable insights into the biological functions of MMP-7 in kidney diseases, how to translate this knowledge into patient care is a daunting task. The revelation of MMP-7 upregulation provides hopes for the application of uMMP-7 as a noninvasive biomarker, and future clinical studies for validation in large and diverse populations of patients are warranted. Developing a therapy to target MMP-7 will rely upon highly selective inhibitors for MMP-7, which are not yet available. Future studies may focus on developing efficient strategies to inhibit MMP-7 expression in vivo for modulating the course of kidney disease. We hope that continuing this line of investigation will improve our understanding of the role of MMP-7 and its mechanism of action in the pathogenesis of various kidney disorders, and eventually translate into improved patient care.

Funding: This research was funded by the National Natural Science Foundation of China (grant 81521003 and 81920108007) and the National Institute of Health grant DK064005.

Conflicts of Interest: The authors declare no conflict of interest.

References

1. Catania, J.M.; Chen, G.; Parrish, A.R. Role of matrix metalloproteinases in renal pathophysiologies. *Am. J. Physiol. Renal Physiol.* **2007**, *292*, F905–F911. [CrossRef] [PubMed]
2. Tan, R.J.; Liu, Y. Matrix metalloproteinases in kidney homeostasis and diseases. *Am. J. Physiol. Renal Physiol.* **2012**, *302*, F1351–F1361. [CrossRef] [PubMed]
3. Amar, S.; Smith, L.; Fields, G.B. Matrix metalloproteinase collagenolysis in health and disease. *BBA-Mol. Cell Res.* **2017**, *1864*, 1940–1951. [CrossRef] [PubMed]
4. Cui, N.; Hu, M.; Khalil, R.A. Biochemical and Biological Attributes of Matrix Metalloproteinases. *Pro. Mol. Biol. Trans. Sci.* **2017**, *147*, 1–73.
5. Kessenbrock, K.; Plaks, V.; Werb, Z. Matrix metalloproteinases: Regulators of the tumor microenvironment. *Cell* **2010**, *141*, 52–67. [CrossRef]
6. Woessner, J.F., Jr.; Taplin, C.J. Purification and properties of a small latent matrix metalloproteinase of the rat uterus. *J. Biol. Chem.* **1988**, *263*, 16918–16925.
7. Tan, R.J.; Li, Y.; Rush, B.M.; Cerqueira, D.M.; Zhou, D.; Fu, H.; Ho, J.; Beer Stolz, D.; Liu, Y. Tubular injury triggers podocyte dysfunction by beta-catenin-driven release of MMP-7. *JCI Insight* **2019**, *4*, e122399. [CrossRef]
8. McGuire, J.K.; Li, Q.; Parks, W.C. Matrilysin (matrix metalloproteinase-7) mediates E-cadherin ectodomain shedding in injured lung epithelium. *Am. J. Pathol.* **2003**, *162*, 1831–1843. [CrossRef]

9. Vargo-Gogola, T.; Crawford, H.C.; Fingleton, B.; Matrisian, L.M. Identification of novel matrix metalloproteinase-7 (matrilysin) cleavage sites in murine and human Fas ligand. *Arch. Biochem. Biophys.* **2002**, *408*, 155–161. [CrossRef]
10. Mitsiades, N.; Yu, W.H.; Poulaki, V.; Tsokos, M.; Stamenkovic, I. Matrix metalloproteinase-7-mediated cleavage of Fas ligand protects tumor cells from chemotherapeutic drug cytotoxicity. *Cancer Res.* **2001**, *61*, 577–581.
11. Fu, H.; Zhou, D.; Zhu, H.; Liao, J.; Lin, L.; Hong, X.; Hou, F.F.; Liu, Y. Matrix metalloproteinase-7 protects against acute kidney injury by priming renal tubules for survival and regeneration. *Kidney Int.* **2019**, *95*, 1167–1180. [CrossRef] [PubMed]
12. Zhou, D.; Tian, Y.; Sun, L.; Zhou, L.; Xiao, L.; Tan, R.J.; Tian, J.; Fu, H.; Hou, F.F.; Liu, Y. Matrix metalloproteinase-7 is a urinary biomarker and pathogenic mediator of kidney fibrosis. *J. Am. Soc. Nephrol.* **2017**, *28*, 598–611. [CrossRef] [PubMed]
13. Yang, X.; Chen, C.; Teng, S.; Fu, X.; Zha, Y.; Liu, H.; Wang, L.; Tian, J.; Zhang, X.; Liu, Y.; et al. Urinary matrix metalloproteinase-7 predicts severe AKI and poor outcomes after cardiac surgery. *J. Am. Soc. Nephrol.* **2017**, *28*, 3373–3382. [CrossRef] [PubMed]
14. Afkarian, M.; Zelnick, L.R.; Ruzinski, J.; Kestenbaum, B.; Himmelfarb, J.; de Boer, I.H.; Mehrotra, R. Urine matrix metalloproteinase-7 and risk of kidney disease progression and mortality in type 2 diabetes. *J. Diabetes Complicat.* **2015**, *29*, 1024–1031. [CrossRef] [PubMed]
15. Yang, X.; Ou, J.; Zhang, H.; Xu, X.; Zhu, L.; Li, Q.; Li, J.; Xie, D.; Sun, J.; Zha, Y.; et al. Urinary matrix metalloproteinase 7 and prediction of IgA nephropathy progression. *Am. J. Kidney Dis.* **2020**, *75*, 384–393. [CrossRef] [PubMed]
16. Nagase, H.; Visse, R.; Murphy, G. Structure and function of matrix metalloproteinases and TIMPs. *Cardiovasc Res.* **2006**, *69*, 562–573. [CrossRef]
17. Van Wart, H.E.; Birkedal-Hansen, H. The cysteine switch: A principle of regulation of metalloproteinase activity with potential applicability to the entire matrix metalloproteinase gene family. *Proc. Natl. Acad. Sci. USA* **1990**, *87*, 5578–5582. [CrossRef]
18. Visse, R.; Nagase, H. Matrix metalloproteinases and tissue inhibitors of metalloproteinases: Structure, function, and biochemistry. *Circ. Res.* **2003**, *92*, 827–839. [CrossRef]
19. Wang, D.; Dai, C.; Li, Y.; Liu, Y. Canonical Wnt/beta-catenin signaling mediates transforming growth factor-beta1-driven podocyte injury and proteinuria. *Kidney Int.* **2011**, *80*, 1159–1169. [CrossRef]
20. Lu, H.; Yang, Z.; Zhang, H.; Gan, M.; Zhou, T.; Wang, S. The expression and clinical significance of matrix metalloproteinase 7 and tissue inhibitor of matrix metalloproteinases 2 in clear cell renal cell carcinoma. *Exp. Ther. Med.* **2013**, *5*, 890–896. [CrossRef]
21. He, W.; Tan, R.J.; Li, Y.; Wang, D.; Nie, J.; Hou, F.F.; Liu, Y. Matrix metalloproteinase-7 as a surrogate marker predicts renal Wnt/beta-catenin activity in CKD. *J. Am. Soc. Nephrol.* **2012**, *23*, 294–304. [CrossRef] [PubMed]
22. Miyata, Y.; Iwata, T.; Ohba, K.; Kanda, S.; Nishikido, M.; Kanetake, H. Expression of matrix metalloproteinase-7 on cancer cells and tissue endothelial cells in renal cell carcinoma: Prognostic implications and clinical significance for invasion and metastasis. *Clin. Cancer Res.* **2006**, *12*, 6998–7003. [CrossRef] [PubMed]
23. Surendran, K.; Simon, T.C.; Liapis, H.; McGuire, J.K. Matrilysin (MMP-7) expression in renal tubular damage: Association with Wnt4. *Kidney Int.* **2004**, *65*, 2212–2222. [CrossRef] [PubMed]
24. Melk, A.; Mansfield, E.S.; Hsieh, S.C.; Hernandez-Boussard, T.; Grimm, P.; Rayner, D.C.; Halloran, P.F.; Sarwal, M.M. Transcriptional analysis of the molecular basis of human kidney aging using cDNA microarray profiling. *Kidney Int.* **2005**, *68*, 2667–2679. [CrossRef]
25. Brabletz, T.; Jung, A.; Dag, S.; Hlubek, F.; Kirchner, T. beta-catenin regulates the expression of the matrix metalloproteinase-7 in human colorectal cancer. *Am. J. Pathol.* **1999**, *155*, 1033–1038. [CrossRef]
26. Crawford, H.C.; Fingleton, B.; Gustavson, M.D.; Kurpios, N.; Wagenaar, R.A.; Hassell, J.A.; Matrisian, L.M. The PEA3 subfamily of Ets transcription factors synergizes with beta-catenin-LEF-1 to activate matrilysin transcription in intestinal tumors. *Mol. Cell. Biol.* **2001**, *21*, 1370–1383. [CrossRef]
27. Reich, H.N.; Landolt-Marticorena, C.; Boutros, P.C.; John, R.; Wither, J.; Fortin, P.R.; Yang, S.; Scholey, J.W.; Herzenberg, A.M. Molecular markers of injury in kidney biopsy specimens of patients with lupus nephritis. *J. Mol. Diagn.* **2011**, *13*, 143–151. [CrossRef]

28. Rodder, S.; Scherer, A.; Korner, M.; Eisenberger, U.; Hertig, A.; Raulf, F.; Rondeau, E.; Marti, H.P. Meta-analyses qualify metzincins and related genes as acute rejection markers in renal transplant patients. *Am. J. Transpl.* **2010**, *10*, 286–297. [CrossRef]
29. Rodder, S.; Scherer, A.; Raulf, F.; Berthier, C.C.; Hertig, A.; Couzi, L.; Durrbach, A.; Rondeau, E.; Marti, H.P. Renal allografts with IF/TA display distinct expression profiles of metzincins and related genes. *Am. J. Transpl.* **2009**, *9*, 517–526. [CrossRef]
30. Keeling, J.; Herrera, G.A. Matrix metalloproteinases and mesangial remodeling in light chain-related glomerular damage. *Kidney Int.* **2005**, *68*, 1590–1603. [CrossRef]
31. Henger, A.; Kretzler, M.; Doran, P.; Bonrouhi, M.; Schmid, H.; Kiss, E.; Cohen, C.D.; Madden, S.; Porubsky, S.; Grone, E.F.; et al. Gene expression fingerprints in human tubulointerstitial inflammation and fibrosis as prognostic markers of disease progression. *Kidney Int.* **2004**, *65*, 904–917. [CrossRef] [PubMed]
32. Jiang, H.; Liang, L.; Qin, J.; Lu, Y.; Li, B.; Wang, Y.; Lin, C.; Zhou, Q.; Feng, S.; Yip, S.H.; et al. Functional networks of aging markers in the glomeruli of IgA nephropathy: A new therapeutic opportunity. *Oncotarget* **2016**, *7*, 33616–33626. [CrossRef] [PubMed]
33. Cohen, C.D.; Lindenmeyer, M.T.; Eichinger, F.; Hahn, A.; Seifert, M.; Moll, A.G.; Schmid, H.; Kiss, E.; Grone, E.; Grone, H.J.; et al. Improved elucidation of biological processes linked to diabetic nephropathy by single probe-based microarray data analysis. *PLoS ONE* **2008**, *3*, e2937. [CrossRef] [PubMed]
34. Zuo, Y.; Liu, Y. New insights into the role and mechanism of Wnt/beta-catenin signalling in kidney fibrosis. *Nephrology* **2018**, *23* (Suppl. 4), 38–43. [CrossRef]
35. Zhou, D.; Tan, R.J.; Fu, H.; Liu, Y. Wnt/beta-catenin signaling in kidney injury and repair: A double-edged sword. *Lab. Investig.* **2016**, *96*, 156–167. [CrossRef]
36. Angers, S.; Moon, R.T. Proximal events in Wnt signal transduction. *Nat. Rev. Mol. Cell Biol.* **2009**, *10*, 468–477. [CrossRef]
37. Zhou, L.; Liu, Y. Wnt/beta-catenin signalling and podocyte dysfunction in proteinuric kidney disease. *Nat. Rev. Nephrol.* **2015**, *11*, 535–545. [CrossRef]
38. Simic, P.; Williams, E.O.; Bell, E.L.; Gong, J.J.; Bonkowski, M.; Guarente, L. SIRT1 suppresses the epithelial-to-mesenchymal transition in cancer metastasis and organ fibrosis. *Cell Rep.* **2013**, *3*, 1175–1186. [CrossRef]
39. Xiao, Z.; Chen, C.; Meng, T.; Zhang, W.; Zhou, Q. Resveratrol attenuates renal injury and fibrosis by inhibiting transforming growth factor-beta pathway on matrix metalloproteinase 7. *Exp. Biol. Med.* **2016**, *241*, 140–146. [CrossRef]
40. Akhmetshina, A.; Palumbo, K.; Dees, C.; Bergmann, C.; Venalis, P.; Zerr, P.; Horn, A.; Kireva, T.; Beyer, C.; Zwerina, J.; et al. Activation of canonical Wnt signalling is required for TGF-beta-mediated fibrosis. *Nat. Commun.* **2012**, *3*, 735. [CrossRef]
41. Nlandu-Khodo, S.; Neelisetty, S.; Phillips, M.; Manolopoulou, M.; Bhave, G.; May, L.; Clark, P.E.; Yang, H.; Fogo, A.B.; Harris, R.C.; et al. Blocking TGF-beta and beta-catenin epithelial crosstalk exacerbates CKD. *J. Am. Soc. Nephrol.* **2017**, *28*, 3490–3503. [CrossRef] [PubMed]
42. Zeng, Y.; Yao, X.; Chen, L.; Yan, Z.; Liu, J.; Zhang, Y.; Feng, T.; Wu, J.; Liu, X. Sphingosine-1-phosphate induced epithelial-mesenchymal transition of hepatocellular carcinoma via an MMP-7/syndecan-1/TGF-β autocrine loop. *Oncotarget* **2016**, *7*, 63324–63337. [CrossRef] [PubMed]
43. Zeng, Y.; Liu, X.; Yan, Z.; Xie, L. Sphingosine 1-phosphate regulates proliferation, cell cycle and apoptosis of hepatocellular carcinoma cells via syndecan-1. *Prog. Biophys. Mol. Biol.* **2019**, *148*, 32–38. [CrossRef]
44. Fink, H.A.; Ishani, A.; Taylor, B.C.; Greer, N.L.; MacDonald, R.; Rossini, D.; Sadiq, S.; Lankireddy, S.; Kane, R.L.; Wilt, T.J. Screening for, monitoring, and treatment of chronic kidney disease stages 1 to 3: A systematic review for the U.S. Preventive Services Task Force and for an American College of Physicians Clinical Practice Guideline. *Ann. Intern. Med.* **2012**, *156*, 570–581. [CrossRef] [PubMed]
45. Rysz, J.; Gluba-Brzózka, A.; Franczyk, B.; Jabłonowski, Z.; Ciałkowska-Rysz, A. Novel Biomarkers in the Diagnosis of Chronic Kidney Disease and the Prediction of Its Outcome. *Int. J. Mol. Sci.* **2017**, *18*, 1702. [CrossRef]
46. Ronco, C.; Bellomo, R.; Kellum, J.A. Acute kidney injury. *Lancet* **2019**, *394*, 1949–1964. [CrossRef]
47. Delanaye, P.; Cavalier, E.; Pottel, H. Serum creatinine: Not so simple! *Nephron* **2017**, *136*, 302–308. [CrossRef]
48. Ronco, C.; Bellomo, R.; Kellum, J. Understanding renal functional reserve. *Inten. Care Med.* **2017**, *43*, 917–920. [CrossRef]

49. Fang, F.; Luo, W.; Yang, M.; Yang, P.; Yang, X. Urinary matrix metalloproteinase-7 and prediction of AKI progression post cardiac surgery. *Dis. Markers* **2019**, *2019*, 9217571. [CrossRef]
50. Parikh, C.R.; Devarajan, P.; Zappitelli, M.; Sint, K.; Thiessen-Philbrook, H.; Li, S.; Kim, R.W.; Koyner, J.L.; Coca, S.G.; Edelstein, C.L.; et al. Postoperative biomarkers predict acute kidney injury and poor outcomes after pediatric cardiac surgery. *J. Am. Soc. Nephrol.* **2011**, *22*, 1737–1747. [CrossRef]
51. Yang, X.; Chen, C.; Tian, J.; Zha, Y.; Xiong, Y.; Sun, Z.; Chen, P.; Li, J.; Yang, T.; Ma, C.; et al. Urinary angiotensinogen level predicts AKI in acute decompensated heart failure: A prospective, two-Stage Study. *J. Am. Soc. Nephrol.* **2015**, *26*, 2032–2041. [CrossRef] [PubMed]
52. Alge, J.L.; Karakala, N.; Neely, B.A.; Janech, M.G.; Tumlin, J.A.; Chawla, L.S.; Shaw, A.D.; Arthur, J.M. Urinary angiotensinogen and risk of severe AKI. *Clin. J. Am. Soc. Nephrol.* **2013**, *8*, 184–193. [CrossRef] [PubMed]
53. Molnar, A.O.; Parikh, C.R.; Sint, K.; Coca, S.G.; Koyner, J.; Patel, U.D.; Butrymowicz, I.; Shlipak, M.; Garg, A.X. Association of postoperative proteinuria with AKI after cardiac surgery among patients at high risk. *Clin. J. Am. Soc. Nephrol.* **2012**, *7*, 1749–1760. [CrossRef] [PubMed]
54. Liu, Y. Cellular and molecular mechanisms of renal fibrosis. *Nat. Rev. Nephrol.* **2011**, *7*, 684–696. [CrossRef]
55. Farris, A.B.; Alpers, C.E. What is the best way to measure renal fibrosis?: A pathologist's perspective. *Kidney Int. Suppl.* **2014**, *4*, 9–15. [CrossRef]
56. Farris, A.B.; Adams, C.D.; Brousaides, N.; Della Pelle, P.A.; Collins, A.B.; Moradi, E.; Smith, R.N.; Grimm, P.C.; Colvin, R.B. Morphometric and visual evaluation of fibrosis in renal biopsies. *J. Am. Soc. Nephrol.* **2011**, *22*, 176–186. [CrossRef]
57. Tan, R.J.; Zhou, D.; Zhou, L.; Liu, Y. Wnt/beta-catenin signaling and kidney fibrosis. *Kidney Int. Suppl.* **2014**, *4*, 84–90. [CrossRef]
58. Dai, C.; Stolz, D.B.; Kiss, L.P.; Monga, S.P.; Holzman, L.B.; Liu, Y. Wnt/beta-catenin signaling promotes podocyte dysfunction and albuminuria. *J. Am. Soc. Nephrol.* **2009**, *20*, 1997–2008. [CrossRef]
59. Nelson, P.J.; von Toerne, C.; Grone, H.J. Wnt-signaling pathways in progressive renal fibrosis. *Expert Opin. Ther. Targets* **2011**, *15*, 1073–1083. [CrossRef]
60. von Toerne, C.; Schmidt, C.; Adams, J.; Kiss, E.; Bedke, J.; Porubsky, S.; Gretz, N.; Lindenmeyer, M.T.; Cohen, C.D.; Grone, H.J.; et al. Wnt pathway regulation in chronic renal allograft damage. *Am. J. Transpl.* **2009**, *9*, 2223–2239. [CrossRef]
61. Huang, C.C.; Chuang, J.H.; Chou, M.H.; Wu, C.L.; Chen, C.M.; Wang, C.C.; Chen, Y.S.; Chen, C.L.; Tai, M.H. Matrilysin (MMP-7) is a major matrix metalloproteinase upregulated in biliary atresia-associated liver fibrosis. *Mod. Pathol.* **2005**, *18*, 941–950. [CrossRef] [PubMed]
62. Lichtinghagen, R.; Michels, D.; Haberkorn, C.I.; Arndt, B.; Bahr, M.; Flemming, P.; Manns, M.P.; Boeker, K.H. Matrix metalloproteinase (MMP)-2, MMP-7, and tissue inhibitor of metalloproteinase-1 are closely related to the fibroproliferative process in the liver during chronic hepatitis C. *J. Hepatol.* **2001**, *34*, 239–247. [CrossRef]
63. Fujishima, S.; Shiomi, T.; Yamashita, S.; Yogo, Y.; Nakano, Y.; Inoue, T.; Nakamura, M.; Tasaka, S.; Hasegawa, N.; Aikawa, N.; et al. Production and activation of matrix metalloproteinase 7 (matrilysin 1) in the lungs of patients with idiopathic pulmonary fibrosis. *Arch. Pathol. Lab. Med.* **2010**, *134*, 1136–1142. [PubMed]
64. Rosas, I.O.; Richards, T.J.; Konishi, K.; Zhang, Y.; Gibson, K.; Lokshin, A.E.; Lindell, K.O.; Cisneros, J.; Macdonald, S.D.; Pardo, A.; et al. MMP1 and MMP7 as potential peripheral blood biomarkers in idiopathic pulmonary fibrosis. *PLoS Med.* **2008**, *5*, e93. [CrossRef]
65. Maher, T.M.; Oballa, E.; Simpson, J.K.; Porte, J.; Habgood, A.; Fahy, W.A.; Flynn, A.; Molyneaux, P.L.; Braybrooke, R.; Divyateja, H.; et al. An epithelial biomarker signature for idiopathic pulmonary fibrosis: An analysis from the multicentre PROFILE cohort study. *Lancet Respir. Med.* **2017**, *5*, 946–955. [CrossRef]
66. Nakatsuka, Y.; Handa, T.; Nakashima, R.; Tanizawa, K.; Kubo, T.; Murase, Y.; Sokai, A.; Ikezoe, K.; Hosono, Y.; Watanabe, K.; et al. Serum matrix metalloproteinase levels in polymyositis/dermatomyositis patients with interstitial lung disease. *Rheumatology* **2019**, *58*, 1465–1473. [CrossRef]
67. Gille, T.; Didier, M.; Boubaya, M.; Moya, L.; Sutton, A.; Carton, Z.; Baran-Marszak, F.; Sadoun-Danino, D.; Israël-Biet, D.; Cottin, V.; et al. Obstructive sleep apnoea and related comorbidities in incident idiopathic pulmonary fibrosis. *Eur. Respir. J.* **2017**, *49*, 1601934. [CrossRef]
68. Lai, K.N.; Tang, S.C.; Schena, F.P.; Novak, J.; Tomino, Y.; Fogo, A.B.; Glassock, R.J. IgA nephropathy. *Nat. Rev. Dis. Primers* **2016**, *2*, 16001. [CrossRef]

69. Herzenberg, A.M.; Fogo, A.B.; Reich, H.N.; Troyanov, S.; Bavbek, N.; Massat, A.E.; Hunley, T.E.; Hladunewich, M.A.; Julian, B.A.; Fervenza, F.C.; et al. Validation of the Oxford classification of IgA nephropathy. *Kidney Int.* **2011**, *80*, 310–317. [CrossRef]
70. Rodrigues, J.C.; Haas, M.; Reich, H.N. IgA nephropathy. *Clin. J. Am. Soc. Nephrol.* **2017**, *12*, 677–686. [CrossRef]
71. Zhao, N.; Hou, P.; Lv, J.; Moldoveanu, Z.; Li, Y.; Kiryluk, K.; Gharavi, A.G.; Novak, J.; Zhang, H. The level of galactose-deficient IgA1 in the sera of patients with IgA nephropathy is associated with disease progression. *Kidney Int.* **2012**, *82*, 790–796. [CrossRef] [PubMed]
72. Berthoux, F.; Suzuki, H.; Thibaudin, L.; Yanagawa, H.; Maillard, N.; Mariat, C.; Tomino, Y.; Julian, B.A.; Novak, J. Autoantibodies targeting galactose-deficient IgA1 associate with progression of IgA nephropathy. *J. Am. Soc. Nephrol.* **2012**, *23*, 1579–1587. [CrossRef] [PubMed]
73. Lundberg, S.; Qureshi, A.R.; Olivecrona, S.; Gunnarsson, I.; Jacobson, S.H.; Larsson, T.E. FGF23, albuminuria, and disease progression in patients with chronic IgA nephropathy. *Clin. J. Am. Soc. Nephrol.* **2012**, *7*, 727–734. [CrossRef] [PubMed]
74. Zhang, J.; Ren, P.; Wang, Y.; Feng, S.; Wang, C.; Shen, X.; Weng, C.; Lang, X.; Chen, Z.; Jiang, H.; et al. Serum matrix metalloproteinase-7 level is associated with fibrosis and renal survival in patients with IgA nephropathy. *Kidney Blood Press. Res.* **2017**, *42*, 541–552. [CrossRef]
75. Yamamoto, T.; Nakagawa, T.; Suzuki, H.; Ohashi, N.; Fukasawa, H.; Fujigaki, Y.; Kato, A.; Nakamura, Y.; Suzuki, F.; Hishida, A. Urinary angiotensinogen as a marker of intrarenal angiotensin II activity associated with deterioration of renal function in patients with chronic kidney disease. *J. Am. Soc. Nephrol.* **2007**, *18*, 1558–1565. [CrossRef] [PubMed]
76. Ju, W.; Nair, V.; Smith, S.; Zhu, L.; Shedden, K.; Song, P.X.K.; Mariani, L.H.; Eichinger, F.H.; Berthier, C.C.; Randolph, A.; et al. Tissue transcriptome-driven identification of epidermal growth factor as a chronic kidney disease biomarker. *Sci. Transl. Med.* **2015**, *7*, 316ra193. [CrossRef]
77. Peters, H.P.; Waanders, F.; Meijer, E.; van den Brand, J.; Steenbergen, E.J.; van Goor, H.; Wetzels, J.F. High urinary excretion of kidney injury molecule-1 is an independent predictor of end-stage renal disease in patients with IgA nephropathy. *Nephrol. Dial. Transpl.* **2011**, *26*, 3581–3588. [CrossRef]
78. Musial, K.; Bargenda, A.; Zwolinska, D. Urine matrix metalloproteinases and their extracellular inducer EMMPRIN in children with chronic kidney disease. *Ren Fail.* **2015**, *37*, 980–984. [CrossRef]
79. Thrailkill, K.M.; Clay Bunn, R.; Fowlkes, J.L. Matrix metalloproteinases: Their potential role in the pathogenesis of diabetic nephropathy. *Endocrine* **2009**, *35*, 1–10. [CrossRef]
80. Bonventre, J.V.; Yang, L. Cellular pathophysiology of ischemic acute kidney injury. *J. Clin. Invest.* **2011**, *121*, 4210–4221. [CrossRef]
81. Kuncewitch, M.; Yang, W.L.; Corbo, L.; Khader, A.; Nicastro, J.; Coppa, G.F.; Wang, P. WNT agonist decreases tissue damage and improves renal function after ischemia-reperfusion. *Shock* **2015**, *43*, 268–275. [CrossRef]
82. Chang-Panesso, M.; Humphreys, B.D. Cellular plasticity in kidney injury and repair. *Nat. Rev. Nephrol.* **2017**, *13*, 39–46. [CrossRef] [PubMed]
83. Boor, P.; Ostendorf, T.; Floege, J. Renal fibrosis. Novel insights into mechanisms and therapeutic targets. *Nat. Rev. Nephrol.* **2010**, *6*, 643–656. [CrossRef] [PubMed]
84. Zeisberg, M.; Neilson, E.G. Mechanisms of tubulointerstitial fibrosis. *J. Am. Soc. Nephrol.* **2010**, *21*, 1819–1834. [CrossRef] [PubMed]
85. Yuan, Q.; Tan, R.J.; Liu, Y. Myofibroblast in kidney fibrosis: Origin, activation, and regulation. *Adv. Exp. Med. Biol.* **2019**, *1165*, 253–283. [PubMed]
86. Tian, X.J.; Zhou, D.; Fu, H.; Zhang, R.; Wang, X.; Huang, S.; Liu, Y.; Xing, J. Sequential Wnt agonist then antagonist treatment accelerates tissue repair and minimizes fibrosis. *iScience* **2020**, *23*, 101047. [CrossRef] [PubMed]
87. Ke, B.; Fan, C.; Yang, L.; Fang, X. Matrix Metalloproteinases-7 and Kidney Fibrosis. *Front. Physiol.* **2017**, *8*, 21. [CrossRef]
88. Kriz, W.; LeHir, M. Pathways to nephron loss starting from glomerular diseases-insights from animal models. *Kidney Int.* **2005**, *67*, 404–419. [CrossRef]
89. Yokoyama, Y.; Grunebach, F.; Schmidt, S.M.; Heine, A.; Hantschel, M.; Stevanovic, S.; Rammensee, H.G.; Brossart, P. Matrilysin (MMP-7) is a novel broadly expressed tumor antigen recognized by antigen-specific T cells. *Clin. Cancer Res.* **2008**, *14*, 5503–5511. [CrossRef]

90. Ehrenschwender, M.; Wajant, H. The role of FasL and Fas in health and disease. *Adv. Exp. Med. Biol.* **2009**, *647*, 64–93.
91. Jiang, M.; Wang, C.Y.; Huang, S.; Yang, T.; Dong, Z. Cisplatin-induced apoptosis in p53-deficient renal cells via the intrinsic mitochondrial pathway. *Am. J. Physiol. Renal Physiol.* **2009**, *296*, F983–F993. [CrossRef] [PubMed]
92. Havasi, A.; Borkan, S.C. Apoptosis and acute kidney injury. *Kidney Int.* **2011**, *80*, 29–40. [CrossRef] [PubMed]
93. Waring, P.; Mullbacher, A. Cell death induced by the Fas/Fas ligand pathway and its role in pathology. *Immunol. Cell Biol.* **1999**, *77*, 312–317. [CrossRef]
94. Nareznoi, D.; Konikov-Rozenman, J.; Petukhov, D.; Breuer, R.; Wallach-Dayan, S.B. Matrix Metalloproteinases Retain Soluble FasL-mediated Resistance to Cell Death in Fibrotic-Lung Myofibroblasts. *Cells* **2020**, *9*, 411. [CrossRef] [PubMed]
95. Zhou, D.; Tan, R.J.; Zhou, L.; Li, Y.; Liu, Y. Kidney tubular beta-catenin signaling controls interstitial fibroblast fate via epithelial-mesenchymal communication. *Sci. Rep.* **2013**, *3*, 1878. [CrossRef] [PubMed]
96. Wadsworth, S.J.; Atsuta, R.; McIntyre, J.O.; Hackett, T.L.; Singhera, G.K.; Dorscheid, D.R. IL-13 and TH2 cytokine exposure triggers matrix metalloproteinase 7-mediated Fas ligand cleavage from bronchial epithelial cells. *J. Allergy Clin. Immunol.* **2010**, *126*, 366–374. [CrossRef] [PubMed]
97. Hu, K.; Lin, L.; Tan, X.; Yang, J.; Bu, G.; Mars, W.M.; Liu, Y. tPA protects renal interstitial fibroblasts and myofibroblasts from apoptosis. *J. Am. Soc. Nephrol.* **2008**, *19*, 503–514. [CrossRef]
98. Roucou, X.; Antonsson, B.; Martinou, J.C. Involvement of mitochondria in apoptosis. *Cardiol. Clin.* **2001**, *19*, 45–55. [CrossRef]
99. Tian, X.; Liu, Z.; Niu, B.; Zhang, J.; Tan, T.K.; Lee, S.R.; Zhao, Y.; Harris, D.C.; Zheng, G. E-cadherin/beta-catenin complex and the epithelial barrier. *J. Biomed. Biotechnol.* **2011**, *2011*, 567305. [CrossRef]
100. Noe, V.; Fingleton, B.; Jacobs, K.; Crawford, H.C.; Vermeulen, S.; Steelant, W.; Bruyneel, E.; Matrisian, L.M.; Mareel, M. Release of an invasion promoter E-cadherin fragment by matrilysin and stromelysin-1. *J. Cell. Sci* **2001**, *114*, 111–118.
101. Liu, Y. New insights into epithelial-mesenchymal transition in kidney fibrosis. *J. Am. Soc. Nephrol.* **2010**, *21*, 212–222. [CrossRef] [PubMed]
102. Zhu, H.; Liao, J.; Zhou, X.; Hong, X.; Song, D.; Hou, F.F.; Liu, Y.; Fu, H. Tenascin-C promotes acute kidney injury to chronic kidney disease progression by impairing tubular integrity via alphavbeta6 integrin signaling. *Kidney Int.* **2020**, *97*, 1017–1031. [CrossRef]
103. Debelec-Butuner, B.; Alapinar, C.; Ertunc, N.; Gonen-Korkmaz, C.; Yörükoğlu, K.; Korkmaz, K.S. TNFα-mediated loss of β-catenin/E-cadherin association and subsequent increase in cell migration is partially restored by NKX3.1 expression in prostate cells. *PLoS ONE* **2014**, *9*, e109868. [CrossRef] [PubMed]
104. Zhang, Q.; Liu, S.; Parajuli, K.R.; Zhang, W.; Zhang, K.; Mo, Z.; Liu, J.; Chen, Z.; Yang, S.; Wang, A.R.; et al. Interleukin-17 promotes prostate cancer via MMP7-induced epithelial-to-mesenchymal transition. *Oncogene* **2017**, *36*, 687–699. [CrossRef]
105. Liu, Y. Epithelial to mesenchymal transition in renal fibrogenesis: Pathologic significance, molecular mechanism, and therapeutic intervention. *J. Am. Soc. Nephrol.* **2004**, *15*, 1–12. [CrossRef] [PubMed]
106. Mendonsa, A.M.; Na, T.Y.; Gumbiner, B.M. E-cadherin in contact inhibition and cancer. *Oncogene* **2018**, *37*, 4769–4780. [CrossRef] [PubMed]
107. Motti, M.L.; Califano, D.; Baldassarre, G.; Celetti, A.; Merolla, F.; Forzati, F.; Napolitano, M.; Tavernise, B.; Fusco, A.; Viglietto, G. Reduced E-cadherin expression contributes to the loss of p27kip1-mediated mechanism of contact inhibition in thyroid anaplastic carcinomas. *Carcinogenesis* **2005**, *26*, 1021–1034. [CrossRef]
108. St Croix, B.; Sheehan, C.; Rak, J.W.; Florenes, V.A.; Slingerland, J.M.; Kerbel, R.S. E-Cadherin-dependent growth suppression is mediated by the cyclin-dependent kinase inhibitor p27(KIP1). *J. Cell Biol.* **1998**, *142*, 557–571. [CrossRef]
109. Watabe, M.; Nagafuchi, A.; Tsukita, S.; Takeichi, M. Induction of polarized cell-cell association and retardation of growth by activation of the E-cadherin-catenin adhesion system in a dispersed carcinoma line. *J. Cell Biol.* **1994**, *127*, 247–256. [CrossRef]
110. Grahammer, F.; Schell, C.; Huber, T.B. The podocyte slit diaphragm—from a thin grey line to a complex signalling hub. *Nat. Rev. Nephrol.* **2013**, *9*, 587–598. [CrossRef]
111. Crabbe, T.; Smith, B.; O'Connell, J.; Docherty, A. Human progelatinase A can be activated by matrilysin. *FEBS Lett.* **1994**, *345*, 14–16. [CrossRef]

112. Barille, S.; Bataille, R.; Rapp, M.J.; Harousseau, J.L.; Amiot, M. Production of metalloproteinase-7 (matrilysin) by human myeloma cells and its potential involvement in metalloproteinase-2 activation. *J. Immunol.* **1999**, *163*, 5723–5728. [PubMed]
113. Wang, F.Q.; So, J.; Reierstad, S.; Fishman, D.A. Matrilysin (MMP-7) promotes invasion of ovarian cancer cells by activation of progelatinase. *Int. J. Cancer* **2005**, *114*, 19–31. [CrossRef] [PubMed]
114. von Bredow, D.C.; Cress, A.E.; Howard, E.W.; Bowden, G.T.; Nagle, R.B. Activation of gelatinase-tissue-inhibitors-of-metalloproteinase complexes by matrilysin. *Biochem J.* **1998**, *331 (Pt 3)*, 965–972. [CrossRef] [PubMed]
115. Imai, K.; Yokohama, Y.; Nakanishi, I.; Ohuchi, E.; Fujii, Y.; Nakai, N.; Okada, Y. Matrix metalloproteinase 7 (matrilysin) from human rectal carcinoma cells. Activation of the precursor, interaction with other matrix metalloproteinases and enzymic properties. *J. Biol. Chem.* **1995**, *270*, 6691–6697. [CrossRef]
116. Cheng, Z.; Limbu, M.H.; Wang, Z.; Liu, J.; Liu, L.; Zhang, X.; Chen, P.; Liu, B. MMP-2 and 9 in chronic kidney disease. *Int. J. Mol. Sci.* **2017**, *18*, 776. [CrossRef]
117. Cheng, S.; Lovett, D.H. Gelatinase A (MMP-2) is necessary and sufficient for renal tubular cell epithelial-mesenchymal transformation. *Am. J. Pathol.* **2003**, *162*, 1937–1949. [CrossRef]

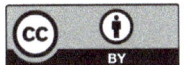

© 2020 by the authors. Licensee MDPI, Basel, Switzerland. This article is an open access article distributed under the terms and conditions of the Creative Commons Attribution (CC BY) license (http://creativecommons.org/licenses/by/4.0/).

MDPI
St. Alban-Anlage 66
4052 Basel
Switzerland
Tel. +41 61 683 77 34
Fax +41 61 302 89 18
www.mdpi.com

Biomolecules Editorial Office
E-mail: biomolecules@mdpi.com
www.mdpi.com/journal/biomolecules

www.ingramcontent.com/pod-product-compliance
Lightning Source LLC
LaVergne TN
LVHW070717100526
838202LV00013B/1115